T0348809

Cushing's Syndrome

Editor

ADRIANA G. IOACHIMESCU

ENDOCRINOLOGY AND METABOLISM CLINICS OF NORTH AMERICA

www.endo.theclinics.com

Consulting Editor
ADRIANA G. IOACHIMESCU

June 2018 • Volume 47 • Number 2

ELSEVIER

1600 John F. Kennedy Boulevard • Suite 1800 • Philadelphia, Pennsylvania, 19103-2899

http://www.theclinics.com

ENDOCRINOLOGY AND METABOLISM CLINICS OF NORTH AMERICA Volume 47, Number 2
June 2018 ISSN 0889-8529, ISBN 13: 978-0-323-61293-7

Editor: Stacy Eastman
Developmental Editor: Meredith Madeira

Endocrinology and Metabolism Clinics of North America (ISSN 0889-8529) is published quarterly by Elsevier Inc., 360 Park Avenue South, New York, NY 10010-1710. Months of issue are March, June, September, and December. Periodicals postage paid at New York, NY and additional mailing offices. Subscription prices are USD 357.00 per year for US individuals, USD 721.00 per year for US institutions, USD 100.00 per year for US students and residents, USD 447.00 per year for Canadian individuals, USD 893.00 per year for Canadian institutions, USD 490.00 per year for international individuals, USD 893.00 per year for international institutions, and USD 245.00 per year for international and Canadian and foreign students/residents. To receive student/resident rate, orders must be accompanied by name of affiliated institution, date of term, and the signature of program/ residency coordinator on institution letterhead. Orders will be billed at individual rate until proof of status is received. Foreign air speed delivery is included in all *Clinics* subscription prices. All prices are subject to change without notice. **POSTMASTER:** Send address changes to *Endocrinology and Metabolism Clinics of North America*, Elsevier Health Sciences Division, Subscription Customer Service, 3251 Riverport Lane, Maryland Heights, MO 63043. **Customer Service: Telephone: 1-800-654-2452** (U.S. and Canada); **1-314-447-8871** (outside U.S. and Canada). **Fax: 1-314-447-8029. E-mail: journalscustomerservice-usa@elsevier.com (for print support); journalsonlinesupport-usa@elsevier.com (for online support).**

Reprints. For copies of 100 or more, of articles in this publication, please contact the Commercial Rights Department, Elsevier Inc., 360 Park Avenue South, New York, NY 10010-1710; phone: +1-212-633-3874; fax: +1-212-633-3820; E-mail: reprints@elsevier.com.

Endocrinology and Metabolism Clinics of North America is covered in *MEDLINE/PubMed (Index Medicus)*, *EMBASE/Excerpta Medica*, *Current Contents/Clinical Medicine*, *Current Contents/Life Sciences*, *Science Citation Index, ISI/BIOMED, BIOSIS*, and *Chemical Abstracts*.

Contributors

CONSULTING EDITOR

ADRIANA G. IOACHIMESCU, MD, PhD, FACE
Associate Professor of Medicine and Neurosurgery, Co-Director, Emory Pituitary Center, Emory University School of Medicine, Atlanta, Georgia, USA

EDITOR

ADRIANA G. IOACHIMESCU, MD, PhD, FACE
Associate Professor of Medicine and Neurosurgery, Co-Director, Emory Pituitary Center, Emory University School of Medicine, Atlanta, Georgia, USA

AUTHORS

BEVERLY M.K. BILLER, MD
Professor of Medicine, Neuroendocrine Unit, Massachusetts General Hospital, Harvard Medical School, Boston, Massachusetts, USA

MARCELLO DELANO BRONSTEIN, MD, PhD
Professor of Endocrinology, Chief of Neuroendocrine Unit, Division of Endocrinology and Metabolism, Hospital das Clinicas, University of São Paulo Medical School, São Paulo, São Paulo, Brazil

CHING-JEN CHEN, MD
Department of Neurological Surgery, University of Virginia Health System, Charlottesville, Virginia, USA

GUIDO DI DALMAZI, MD
Division of Endocrinology, Department of Medical and Surgical Sciences, Alma Mater Studiorum University of Bologna, S. Orsola-Malpighi Hospital, Bologna, Italy

DAISY DUAN, MD
Department of Medicine, Division of Endocrinology, Diabetes, and Bone Disease, Icahn School of Medicine at Mount Sinai, The Mount Sinai Hospital, New York, New York, USA

ELIZABETH FOULKES, BMedSci
Department of Oncology and Metabolism, The Medical School, The University of Sheffield, Sheffield, United Kingdom

MARIA CANDIDA BARISSON VILARES FRAGOSO, MD, PhD
Professor of Endocrinology, Chief of Adrenal Unit, Assistant Physician, Neuroendocrine Unit, Division of Endocrinology and Metabolism, Hospital das Clínicas, University of São Paulo Medical School, São Paulo, São Paulo, Brazil

ELIZA B. GEER, MD
Associate Professor, Department of Medicine, Medical Director, Division of Endocrinology, Multidisciplinary Pituitary and Skull Base Tumor Center, Memorial Sloan Kettering Cancer Center, New York, New York, USA

ASHLEY B. GROSSMAN, BA, BSc, MD, FRCP, FMedSci
Neuroendocrine Tumour Unit, Royal Free Hospital, London, United Kingdom

AIMEE R. HAYES, BSc, MBBS (Hons), MMed (Clin Epi), FRACP
Neuroendocrine Tumour Unit, Royal Free Hospital, London, United Kingdom

LAURA C. HERNÁNDEZ-RAMÍREZ, MD, PhD
Section on Endocrinology and Genetics, *Eunice Kennedy Shriver* National Institute of Child Health and Human Development (NICHD), National Institutes of Health (NIH), Bethesda, Maryland, USA

ADRIANA G. IOACHIMESCU, MD, PhD, FACE
Associate Professor of Medicine and Neurosurgery, Co-Director, Emory Pituitary Center, Emory University School of Medicine, Atlanta, Georgia, USA

NATASHA IRONSIDE, MBChB
Department of Neurosurgery, Auckland City Hospital, Auckland, New Zealand

PEDRAM JAVANMARD, MD
Department of Medicine, Division of Endocrinology, Diabetes, and Bone Disease, Icahn School of Medicine at Mount Sinai, The Mount Sinai Hospital, New York, New York, USA

MARGARET F. KEIL, PhD, CRNP
Section on Endocrinology and Genetics, *Eunice Kennedy Shriver* National Institute of Child Health and Human Development (NICHD), National Institutes of Health (NIH), NIH Clinical Research Center, Bethesda, Maryland, USA

CHENG-CHIA LEE, MD
Department of Neurosurgery, Taipei Veterans General Hospital, Taipei, Taiwan

MAYA B. LODISH, MD, MHSc
Section on Endocrinology and Genetics, *Eunice Kennedy Shriver* National Institute of Child Health and Human Development (NICHD), National Institutes of Health (NIH), NIH Clinical Research Center, Bethesda, Maryland, USA

MARCIO CARLOS MACHADO, MD, PhD
Assistant Physician, Neuroendocrine Unit, Division of Endocrinology and Metabolism, Hospital das Clínicas, Physical Assistant, Endocrinology Service, AC Camargo Cancer Center, Laboratory for Endocrinology Cellular and Molecular – LIM25, University of São Paulo Medical School, São Paulo, São Paulo, Brazil

JOHN NEWELL-PRICE, MA, PhD, FRCP
Professor, Department of Oncology and Metabolism, The Medical School, The University of Sheffield, Sheffield, United Kingdom

LYNNETTE KAYE NIEMAN, MD
Senior Investigator, Diabetes, Endocrine, and Obesity Branch, The National Institute of Diabetes and Digestive and Kidney Diseases (NIDDK), National Institutes of Health, Bethesda, Maryland, USA

PAOLA PEROTTI, BS
Internal Medicine, Department of Clinical and Biological Sciences, San Luigi Gonzaga Hospital, Orbassano, Italy

ANNA PIA, MD
Internal Medicine, Department of Clinical and Biological Sciences, San Luigi Gonzaga Hospital, Orbassano, Italy

SORAYA PUGLISI, MD
Internal Medicine, Department of Clinical and Biological Sciences, San Luigi Gonzaga Hospital, Orbassano, Italy

GIUSEPPE REIMONDO, MD, PhD
Internal Medicine, Department of Clinical and Biological Sciences, San Luigi Gonzaga Hospital, Orbassano, Italy

MARTIN REINCKE, MD
Department of Medicine IV, Klinikum der Universität, Ludwig-Maximilians-Universität München, München, Germany

JASON P. SHEEHAN, MD, PhD
Department of Neurological Surgery, University of Virginia Health System, Charlottesville, Virginia, USA

CONSTANTINE A. STRATAKIS, MD, D(Med)Sci
Section on Endocrinology and Genetics, *Eunice Kennedy Shriver* National Institute of Child Health and Human Development (NICHD), National Institutes of Health (NIH), NIH Clinical Research Center, Bethesda, Maryland, USA

MASSIMO TERZOLO, MD
Internal Medicine, Department of Clinical and Biological Sciences, San Luigi Gonzaga Hospital, Orbassano, Italy

DANIEL M. TRIFILETTI, MD
Department of Radiation Oncology, Mayo Clinic, Jacksonville, Florida, USA

NICHOLAS A. TRITOS, MD, DSc
Associate Professor of Medicine, Neuroendocrine Unit, Neuroendocrine Clinical Center, Massachusetts General Hospital, Harvard Medical School, Boston, Massachusetts, USA

ELENA VALASSI, MD, PhD
Departments of Endocrinology and Medicine, Hospital Sant Pau, Universitat Autònoma de Barcelona, Centro de Investigación Biomédica en Red de Enfermedades Raras (CIBER-ER, Unidad 747), IIB-Sant Pau, ISCIII, Barcelona, Spain

MARY LEE VANCE, MD
Division of Endocrinology and Metabolism, University of Virginia Health System, Charlottesville, Virginia, USA

SUSAN M. WEBB, MD, PhD
Departments of Endocrinology and Medicine, Hospital Sant Pau, Universitat Autònoma de Barcelona, Centro de Investigación Biomédica en Red de Enfermedades Raras (CIBER-ER, Unidad 747), IIB-Sant Pau, ISCIII, Barcelona, Spain

GUIDO ZAVATTA, MD
Division of Endocrinology, Department of Medical and Surgical Sciences, Alma Mater Studiorum University of Bologna, S. Orsola-Malpighi Hospital, Bologna, Italy

Contents

Four challenges complicate the evaluation for Cushing's syndrome. These challenges include increasing global prevalence of obesity and diabetes; increasing use of exogenous glucocorticoids, which cause a Cushing's syndrome phenotype; the confusion caused by nonpathologic hypercortisolism not associated with Cushing's syndrome, which may present with symptoms consistent with Cushing's syndrome; and difficulty identifying pathologic hypercortisolism when it is extremely mild or cyclic or in renal failure, incidental adrenal masses, and pregnancy. Careful choice of screening tests, consideration of confounding conditions, and repeated testing when the results are ambiguous improve the accuracy of diagnosis.

The knowledge on the molecular and genetic causes of Cushing's syndrome (CS) has greatly increased in the recent years. Somatic mutations leading to overactive 3',5'-cyclic adenosine monophosphate/protein kinase A and wingless-type MMTV integration site family/beta-catenin pathways are the main molecular mechanisms underlying adrenocortical tumorigenesis. Corticotropinomas are characterized by resistance to glucocorticoid negative feedback, impaired cell cycle control, and overexpression of pathways sustaining adrenocorticotropic hormone secretion. Recognizing the genetic defects behind corticotroph and adrenocortical tumorigenesis proves crucial for tailoring the clinical management of patients with CS and for designing strategies for genetic counseling and clinical screening to be applied in routine medical practice.

Cortisol excess in Cushing's syndrome is associated with metabolic, cardiovascular, and cognitive alterations, only partially reversible after resolution of hypercortisolism. Elevated cardiovascular risk may persist after eucortisolism has been achieved. Fractures and low bone mineral density are also described in Cushing's syndrome in remission. Hypercortisolism may induce irreversible structural and functional changes in the brain, leading to neuropsychiatric disorders in the active phase of the disease, which persist. Sustained deterioration of the cardiovascular system, bone remodeling, and cognitive function along with neuropsychological impairment are associated with high morbidity and poor quality of life before and after remission.

Cushing's syndrome is associated with increased morbidity and mortality. Cardiovascular events, sepsis, and thromboembolism are the leading causes of mortality. Patients with Cushing's syndrome due to a pituitary adenoma or due to benign adrenal adenoma have relatively good survival outcomes, often mirroring that of the general population. Persistent or recurrent disease is associated with high mortality risk. Ectopic Cushing's syndrome and that due to adrenocortical carcinoma confer the highest mortality risk among the causes of Cushing's syndrome. Prompt diagnosis and treatment and specific monitoring for and treatment of associated comorbidities are essential to decrease the burden of mortality from Cushing's syndrome.

Transsphenoidal surgery is the main treatment of patients with adrenocorticotropic hormone (ACTH)–secreting pituitary adenomas. Although biochemical remission occurs in most patients undergoing operations at specialized centers, the recurrence risk is significant. Visualization of microadenomas on preoperative imaging and confirmation of ACTH-positive adenomas have been associated with higher remission rates. Low cortisol levels in the first 2 weeks postoperatively have been associated with durable remission; however, recurrence cannot be excluded by any cortisol threshold. The decision to perform a pituitary reoperation is based on this parameter; the protocols are institution specific. Patients with Cushing's disease warrant lifelong endocrinologic surveillance.

Achievement of biochemical remission with preservation of normal pituitary function is the goal of treatment for Cushing's disease. For patients with persistent or recurrent Cushing's disease after transsphenoidal resection, radiation therapy may be a safe and effective treatment. Stereotactic radiosurgery is favored over conventional fractionated external beam radiation. Hormonal recurrence rates range from 0% to 36% at 8 years after treatment. Tumor control rates are high. New pituitary hormone deficiency is the most common adverse effect after stereotactic radiosurgery and external beam radiation. The effects of radiation planning optimization and use of adjuvant medication on endocrine remission rates warrant investigation.

Despite the best outcomes from transsphenoidal surgery, approximately one-third of patients with Cushing's disease will need medical therapy. Current treatments have drawbacks, and there is a clear clinical need for new therapies. Recent understanding of molecular pathways leading to excess ACTH secretion has identified key components that may be targeted with the aim of providing novel effective treatment for this devastating disease. These components include testicular orphan nuclear receptor 4, heat shock protein 90, and epidermal growth factor receptor. Based on data from preclinical studies, clinical trials are seeking to assess whether targeting these novel pathways can translate into patient benefit.

During the last 20 years, a significant body of literature has accumulated regarding subclinical hypercortisolism in patients with adrenal incidentalomas. Retrospective studies have indicated these patients have an increase in cardiovascular events and mortality. Current recommendations for patients with adrenal incidentalomas include an overnight low-dose dexamethasone suppression test and a thorough evaluation of cardiovascular and metabolic risk factors. Further hormonal testing and close monitoring are necessary in patients with incomplete suppression. Unilateral adrenalectomy may be beneficial in cases with abnormal suppression and comorbidities related to hypercortisolemia. Prospective studies are needed for a better risk stratification and tailored therapy.

Recent advances in the molecular pathogenesis and the natural history of Cushing's syndrome have improved the understanding of the management of this disease. The long-term efficacy of several cortisol-lowering medical treatments is currently under evaluation. However, adrenalectomy is a safe option for the treatment of patients affected by Cushing's syndrome. Unilateral adrenalectomy is the gold standard for treatment of adrenocortical adenomas associated with hypercortisolism. Bilateral adrenalectomy has been widely used in the past as definitive treatment of bilateral macronodular hyperplasia and persistent or recurrent Cushing's disease. The indication and the potential applications of this technique have been recently critically analyzed.

Adrenocortical carcinoma (ACC) is a rare and aggressive tumor. ACC may be associated with different syndromes of hormone excess, most frequently Cushing's syndrome with or without hypersecretion of androgens. Recent data suggest that cortisol excess is a negative prognostic factor in advanced and localized ACC. Surgery with radical intent, when feasible, is the most effective treatment for ACC with hypercortisolism. Mitotane is the medical treatment of choice, both postoperatively and in inoperable or metastatic cases. Because of its slow onset of action, combination with other antisecretory agents (ie, metyrapone) is helpful to achieve more rapid and effective control of hypercortisolism.

the typical presentation is height deceleration concomitant with weight gain. Endogenous and ectopic causes are rare. CS in children may be associated with distinct germline and somatic mutations. Clinical practice guidelines are available to assist clinicians. Patients should be referred to multidisciplinary centers of excellence with experience in endocrinology and surgery. Early detection and treatment is essential to reduce associated acute and long-term morbidity and potential death.

ENDOCRINOLOGY AND METABOLISM CLINICS OF NORTH AMERICA

ISSUE OF RELATED INTEREST

Surgical Clinics, June 2014 (Vol. 94, Issue 3)
Endocrine Surgery
Peter J. Mazzaglia, *Editor*

VISIT THE CLINICS ONLINE!
Access your subscription at:
www.theclinics.com

Preface

Cushing's Syndrome 2018: Best Practices and Looking Ahead

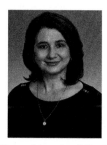

Adriana G. Ioachimescu, MD, PhD, FACE
Editor

Endogenous Cushing's syndrome is a rare endocrine disorder with serious health implications. The June 2018 *Endocrinology and Metabolism Clinics of North America* issue is an update on pathogenesis, diagnosis, management, and prognosis of this challenging condition. The articles were written with a clinical focus by a group of international experts in the field.

A review on Cushing's syndrome is timely as more patients are screened for hypercortisolism in context of increased prevalence of obesity, diabetes, and adrenal incidentaloma. Differentiation of mild Cushing's syndrome from reactive hypercortisolism (or "pseudo-Cushing") entails a thorough understanding of the available tests and their caveats. Substantial evidence has accumulated regarding outcomes of patients with "subclinical Cushing's syndrome." Several factors must be considered when identifying patients who might benefit from surgical removal of adrenal incidentalomas. Children and pregnant women are rarely affected by Cushing's syndrome; however, these patient categories pose urgent and unique diagnostic and management problems.

Cushing's syndrome is classified in two main categories: ACTH dependent (Cushing's disease and ectopic Cushing's syndrome) and ACTH independent. Syndromic presentation of hypercortisolism is infrequent and may affect patients with McCune-Albright syndrome, Carney complex, and multiple endocrine neoplasia. Recognizing these entities has implications for clinical management and genetic counseling. In addition, Cushing's disease can rarely occur in the setting of familial isolated pituitary adenomas. Recent studies point to germline loss-of-function mutations in the aryl hydrocarbon receptor interacting protein gene as the most frequent abnormality in these cases.

Cushing's disease, the most frequent type of Cushing's syndrome, is caused by an ACTH-secreting pituitary adenoma. Transsphenoidal adenomectomy by an expert neurosurgeon leads to biochemical remission in most cases, but carries a substantial risk of recurrence. Additional treatments with curative intent include pituitary reoperation and radiation (which both carry a risk of permanent pituitary deficiencies) and bilateral adrenalectomy. The latter associates lifelong glucocorticoid and mineralocorticoid deficiency and a risk for Nelson syndrome. Several parameters have been proposed for risk stratification, which may be useful to design individualized treatment plans and improve long-term outcomes.

The main cause of ectopic Cushing's syndrome consists of the ACTH-producing pulmonary carcinoid tumor. The differentiation from Cushing's disease is difficult because patients harbor similar clinical and biochemical features, while pituitary and body imaging might be unrevealing. The recent introduction of ^{68}Ga-DOTA-somatostatin analogue PET/computed tomography (CT) is an additional tool for localization of tumors not detected by CT or MRI.

ACTH-independent Cushing's is usually caused by cortisol-secreting adrenal adenomas and less frequently by adrenocortical carcinomas or bilateral adrenal hyperplasia. Surgical resection of the adrenal adenoma usually provides long-lasting relief from hypercortisolism with temporary corticoadrenal insufficiency. Adrenocortical carcinoma with cortisol hypersecretion is a grave illness that necessitates urgent treatment of both malignancy and hypercortisolism.

Medical treatment of Cushing's syndrome has made significant progress in recent years when the US Food and Drug Administration approved two drugs for this indication: a somatostatin receptor ligand for Cushing's disease and a cortisol receptor blocker for Cushing's syndrome associated with hyperglycemia. In addition, steroidogenesis inhibitors continue to be used off label to alleviate consequences of hypercortisolism until surgery is performed or while awaiting effect of pituitary radiation. Cabergoline has also been used off label in some patients with Cushing's disease. Long-term outcomes of medications used in Cushing's syndrome are still to be determined. Recent advances in molecular biology of corticotroph tumorigenesis identified new potential targets for therapy, including the ubiquitin-specific protease 8 (USP8), testicular orphan nuclear receptor 4, heat shock protein 90, and epithelial growth factor receptor. The somatic gain-of-function mutation in the USP8 gene is currently thought to be the most common genetic defect in ACTH-secreting pituitary tumors.

Untreated Cushing's syndrome significantly increases mortality by cardiovascular and thromboembolic events, as well as infection. Therefore, prompt diagnosis and treatment of hypercortisolism are essential. Patients with ectopic ACTH-secreting tumors and adrenocortical carcinomas have the highest mortality. Patients with Cushing's disease who achieved durable remission after transsphenoidal surgery may have a better survival compared with those requiring multimodality therapies.

Cushing's syndrome causes a large array of metabolic, cardiovascular, musculoskeletal, and cognitive alterations that are only partially reversible after normocortisolism is achieved. These warrant early recognition and multispecialty management.

I would like to conclude by acknowledging all the authors and the *Endocrinology and Metabolism Clinics of North America* staff for their diligent work. I am honored to have served as guest editor for the Cushing's syndrome issue. I hope readers will find it informative and useful in their practice.

Adriana G. Ioachimescu, MD, PhD, FACE
Emory University School of Medicine
The Emory Pituitary Center
1365 B Clifton Road, Northeast, B6209
Atlanta, GA 30322, USA

E-mail address:
aioachi@emory.edu

Diagnosis of Cushing's Syndrome in the Modern Era

Lynnette Kaye Nieman, MD

KEYWORDS

- Cushing's syndrome • Cortisol • Urine free cortisol • Salivary cortisol

KEY POINTS

- Patients with a clinical phenotype of Cushing's syndrome should be questioned and possibly screened for exogenous glucocorticoid exposure.
- The choice of screening tests for the diagnosis of Cushing's syndrome should be individualized, taking into account potential confounding conditions.
- Physiologic states of hypercortisolism must be considered in the differential diagnosis of Cushing's syndrome.

INTRODUCTION

Cushing's syndrome (CS) is a group of signs and symptoms caused by chronic exposure to excess glucocorticoids. It is important to identify the syndrome at an early stage, so that treatment may be started to prevent symptom progression, morbidity, and potentially death. The diagnosis relies on laboratory confirmation using screening tests.

In the modern era, there are 5 major challenges associated with the diagnosis of CS:

- There is an increasing global prevalence of obesity and diabetes. These signs of CS, which are rarely caused by glucocorticoid excess, raise the question of whether to screen for the syndrome.
- There is increasing use of exogenous glucocorticoids, either for the treatment of disease or surreptitiously. This use leads to a CS phenotype without an endogenous cause.
- There is confusion caused by nonpathologic hypercortisolism not associated with CS, which may present with symptoms consistent with CS. This entity, termed pseudo-CS, may be difficult to distinguish from mild endogenous CS.

Disclosure Statement: The author has nothing to disclose.
Diabetes, Endocrine, and Obesity Branch, The National Institute of Diabetes and Digestive and Kidney Diseases (NIDDK), National Institutes of Health, Building 10, CRC, 1 East, Room 1-3140, 10 Center Drive, MSC 1109, Bethesda, MD 20892-1109, USA
E-mail address: NiemanL@nih.gov

Endocrinol Metab Clin N Am 47 (2018) 259–273
https://doi.org/10.1016/j.ecl.2018.02.001
0889-8529/18/Published by Elsevier Inc.

- There is uncertainty about the best screening test for CS and how to individualize the choice of tests to prevent false-positive interpretation of the results.
- There is difficulty in identifying pathologic hypercortisolism in certain conditions: when it is extremely mild or cyclic, in renal failure, in incidental adrenal masses, and in pregnancy.
  - These difficulties are mitigated in part by
  - The availability of assays for synthetic glucocorticoids
  - Increased understanding of the caveats and confounding factors that can cause false-positive and false-negative tests
  - Increased understanding of the physiologic underpinning of pseudo-CS states, adrenal masses, and pregnancy

Unfortunately, it is still often difficult to be certain about the diagnosis; in such cases, watchful waiting for clinical and biochemical progression may be the safest approach for patients, although frustrating for both patients and clinicians.

DISCUSSION
The Influence of the Clinical Presentation, Particularly Obesity and Diabetes, on the Need to Screen for Cushing's Syndrome

In most cases, patients are screened for CS based on their clinical presentation (rather than a randomly obtained laboratory test). The clinical presentation of patients with the syndrome varies widely in terms of the type, number, and severity of the signs and symptoms. **Table 1** lists the signs and symptoms grouped by system. Several of these features are prevalent in the general population, whereas others are expected only at certain ages.

Given the recent global increases in diabetes mellitus and weight gain/overweight/obesity, it is important to consider whether to screen these patients without considering other factors. The age-standardized global prevalence of adult diabetes is shown in **Fig. 1**. The worldwide number of people with diabetes was estimated to increase from 153 million in 1980 to 347 million in 2008, largely because of an aging and growing population.[9] The age-standardized prevalence of worldwide obesity is also increasing (see **Fig. 1**) and is estimated to reach 18% in men and to surpass 21% of women by 2025.[10] Because hypercortisolism is a treatable cause of secondary obesity and diabetes, the increased prevalence of these conditions may lead an increased need for screening.

Previous reports show a large range in the prevalence of unrecognized CS in patients with type 2 diabetes mellitus, from 0% to 9.4%.[11] Similarly, the prevalence of unrecognized CS in patients with obesity was 0% to 9.3% in 3 studies.[12–14] These data led to conflicting recommendations to screen, or not to screen, for CS in these populations.

How should clinicians approach the evaluation of patients with obesity and/or diabetes? As endocrinologists, what do we need to consider when patients are referred (with these or other features) to exclude/include the diagnosis CS? There is no one-size-fits-all approach to these patients. Rather, the pertinent history should be collected, using the questions in **Box 1**.

How do the answers to the questions in **Box 1** help?

- CS is generally a progressive disorder, so that signs and symptoms accumulate and worsen over time. A very long history of mild symptoms that are common in the patients' population cohort and do not increase in severity or number is

Table 1
Signs and symptoms associated with Cushing's syndrome grouped by system

System	Comments
General	
Fatigue	
Growth	In children, typically a decrease in height percentile as weight percentile increases
Adipose	
Increased weight from baseline	BMI may be normal, overweight or obese
Changes in adipose distribution	Increased temporal, supraclavicular or dorso-cervical adipose; may lead to moon facies or central adiposity
Skin/Hair	
Striae	Often with more severe hypercortisolism; significant if >1 cm and purple color; occur on abdomen, buttocks, upper arm/leg, breasts
Thin skin	Compare with age/sex controls (skin is thinnest in older women)
Hyperpigmentation	May be present in ACTH-dependent forms
Hirsutism (women)	Not typical for ACTH-independent adenomas
Balding (women)	Not typical for ACTH-independent adenomas
Acne	May be glucocorticoid (red) or androgen (pustular) related
Poor wound healing	
Increased bruising	
Flushed face	
Psychiatric/Cognitive	
Accentuation of previous personality/disorder	Up to 80% of patients may have previous diagnosis[1]
Increased irritability	Present in up to 86% of patients[2]
Development of new psychiatric disorder	
Decreased memory	Short-term memory is particularly affected; may be assessed at bedside by recall of 3 cities or objects[2,3]
Decreased cognitive ability	May be assessed at bedside by serial 7s (consecutive subtraction of 7 from 100)[2,3]
Infectious	
Increased number of infections	Including typical community-acquired infections as well as those seen more often in immunocompromised individuals; the latter most frequently in patients with more severe hypercortisolism[4]
Renal	
Increased incidence of stones	
Metabolic	
Glucose intolerance/diabetes	Both new and exacerbation of existing glucose intolerance seen

(continued on next page)

Table 1 (continued)	
System	Comments
Cardiovascular/thrombotic	
Hypertension	Greatest diagnostic weight in children and older patients in whom it is difficult to control, as both are unexpected in the general population
Increased incidence CVA[5]	
Increased incidence myocardial infarction[5]	
Increased clotting	May result in deep venous thrombosis and pulmonary embolism, more common in severe hypercortisolism[6]
Edema	
Reproductive	
Decreased libido	
Delayed or stuttering puberty (children)	
Infertility	Presumed to result from anovulation; role of hyperandrogenism not well-studied
Hypogonadism	Results from cortisol suppression of hypothalamic-pituitary function
Ophthalmologic	
Central serous chorioretinopathy	An uncommon feature of CS[7]
Musculoskeletal	
Proximal muscle weakness	Tested by asking patients to rise from a chair without using upper extremities
Back pain	
Decreased BMD/fracture	Greatest diagnostic weight' if occurs at an early age (<35 y)
Sleep	
Insomnia	May present as difficulty falling asleep, frequent wakening, or early wakening[2]
Vivid dreams	
Obstructive sleep apnea	In one study, 50% prevalence in CS compared with 23% in controls[8]

Abbreviations: ACTH, adrenocorticotropic hormone; BMD, bone mineral density; BMI, body mass index; CVA, cerebrovascular accident.

against CS. An example might be a 60-year-old woman who has been over-weight with easily controlled hypertension since 45 years of age. Conversely, a history of an increasing number and severity of features is more concerning.

- New or unexplained changes in cognition (difficulty with comprehension and synthesis), memory (especially short-term), mood (enhancement of previous, a new diagnosis of anxiety or depression, or new lability/irritability of mood) enhance the probability of CS.
- Features that are unusual for their age or for the patients' population cohort increase the pretest probability of CS. In a younger person, this includes unexplained fracture, easy bruising (especially in men), hypertension, thin skin, infections consistent with immunosuppression, or unexplained amenorrhea in

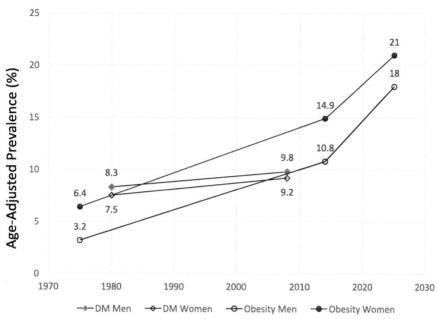

Fig. 1. Age-adjusted global prevalence of adult diabetes. DM, diabetes mellitus.

a normal-weight woman with a history of regular cycles. Such features are more likely to occur in older individuals and do not carry as much weight in that population.

- Changes in regional fat distribution that suggest CS include increased supraclavicular and temporal fat but not increased dorso-cervical or central deposition, as these are common in simple obesity. Some investigators cite personal

---

Box 1
Historical clinical data to obtain during the evaluation of possible Cushing's syndrome

What signs/symptoms of CS are currently present?

What is the duration of the signs/symptoms?

Have the number of signs/symptoms increased? Are they progressing in severity?

Do all of the signs/symptoms fall into a single systemic category (eg, reproductive) or are many systems affected?

Are there cognitive/memory/psychiatric features not usually associated with the other signs or symptoms?

Are the signs/symptoms common at this age or in this population cohort?

Are any of the conditions associated with physiologic hypercortisolism or pseudo-Cushing's state present?

In children
  If appropriate for age, what is the status of pubertal development: did it occur at the normal age and with the usual tempo of progression?
  What does the growth curve show? Is the child crossing percentile lines with increasing weight and decreased linear growth?

experience that purple striae more than 1 cm in diameter are suggestive of the syndrome, but at least one study showed a prevalence of nearly 40% in a pseudo-CS population.[15,16]

- If the history suggests conditions that are independently associated with hypercortisolism in the absence of CS, this should be taken into account when choosing the screening tests (see later discussion).
- Children with significant hypercortisolism have a characteristic growth curve in which the weight percentile increases while the height percentile decreases. They also tend to have a late puberty or a stuttering/stopping of pubertal progression.[17,18]

When a Cushing's Syndrome Phenotype Is Present, Exogenous Exposure to Glucocorticoids Should Be Excluded

This article primarily discusses endogenous CS, caused by cortisol excess. However, exposure to exogenous glucocorticoids, whether surreptitious, unknowing, or prescribed, also causes the clinical features of CS and must be distinguished from the endogenous forms so as to treat patients appropriately and avoid screening for endogenous hypercortisolism.

The medical history should include a question on what medications patients take, and this should be supplemented by review of the electronic health record. In the United States, many of these medication names end in *one* or *ide*; this may be a useful verbal prompt, as is a question about whether they have received any injections for joint or back pain. In addition to asking for the names of medications, it is useful to ask about medications administered via nonoral routes, such as inhalers, rectal suppositories or enemas, ointments, injections; in combination with knowledge of other associated diagnoses, this may lead to a suspicion of exogenous administration. Over-the-counter agents, such as herbal preparations, tonics, and skin-bleaching creams, may contain glucocorticoids; the use of these products should be evaluated.[19–22] However, in some cases, patients are not good historians and/or the records are not available. Additionally, occasionally patients are not aware that they have received a glucocorticoid, particularly if it was a short-term exposure or an injection.

When exposure to exogenous glucocorticoids cannot be confirmed by history, screening for synthetic glucocorticoids, along with measurement of adrenocorticotropic hormone (ACTH) and/or dehydroepiandrosterone sulfate (DHEAS), may help to confirm a high suspicion of exposure. In this setting, ACTH, DHEAS, and endogenous cortisol (unless hydrocortisone is taken) are all low, despite the clinical features of CS; usually the screen for exogenous substances is positive.

Biochemical Screening Tests for Cushing's Syndrome

When the pretest probability of CS is high, and exogenous steroid exposure has been excluded, patients should undergo recommended first- and (as appropriate) second-line biochemical tests to screen for CS (**Table 2**).[15] In general, these tests either measure baseline levels of cortisol (urine, saliva, serum) or evaluate the response of the hypothalamic-pituitary-adrenal axis to stimulatory (corticotropin-releasing hormone [CRH], desmopressin) or suppressive (dexamethasone [Dex]) agents. Interpretation of these tests relies on reference ranges for normal basal values and known responses to each of the provocative agents. The results also must be interpreted in light of the specific assay that is used for the outcome measure[26] and with knowledge of confounding factors that result in abnormal (or falsely normal) results.

Table 2
Recommended first- and second-line screening tests for the diagnosis of Cushing's syndrome

Measurement (Name of Test)	Stimulus/Suppressive Agent	Time of Day of Collection or Administration	Measurement Time after Administration	Cutoff Point for Normal Response	Confounders
First-line tests					
Urine cortisol (UFC)	None	24 h	N/A	Assay ULN	Incomplete/overcollection, renal failure, mild/cyclic hypercortisolism, excess fluid intake
Salivary cortisol (bedtime or late night salivary cortisol test)	None	Bedtime	N/A	Assay ULN	Older age, hypertension, diabetes, smoking, variable bedtime, mild/cyclic hypercortisolism
Serum cortisol (1 mg overnight Dex test)	Dex 1 mg po	2300–0000 h	8 h (0700–0800 h)	1.8 µg/dl (50 nmol/L)	CBG abnormalities, abnormal Dex metabolism, mild/cyclic hypercortisolism
Alternative approaches to first-line tests					
Serum cortisol (bedtime or late night serum cortisol test)	None	Bedtime	N/A	7.5 µg/dL if awake	CBG abnormalities, variable bedtime, mild/cyclic hypercortisolism
Serum cortisol (2 mg, 2-d or low-dose Dex test, LDDST)	Dex 0.5 mg po	q6h × 8 doses, begin at noon	2 h after last dose	1.4 (38 nmol/L)	CBG abnormalities, abnormal Dex metabolism, mild/cyclic hypercortisolism
Second-line tests					
Serum cortisol (Dex-CRH test)[23]	Dex 0.5 mg po & ovine CRH 1 µg/kg up to 100 µg IV	Dex q6h × 8 doses, begin at noon; give CRH at 0900 after 0600 h Dex	−5, 0, 15 min relative to CRH administration	1.4 (38 nmol/L)	Mild/cyclic hypercortisolism, use of medications that affect Dex metabolism[24]
Plasma ACTH ±cortisol (desmopressin test)[25]	Desmopressin 10 µg IV	Morning	0, 10, 20, 30 min	Varies, see text	Ectopic ACTH secretion may respond, mild/cyclic hypercortisolism

Abbreviations: CRH, corticotropin-releasing hormone; Dex, dexamethasone; IV, intravenous; LDDST, low-dose dexamethasone suppression test; N/A, not applicable; UFC, urine free cortisol; ULN, upper limit of normal.

Most screening tests require that samples be collected at a specific time of day and that measurement of the response to a stimulatory/suppressive agent occurs at a fixed interval after its administration. Failure to adhere to strict timing can lead to false-positive or false-negative results. For example, a 24-hour urine is typically collected beginning in the morning after the first void, continues throughout the day, and includes the next morning's void. The inclusion or exclusion of both voids may lead to overcollection or undercollection and a false result. The adequacy of collection can be judged by the measurement of the total volume, which generally is less than 3 L/d; overhydration and overcollection may increase urine cortisol, and very low values suggest incomplete collection. In addition, the measurement of urine creatinine is helpful, as it does not vary by more than 15% or so in healthy individuals, allowing for comparison between samples. Similarly, time-of-day–specific measurements of salivary or serum cortisol depend on a physiologic nadir just before sleep, as is expected in healthy individuals with a normal circadian rhythm of cortisol. Collection at other times of day results in an increased value compared with the expected bedtime result.

Guidelines on the diagnosis of CS suggest using at least 2 of the first-line tests, with 2 or more measurements of basal cortisol tests, if those are chosen.[15] By reviewing the confounders in **Table 2**, the choice of tests can be individualized to minimize potential false results. As examples, the following are common conditions that might influence the choice of tests, along with ways to determine if the result is correct:

- The Dex tests might be abnormal in a woman taking oral contraceptive agents (if corticosteroid-binding globulin [CBG] is increased, causing increased serum cortisol) or in patients on medications that alter its metabolism.[24] In these settings, other tests might be more reliable, or CBG or Dex can be measured. These false-positive cortisol values are usually less than 7 μg/dL. Thus, if a cortisol value returns more than 10 μg/dL, and the pretest probability is high, measurement of CBG or Dex is not likely to reverse the interpretation.
- Bedtime testing for serum or salivary cortisol might be abnormal in a shift worker, and bedtime serum values may be increased in a woman taking oral estrogens. With shift work, if the bedtime changes frequently, the test should not be used. However, the result is reliable if the shift worker has the same bedtime every day and provides saliva/serum at that time. Measurement of bedtime salivary cortisol, which represents the free fraction, is a better choice than serum cortisol in a woman taking estrogen.
- A urine free cortisol (UFC) result may incorrectly exclude hypercortisolism in patients with a glomerular filtration rate less than 30 mL/min[27] but might falsely diagnose hypercortisolism in individuals drinking more than 5 L of fluid daily. In the former situation, UFC should not be chosen as a screening test. In the latter group of individuals, urinary cortisone and cortisol both increase, so that the effect may be more accentuated in immunoassays in which cortisone cross-reacts with the antibody.[28] Thus, 2 ways of addressing this are to use tandem mass spectroscopy assays (or immunoassays with minimal cross-reactivity) and to ask patients to restrict fluids to 2 L/d.

Unfortunately, except for a few reports, there is little information on the sensitivity and specificity of these tests; a literature review taking pretest probability of CS into account found similar diagnostic accuracy for the tests but did not evaluate confounding factors and did not analyze head-to-head comparisons.[29]

There is less information, and more conflicting results, about the second-line tests, the combined 2 mg-2 day Dex suppression (low-dose Dex suppression test [LDDST]), the CRH stimulation test (Dex-CRH test), and the desmopressin stimulation test. The

Dex-CRH test had 100% diagnostic accuracy when first published on a group of 58 adults referred for evaluation of mild hypercortisolism (UFC level <1000 nmol/d). CS was confirmed in 39 patients; the remaining 19 had a pseudo-Cushing's state.[23] A subsequent study of similar size (32 patients with CS and 23 with pseudo-Cushing's state) reported 100% sensitivity for Dex-CRH and 82% for desmopressin. However, the desmopressin test had better specificity compared with the Dex-CRH test: 90.0% versus 62.5%.[16]

Additional studies failed to find a high diagnostic accuracy using the Dex-CRH test, and often the result of the LDDSTs were similar to those found after CRH. Several potential confounders complicate comparison of the various studies. Most were small, potentially limiting generalizability. None measured Dex levels, so that possible fast metabolizers were not detected. Some used cortisol assays whose functional limit of detection was very close to the interpretative criterion; others used different protocol regimens. Thus, use of the Dex-CRH test should include measurement of Dex levels at baseline, a cortisol assay with very low functional limit of detection, and strict adherence to timing of the study. Overall, when combining data from all studies, the specificity of the LDDST was 79% (95% confidence interval [CI], 70%–86%) and the Dex-CRH specificity was 70% (60%–78%). The sensitivity was also similar, 96% and 98%.[30]

As reviewed by Rollin and colleagues,[25] the diagnostic accuracy of the desmopressin test depends on the criteria used for its interpretation. That study included 68 patients with Cushing's disease and 56 with a presumed pseudo-Cushing's state. The highest area under the curve in a receiver operating characteristic curve analysis (98%) was achieved using an ACTH peak of 71.8 pg/mL, resulting in a sensitivity of 91% and specificity of 95%. A comparison with previous criteria using lower increases in ACTH after desmopressin (37 or 27 pg/mL) yielded lower sensitivities with overlapping CIs, of 82% to 94%. At the more stringent ACTH criterion (37 pg/mL increase), specificity was 96.4 and CIs did not overlap with the specificity at the less conservative ACTH criterion (27 pg/mL increase), which was 86%. Using a combined criterion of an absolute cortisol response of greater than 12 μg/dL and an increase of ACTH of at least 18.18 pg/mL, the sensitivity and specificity of the current and previous studies were 91% to 97% and 84% to 100%.

Additional information regarding conditions associated with false-positive and false-negative screening test results is provided in **Table 3**.

Nonpathologic Hypercortisolism Not Associated with Cushing's Syndrome: Pseudo-Cushing's Syndrome and Physiologic Hypercortisolism

Both clinical and/or biochemical features of endogenous CS occur in individuals without the condition (**Box 2**). The term *pseudo-CS* has been used to characterize individuals who exhibit both features. Individuals with physiologic hypercortisolism may or may not exhibit clinical features. If patients with these conditions also have features of CS, an evaluation for pathologic hypercortisolism often ensues. In both cases, the most common overlapping clinical features include weight gain, increased dorsocervical fat, type 2 diabetes mellitus, hypertension, acne, hirsutism, myopathy, purple striae, and depression.[16,34] In one comparison of patients with proven CS and those without, ecchymoses and osteoporosis were more common in the former and polycystic ovary syndrome was more common in the latter group.

In general, patients with nonpathologic hypercortisolism tend to have urine cortisol excretion less than 3 times normal; values greater than this likely indicate CS.[38] This restriction of UFC to less than three times normal is thought to occur because the hypothalamic-pituitary-adrenal axis is intrinsically able to respond to glucocorticoid

Table 3
Conditions associated with false-positive and false-negative results when screening for Cushing's syndrome

Condition	1 mg DST	UFC	Dex-CRH	Bedtime Serum Cortisol	Bedtime Salivary Cortisol
False-positive results					
Obesity	Y	Y; N	N	N	N
Psychiatric disorder	Y	Y	?	Y; N	?
Alcohol abuse	Y	Y	?	Y	?
Acute illness[31]	Y	Y	?	?	?
Shift work[32]	N	Usu N	?	Y	Y
Estrogen (inc CBG)	Y	N	Y[14]	?	?
Multiple medications (CYP3A4 induction)	Y	N	Y	?	(N)
False-negative results					
Periodic/cyclic CS	Y	Y	?	?	Y
Abn Dex clearance[33]	Y	N	(Y)	N	Y

Abbreviations: ?, not known or unclear; Abn, abnormal; DST, dexamethasone suppression test; inc, increased; N, no; Usu, usually; Y, yes.

restraint, albeit at a somewhat higher-than-usual level. Hence, the stimulus to ACTH overproduction is attenuated by the resulting transient hypercortisolism.

Another feature helps to exclude CS in patients with the nonpathologic hypercortisolism: hypercortisolism reverts with avoidance of a trigger or treatment of the underlying condition.[34] As examples, cortisol normalizes with treatment of pain, sleep apnea, psychiatric disorders, and with avoidance of alcohol and obligate exercise.

When patients present with clinical features that are common in the general population, along with one of the conditions in **Box 2**, the results of screening tests should be interpreted with caution if they are mildly elevated; repeat testing is warranted after withdrawal of a stimulus (eg, a 5-mile daily run) or treatment of a disorder. Conversely, a normal result, assuming that no confounding conditions are present, excludes CS (except for cyclic disease).

Severe, clinically overt CS is easier to diagnose than mild or cyclic cases or when underlying physiology changes the interpretation of tests. Such patients with a classic presentation of severe CS usually have similarly extreme abnormalities in cortisol, and there is little ambiguity in the diagnosis.

Conditions in Which It Is Often Difficult to Identify Pathologic Hypercortisolism

- When it is extremely mild or cyclic
- In renal failure
- In the setting of incidental adrenal masses
- In pregnancy

Patients with mild hypercortisolism tend to have a more subtle clinical presentation and may be difficult to distinguish from those with physiologic hypercortisolism or pseudo-Cushing's states. Those with cyclic hypercortisolism may seem to be normal if studied during a nadir (normal) period. Sometimes they can identify when they are hypercortisolemic, by recrudescence of symptoms, such as weakness, glucose intolerance, or hypertension. In these cases, as well as those in which there is no subjective sense of change over time, multiple measurements of 24-hour urine cortisol, with bedtime salivary cortisol on the same day, may reveal cyclicity.[39,40] Given that the interpretation of differential diagnostic testing requires suppression of normal cortico-trope ACTH secretion, it is probably wise to monitor until patients are consistently hypercortisolemic for 4 to 6 weeks before initiating evaluation of the cause of CS. Although few studies address the response to Dex in this setting, theoretically it would be falsely negative during a nadir period. Hence, the Dex suppression test would not be recommended if cyclic CS is suspected.

Urine cortisol excretion is reduced in moderate and severe chronic kidney disease (creating clearance [CrCl] <50 mL/min), and serum and 2300-hour salivary cortisol increase when CrCl is greater than 20 mL/min.[27] Furthermore, Dex metabolism may be increased, leading to insufficient suppressive doses. When choosing a screening test in these patients, the effect of diabetes, hypertension, and age to increase bedtime salivary cortisol[41,42] should be taken into consideration. Given that all screening test results may be altered by renal failure, one approach is to perform them as usual (except for UFC) and accept the result as correct if it is normal. With an abnormal response to Dex, the test could be repeated with the measurement of a Dex level when cortisol is drawn or with a 2-mg dose for the overnight test,[27,43] which in one study converted abnormal responses to normal ones.

Multiple recent clinical practice guidelines (CPGs) advocate for the evaluation of CS in patients with incidentally discovered adrenal masses.[44,45] Although overt hypercortisolism is evident in a minority of these patients, a larger fraction seem to have dysregulated function of the hypothalamic-pituitary-adrenal axis. This dysfunction can be construed as a spectrum, with incomplete suppression after glucocorticoid feedback (ie, the 1-mg Dex suppression test), to increased late night salivary cortisol,[46] and finally abnormal urine cortisol excretion with suppression of plasma ACTH and DHEAS.[44] Most current CPGs suggest use of the 1-mg overnight Dex suppression test to evaluate whether there is dysregulated or autonomous cortisol secretion, judging a cortisol less than 50 nmol/L (1.8 μg/dL) to be normal, and values greater than 138 nmol/L (>5.0 μg/dL) to indicate autonomous cortisol secretion. Patients with normal responses do not need further evaluation, but those with values greater than 51 nmol/L (1.9 μg/dL) would be evaluated for the presence of cortisol-related comorbidities, such as osteoporosis, diabetes, and hypertension. This strategy allows for consideration of adrenalectomy, which might cure or improve the comorbidities.

Box 2
Examples of nonpathologic hypercortisolism not associated with Cushing's syndrome

Obligate exercise[35]

Pregnancy[36]

Uncontrolled diabetes

Sleep apnea[37]

Pain

Alcoholism, especially withdrawal

Psychiatric disorders

Stress

Extreme obesity

Glucocorticoid resistance syndromes

Most CPGs now emphasize the inability to draw sharp distinctions between any degree of cortisol dysregulation and the need for surgical treatment and emphasize the need for individualization of approach.[44,45]

CS is rare in pregnancy, probably because significant hypercortisolism leads to anovulation and infertility. However, it is important to identify the condition, as it is associated with increased fetal and maternal mortality and morbidity.[36] Pregnancy alters both the clinical and biochemical assessment: certain signs of CS are present (edema, weight gain, full face), coupled with physiologic increases in UFC and ACTH, particularly in the second and third trimesters. The reference range for normal urine and salivary cortisol levels must be adjusted for the stage of pregnancy, and recent reports will likely prove useful in this assessment.[47,48]

SUMMARY AND STRATEGIES

A clear understanding of the pathophysiology of cortisol excess states helps to inform the choice of screening tests for patients with a high pretest clinical probability of having CS. When the results of these tests are consistently abnormal, patients likely have the syndrome and should proceed to tests for the differential diagnosis. When patients have discordant results, reasons for inconsistency should be sought: was a test chosen that carries a high likelihood of a falsely abnormal result in that specific patient? When patients have normal results, but the clinical suspicion is quite high, repeat testing should be done to evaluate for cyclic disease.[15]

Unfortunately, it is still often difficult to be certain about the diagnosis; in such cases, watchful waiting for clinical and biochemical progression may be the safest approach for patients, although frustrating for both patients and clinicians.

REFERENCES

1. Bourdeau I, Bard C, Forget H, et al. Cognitive function and cerebral assessment in patients who have Cushing's syndrome. Endocrinol Metab Clin North Am 2005; 34:357–69.
2. Starkman MN, Schteingart DE. Neuropsychiatric manifestations of patients with Cushing's syndrome. Relationship to cortisol and adrenocorticotropic hormone levels. Arch Intern Med 1981;141:215–9.
3. Starkman MN, Schteingart DE, Schork MA. Correlation of bedside cognitive and neuropsychological tests in patients with Cushing's syndrome. Psychosomatics 1986;27:508–11.
4. Sarlis NJ, Chanock SJ, Nieman LK. Cortisolemic indices predict severe infections in Cushing syndrome due to ectopic production of adrenocorticotropin. J Clin Endocrinol Metab 2000;85:42–7.
5. Dekkers OM, Horváth-Puhó E, Jørgensen JO, et al. Multisystem morbidity and mortality in Cushing's syndrome: a cohort study. J Clin Endocrinol Metab 2013; 98:2277–84.
6. Van der Pas R, Leebeek FW, Hofland LJ, et al. Hypercoagulability in Cushing's syndrome: prevalence, pathogenesis and treatment. Clin Endocrinol (Oxf) 2013;78:481–8.
7. van Dijk EH, Dijkman G, Biermasz NR, et al. Chronic central serous chorioretinopathy as a presenting symptom of Cushing syndrome. Eur J Ophthalmol 2016;26: 442–8.
8. Gokosmanog Lu F, Güzel A, Kan EK, et al. Increased prevalence of obstructive sleep apnea in patients with Cushing's syndrome compared with weight- and age-matched controls. Eur J Endocrinol 2017;176:267–72.

9. Danaei G, Finucane MM, Lu Y, et al, Global Burden of Metabolic Risk Factors of Chronic Diseases Collaborating Group (Blood Glucose). National, regional, and global trends in fasting plasma glucose and diabetes prevalence since 1980: systematic analysis of health examination surveys and epidemiological studies with 370 country-years and 2·7 million participants. Lancet 2011;378:31–40.

10. NCD Risk Factor Collaboration (NCD-RisC). Trends in adult body-mass index in 200 countries from 1975 to 2014: a pooled analysis of 1698 population-based measurement studies with 19·2 million participants. Lancet 2016;387: 1377–96.

11. Krarup T, Krarup T, Hagen C. Do patients with type 2 diabetes mellitus have an increased prevalence of Cushing's syndrome? Diabetes Metab Res Rev 2012; 28:219–27.

12. Sahin SB, Sezgin H, Ayaz T, et al. Routine screening for Cushing's syndrome is not required in patients presenting with obesity. ISRN Endocrinol 2013;2013: 321063.

13. Tiryakioglu O, Ugurlu S, Yalin S, et al. Screening for Cushing's syndrome in obese patients. Clinics (Sao Paulo) 2010;65:9–13.

14. Baid SK, Rubino D, Sinaii N, et al. Specificity of screening tests for Cushing's syndrome in an overweight and obese population. J Clin Endocrinol Metab 2009;94: 3857–64.

15. Nieman LK, Biller BM, Findling JW, et al. The diagnosis of Cushing's syndrome: an Endocrine Society Clinical Practice Guideline. J Clin Endocrinol Metab 2008;93:1526–40.

16. Pecori Giraldi F, Pivonello R, Ambrogio AG, et al. The dexamethasone-suppressed corticotropin-releasing hormone stimulation test and the desmopressin test to distinguish Cushing's syndrome from pseudo-Cushing's states. Clin Endocrinol (Oxf) 2007;66:251–7.

17. Storr HL, Chan LF, Grossman AB, et al. Paediatric Cushing's syndrome: epidemiology, investigation and therapeutic advances. Trends Endocrinol Metab 2007; 18:167–74.

18. Magiakou MA, Mastorakos G, Oldfield EH, et al. Cushing's syndrome in children and adolescents. Presentation, diagnosis, and therapy. N Engl J Med 1994;331: 629–36.

19. Ching CK, Chen SPL, Lee HHC, et al. Adulteration of proprietary Chinese medicines and health products with undeclared drugs: experience of a tertiary toxicology laboratory in Hong Kong. Br J Clin Pharmacol 2018;84(1):172–8.

20. Chong YK, Ching CK, Ng SW, et al. Corticosteroid adulteration in proprietary Chinese medicines: a recurring problem. Hong Kong Med J 2015;21:411–6.

21. Klinsunthorn N, Petsom A, Nhujak T. Determination of steroids adulterated in liquid herbal medicines using QuEChERS sample preparation and high-performance liquid chromatography. J Pharm Biomed Anal 2011;55:1175–8.

22. Olumide YM. Use of skin lightening creams. BMJ 2010;341:c6102.

23. Yanovski JA, Cutler GB Jr, Chrousos GP, et al. The dexamethasone-suppressed corticotropin-releasing hormone stimulation test differentiates mild Cushing's disease from normal physiology. J Clin Endocrinol Metab 1998;83:348–52.

24. Valassi E, Swearingen B, Lee H, et al. Concomitant medication use can confound interpretation of the combined dexamethasone-corticotropin releasing hormone test in Cushing's syndrome. J Clin Endocrinol Metab 2009;94:4851–9.

25. Rollin GA, Costenaro F, Gerchman F, et al. Evaluation of the DDAVP test in the diagnosis of Cushing's disease. Clin Endocrinol (Oxf) 2015;82:793–800.

26. Miller R, Plessow F, Rauh M, et al. Comparison of salivary cortisol as measured by different immunoassays and tandem mass spectrometry. Psychoneuroendocrinology 2013;38:50–7.
27. Chan KC, Lit LC, Law EL, et al. Diminished urinary free cortisol excretion in patients with moderate and severe renal impairment. Clin Chem 2004;50:757–9.
28. Fenske M. Urinary free cortisol and cortisone excretion in healthy individuals: influence of water loading. Steroids 2006;71:1014–8.
29. Elamin MB, Murad MH, Mullan R, et al. Accuracy of diagnostic tests for Cushing's syndrome: a systematic review and meta-analyses. J Clin Endocrinol Metab 2008;93:1553–62.
30. Nieman L. Editorial: the dexamethasone-suppressed corticotropin-releasing hormone test for the diagnosis of Cushing's syndrome: what have we learned in 14 years? J Clin Endocrinol Metab 2007;92:2876–8.
31. Reincke M, Allolio B, Würth G, et al. The hypothalamic-pituitary-adrenal axis in critical illness: response to dexamethasone and corticotropin-releasing hormone. J Clin Endocrinol Metab 1993;77:151–6.
32. Gumenyuk V, Roth T, Drake CL. Circadian phase, sleepiness, and light exposure assessment in night workers with and without shift work disorder. Chronobiol Int 2012;29:928–36.
33. Findling JW, Raff H, Aron DC. The low-dose dexamethasone suppression test: a reevaluation in patients with Cushing's syndrome. J Clin Endocrinol Metab 2004; 89:1222–6.
34. Alwani RA, Schmit Jongbloed LW, de Jong FH, et al. Differentiating between Cushing's disease and pseudo-Cushing's syndrome: comparison of four tests. Eur J Endocrinol 2014;170:477–86.
35. Loucks AB, Mortola JF, Girton L, et al. Alterations in the hypothalamic-pituitary-ovarian and the hypothalamic-pituitary-adrenal axes in athletic women. J Clin Endocrinol Metab 1989;68:402–11.
36. Lindsay JR, Nieman LK. The hypothalamic-pituitary-adrenal axis in pregnancy: challenges in disease detection and treatment. Endocr Rev 2005;26:775–99.
37. Kritikou I, Basta M, Vgontzas AN, et al. Sleep apnoea and the hypothalamic-pituitary-adrenal axis in men and women: effects of continuous positive airway pressure. Eur Respir J 2016;47:531–40.
38. Papanicolaou DA, Mullen N, Kyrou I, et al. Nighttime salivary cortisol: a useful test for the diagnosis of Cushing's syndrome. J Clin Endocrinol Metab 2002;87: 4515–21.
39. Atkinson B, Mullan KR. What is the best approach to suspected cyclical Cushing syndrome? Strategies for managing Cushing's syndrome with variable laboratory data. Clin Endocrinol (Oxf) 2011;75:27–30.
40. Alexandraki KI, Kaltsas GA, Isidori AM, et al. The prevalence and characteristic features of cyclicity and variability in Cushing's disease. Eur J Endocrinol 2009; 160:1011–8.
41. Raff H, Raff JL, Duthie EH, et al. Elevated salivary cortisol in the evening in healthy elderly men and women: correlation with bone mineral density. J Gerontol A Biol Sci Med Sci 1999;54:M479–83.
42. Liu H, Bravata DM, Cabaccan J, et al. Elevated late-night salivary cortisol levels in elderly male type 2 diabetic veterans. Clin Endocrinol (Oxf) 2005;63:642–9.
43. Kawai S, Ichikawa Y, Homma M. Differences in metabolic properties among cortisol, prednisolone, and dexamethasone in liver and renal diseases: accelerated metabolism of dexamethasone in renal failure. J Clin Endocrinol Metab 1985;60:848–54.

44. Fassnacht M, Arlt W, Bancos I, et al. Management of adrenal incidentalomas: European Society of Endocrinology clinical practice guideline in collaboration with the European Network for the Study of Adrenal Tumors. Eur J Endocrinol 2016; 175:G1–34.
45. Terzolo M, Stigliano A, Chiodini I, et al, Italian Association of Clinical Endocrinologists. AME position statement on adrenal incidentaloma. Eur J Endocrinol 2011; 164:851–70.
46. Palmieri S, Morelli V, Polledri E, et al. The role of salivary cortisol measured by liquid chromatography-tandem mass spectrometry in the diagnosis of subclinical hypercortisolism. Eur J Endocrinol 2013;168:289–96.
47. Lopes LM, Francisco RP, Galletta MA, et al. Determination of nighttime salivary cortisol during pregnancy: comparison with values in non-pregnancy and Cushing's disease. Pituitary 2016;19:30–8.
48. Jung C, Ho JT, Torpy DJ, et al. A longitudinal study of plasma and urinary cortisol in pregnancy and postpartum. J Clin Endocrinol Metab 2011;96:1533–40.

Genetics of Cushing's Syndrome

Laura C. Hernández-Ramírez, MD, PhD, Constantine A. Stratakis, MD, D(Med)Sci*

KEYWORDS

- Cushing's syndrome • Glucocorticoids • ACTH • Corticotropinoma
- Pituitary adenoma • Adrenal hyperplasia • cAMP • *USP8*

KEY POINTS

- Cushing's syndrome (CS) of pituitary or adrenal origin usually presents as a sporadic entity and is most commonly due to somatic gene defects.
- Cortisol-producing adenomas are the most common cause of adrenal CS and these lesions are frequently caused by somatic activating mutations in the *PRKACA* gene.
- Somatic gain-of-function mutations in the *USP8* gene constitute the most common genetic defect in corticotropinomas.
- Although infrequent, familial forms of CS may present either isolated or in association with various familial syndromes of multiple endocrine and nonendocrine neoplasia.
- Understanding the genetic defects that drive corticotroph and adrenocortical tumorigenesis should lead to unraveling novel therapeutic targets, which will hopefully be translated into more efficient strategies for the medical treatment of patients with CS.

INTRODUCTION

Characterized by multisystemic manifestations of hypercortisolemia, endogenous Cushing's syndrome (CS) is caused in two-thirds of cases by an adrenocorticotropic hormone (ACTH)-secreting pituitary adenoma (corticotropinoma), and in up to one-quarter of cases by benign adrenal lesions, whereas other causes are more infrequent.[1] CS may have a familial presentation, as part of various syndromes of multiple neoplasia, or present sporadically in the presence of specific germline and/or somatic gene defects (**Table 1**). Vast progress has been achieved in recent years on identifying the molecular and genetic causes of CS of adrenal and pituitary (Cushing's disease [CD]) origin. In this review, we have compiled and summarized the most relevant genetic causes of adrenal and pituitary CS so far described.

Disclosure: The authors have nothing to disclose.
Section on Endocrinology and Genetics (SEGEN), *Eunice Kennedy Shriver* National Institute of Child Health and Human Development (NICHD), National Institutes of Health (NIH), 10 Center Drive, CRC, Room 1E-3216, Bethesda, MD 20892-1862, USA
* Corresponding author.
E-mail address: stratakc@mail.nih.gov

Table 1
Causes of endogenous Cushing's syndrome and their genetic bases

Origin	Lesion Type	General Molecular Mechanisms	Clinical Presentation	Known Genetic Causes
Cushing's disease (60%–70% of cases)	Corticotropinoma	Resistance to glucocorticoid negative feedback, cell-cycle dysregulation, overexpression of membrane receptors (arginine-vasopressin receptors, epidermal growth factor receptor)	Sporadic Cushing's disease, no associated manifestations	Somatic *USP8* GOF hotspot mutations; Somatic *GNAS* GOF mutations (codon 201 or 227); Somatic *RASD1* LOF mutation
			Carney complex	Germline *PRKAR1A* LOF mutations/deletions, uncharacterized defect in 2p16, *PRKACB* amplification
			Familial isolated pituitary adenoma	Germline *AIP* LOF mutations/deletions, unknown genetic defect in 80% of cases
			Familial Cushing's disease with very low penetrance?	Germline *CABLES1* LOF mutations
			Multiple endocrine neoplasia type 1	Germline *MEN1* LOF mutations/deletions
			Multiple endocrine neoplasia type 2	Germline *RET* GOF mutations
			Pheochromocytoma/paraganglioma and pituitary adenoma	
			Multiple endocrine neoplasia type 4	Germline *CDKN1B* LOF mutations/deletions
			Tuberous sclerosis	Germline *TSC1* or *TSC2* LOF mutations

Ectopic ACTH secretion (5%–10% of cases) and ectopic CRH secretion (rare)		Production of ACTH or CRH by tumoral neuroendocrine tissue		
	Medullary thyroid carcinoma		Isolated medullary thyroid carcinoma	RET LOF mutations
			Multiple endocrine neoplasia type 2	
	Other malignant neuroendocrine tumors (bronchial endocrine tumor, small-cell lung cancer, others)		Isolated small-cell lung cancer	Loss of 3p23-p21, somatic TP53 and RB1 LOF mutations, others
			Multiple endocrine neoplasia type 1	Germline MEN1 LOF mutations/deletions
	Benign neuroendocrine tumors (pheochromocytoma, others)		Multiple endocrine neoplasia type 2	Germline RET GOF mutations
			Neurofibromatosis type 1	Germline NF1 LOF mutations
			Von Hippel-Lindau disease	Germline VHL LOF mutations
			Isolated paraganglioma/ pheochromocytoma	SDHA, SDHB, SDHC, SDHD, SDHAF2, FH, MAX, TMEM127 LOF mutations

(continued on next page)

Table 1
(continued)

Origin	Lesion Type	General Molecular Mechanisms	Clinical Presentation	Known Genetic Causes
Adrenal (primary) (20%–30% of cases)	Cortisol-producing adenoma	Overactivation of the cAMP and WNT/CTNNB1 pathways, overexpression of steroidogenic enzymes	Sporadic Cushing's syndrome, no associated manifestations	Somatic *PRKACA* GOF hotspot mutations, somatic *CTNNB1* LOF mutations
			Multiple endocrine neoplasia type 1	*MEN1* LOF mutations/deletions
	Primary macronodular adrenal hyperplasia (PMAH)	Ectopic GPCR and ACTH expression, overactivation of the cAMP and WNT/CTNNB1 pathways, overexpression of steroidogenic enzymes	Familial adenomatous polyposis and Gardner syndrome	Germline *APC* LOF mutations
			Sporadic Cushing's syndrome, no associated manifestations	Germline and somatic *ARMC5* LOF mutations
				Somatic *GIPR* amplification
				Somatic *MC2R* mutations
				Germline *PRKACA* amplification
	Primary pigmented nodular adrenocortical disease (PPNAD)	Overactivation of the cAMP pathway	Sporadic Cushing's syndrome, no associated manifestations (isolated PPNAD)	Germline *PRKAR1A* LOF mutations/deletions, uncharacterized defect in 2p16, germline *PDE11A* LOF mutations
			Carney complex	Germline *PRKAR1A* LOF mutations/deletions, uncharacterized defect in 2p16, *PRKACB* amplification

Disease	Mechanism	Syndrome/Manifestation	Mutation
Isolated micronodular adrenal disease (iMAD)		Sporadic Cushing's syndrome, no associated manifestations	Germline PDE8B LOF mutation; Germline PDE11A LOF mutations
Primary bimorphic adrenocortical disease		McCune-Albright syndrome	Germline PRKACA amplifications; Mosaic GNAS GOF mutation (codon 201)
Adrenocortical carcinoma	Impaired TP53/RB1 signaling and chromatin remodeling, overactivation of the WNT/CTNNB1 pathway	Familial adenomatous polyposis; Sporadic Cushing's syndrome, no associated manifestations	Germline APC LOF mutations; Somatic ZNRF3, APC, CTNNB1, CDKN2A, CDK4, RB1, MDM2, TP53, MEN1, DAXX, and ATRX mutations
		Beckwith-Wiedemann syndrome	11p15.5 maternal rearrangements, paternal uniparental disomy, abnormal methylation, germline CDKN1C and WTX LOF mutations
		Li-Fraumeni syndrome	Germline TP53 LOF mutations
		Multiple endocrine neoplasia type 1	MEN1 LOF mutations/deletions
		Rubinstein-Taybi syndrome	Germline CREBBP or EP300 LOF mutations

See references in text.

Abbreviations: ACTH, adrenocorticotropic hormone; CRH, corticotropic-releasing hormone; CTNNB1, beta-catenin; GOF, gain-of-function; GPCR, G-protein–coupled receptor; LOF, loss-of-function; WNT, wingless-type MMTV integration site family.

GENETIC ALTERATIONS IN CUSHING'S SYNDROME OF ADRENAL ORIGIN
Somatic Activating CTNNB1 Mutations

In mice, beta-catenin (*CTNNB1*) has an important role in driving embryonic adrenocortical cell proliferation, and its constitutive activation results in adrenocortical hyperplasia.[2] Nuclear and cytoplasmic accumulation of the CTNNB1 protein is a common finding in human benign and malignant adrenocortical tumors of various types, and these lesions often display somatic mutations in the *CTNNB1* gene (located on chromosome 3p22.1).[3–5] Within cortisol-producing adenomas (CPAs), the frequency of *CTNNB1* mutations is approximately 15%, whereas two-thirds of nonfunctioning adenomas and one-third of adrenocortical carcinomas carry these genetic defects, which are apparently associated with a more aggressive phenotype.[3,4,6] Most of the patients carry a missense mutation affecting the residue S45, which prevents phosphorylation of the protein by the "destruction complex" (see later in this article), resulting in protein accumulation and activation of its target genes, and therefore resulting in constitutive activation of the wingless-type MMTV integration site family (WNT)/CTNNB1 pathway.[6] Beyond *CTNNB1* sequence mutations, CTNNB1 accumulation also may be due to overactivation of the 3′,5′-cyclic adenosine monophosphate (cAMP)/protein kinase A (PKA) pathway, as it occurs in most adrenocortical lesions.[3]

Familial Adenomatous Polyposis

Germline loss-of-function mutations in the *APC* gene (on chromosome 5q22.2) are associated with adrenocortical adenomas or primary macronodular adrenal hyperplasia (PMAH) in patients with familial adenomatous polyposis; however, this gene does not seem to play a significant role in sporadic CS.[7,8] *APC*-mutated tumors display cytoplasmic and nuclear CTNNB1 accumulation. The APC protein forms part, together with other tumor suppressors and protein kinases, of the "destruction complex," which regulates the WNT/CTNNB1 signaling pathway by targeting and directing CTNNB1 to proteasomal degradation.[2] Therefore, *APC* loss-of-function results in constitutive activation of the WNT/CTNNB1 pathway, in a way that is similar to that of *CTNNB1* mutations.

Activating Somatic PRKACA Hotspot Mutations

Adrenal CS is most often caused by CPAs, and one-third to two-thirds of these tumors bear the somatic recurrent mutation p.L206R in the *PRKACA* gene (on chromosome 19p13.12), encoding the catalytic subunit alpha of PKA.[9–12] The functional effect of the p.L206R mutation is constitutive activation of the cAMP/PKA molecular pathway and therefore increased steroidogenesis, given that these mutations affect a site of the protein that is essential for its interaction with the regulatory subunits of PKA.[9,10,12] The mutation p.L199_C200insW, found in one CPA case, has a similar effect.[9] In addition, germline amplification of the 19p13.2-p13.12 chromosomal region was identified in 5 cases of CS from 4 different families.[9] In these patients, an apparent dosage-dependent effect on the phenotype was observed, as gene triplications were associated with a younger age at disease onset, compared with duplications. These patients developed different types of adrenocortical lesions, including primary pigmented nodular adrenocortical disease (PPNAD), isolated micronodular adrenocortical disease (iMAD), and PMAH, and 1 patient developed breast cancer.[13]

Germline Defects in Phosphodiesterases

Phosphodiesterases are negative regulators of cAMP and 3′,5′-cyclic guanosine monophosphate (cGMP)-dependent intracellular signaling, with multiple isoforms that display differential tissue and substrate specificity. A genome-wide association study identified germline inactivating mutations in the phosphodiesterase 11A gene (*PDE11A*, 2q31.2) in 4 patients with CS due to iMAD, including 2 affected individuals from the same kindred.[14] Later on, a germline missense mutation in the *PDE8B* gene was identified in an additional patient with iMAD. PDE11A is a dual-specificity phosphodiesterase (ie, it hydrolyzes both cAMP and cGMP), whereas PDE8B is cAMP-specific.[15] Both phosphodiesterases are highly expressed (although not exclusively) in the adrenal tissue, and the mutations found in iMAD lead to increased cAMP signaling, in a way similar to *PRKACA* gain-of-function and other cAMP defects identified in adrenal tumors.[16]

Germline and Somatic ARMC5 Mutations

Loss-of-function mutations in the armadillo repeat containing 5 gene (*ARMC5*) are the most common genetic cause of CS due to PMAH. Approximately 26% to 55% patients bear *ARMC5* mutations (on chromosome 16p11.2) at both the somatic and the germline levels; within the PMAH tissue, different *ARMC5* mutations can be found in each nodule.[17–20] ARMC5 encodes a ubiquitously expressed proapoptotic protein, with an additional role as a regulator of steroidogenesis, as demonstrated in vitro.[17,21] In mice, Armc5 is required for gastrulation, and its knockout is lethal, whereas haploinsufficiency leads to late-onset CS.[22] Presentation in *ARMC5* mutation-associated PMAH may be sporadic or familial (autosomal dominant).[23,24] Patients with *ARMC5* mutations have higher midnight serum cortisol, as well as higher urinary 17-hydroxycorticosteroids and free cortisol levels during the 6-day Liddle's test, and their nodules are larger and more numerous, compared with other patients with PMAH.[18,19]

Hereditary Leiomyomatosis and Renal Cell Carcinoma

Fumarate accumulation, as a result of fumarate hydratase (FH) deficiency, leads to pseudohypoxia, a well-known protumorigenic stimulus.[25,26] Loss-of-function mutations in the *FH* gene (1q43) cause an autosomal dominant syndrome characterized by the association of cutaneous leiomyomatosis and renal cell carcinoma. Other tumors less frequently observed in these patients are leiomyosarcomas, uterine leiomyomas, and papillary renal carcinomas, and, occasionally, PMAH (8% of patients).[27,28] Loss of the normal allele has been demonstrated in the PMAH tissue, supporting the causative role of FH in these lesions; however, *FH* mutations have not been associated with sporadic PMAH.[7,27]

Somatic GIPR Microduplications

The finding of local ACTH production and aberrant G-protein–coupled receptor (GPCR) expression as stimuli driving steroidogenesis in PMAH brings attention to the role of ectopic hormone signaling in adrenal tumorigenesis.[26,29] Glucose-dependent insulinotropic polypeptide (GIP)-dependent CS is a rare condition in which ectopic GIP receptor (GIPR) expression in PMAH or CPA tissue leads to hypercortisolemia in response to the physiologic postprandial release of GIP by the small bowel. A recent study identified somatic duplications of the 19q13.32 chromosomal region, including the *GIPR* gene, in 3 of 14 patients with GIP-dependent CS.[30] In 2 of these cases, rearrangements favoring the monoallelic expression of *GIPR* were identified, and among the genes contained in the amplified region, only *GIPR* was consistently overexpressed in the adrenocortical lesions. GIPR overexpression leads to increased steroidogenesis via overactivation of the cAMP/PKA pathway.

Gain-of-Function Germline MC2R Mutations

A germline mutation (p.F278C), in the *MC2R* gene (on chromosome 18p11.21), encoding the ACTH receptor MC2R, was identified in a single patient with PMAH and resulted in constitutive receptor activation in vitro.[31] Two additional *MC2R* mutations (p.C21R and p.S247G) found in a patient with hypersensitivity to ACTH, had the same effect.[32] *MC2R* mutations appear to be a very rare cause of CS, if at all contributory.

GENETIC ALTERATIONS COMMON TO CUSHING'S SYNDROME OF ADRENAL AND PITUITARY ORIGIN
Mosaic or Somatic GNAS Mutations

Early postzygotic mutations in the guanine nucleotide binding protein, alpha stimulating complex locus gene (*GNAS*, on chromosome 20q13.32) affecting the amino acid 201 its best-known product, the G stimulatory protein subunit alpha, cause the McCune-Albright syndrome (MAS).[33] MAS consists of monostotic or polyostotic fibrous dysplasia presenting together with 1 or more manifestations of endocrine hyperfunction (most frequently, primary precocious puberty) and/or dermal café-au-lait spots. Such mutations cause loss of the GTPase function of the protein, resulting in constitutively active GNAS (*gsp* oncogene).[34] CS is an infrequent component of MAS (4% of patients), occurring most often in patients with multiple other manifestations of the syndrome.[33,35] Hypercortisolism in this setting is due to bilateral primary bimorphic (diffuse/nodular hyperplasia and cortical atrophy with apparent *zona glomerulosa* hyperplasia) adrenocortical disease.[36] Besides MAS, somatic mutations in *GNAS* codons 201 and 227 (which have the same functional effects) can also be found as somatic changes in 4% to 15% of CPAs.[10–12] The same mutations are a common finding in sporadic pituitary adenomas (mainly somatotropinomas), although they are rarely found in corticotropinomas, with only 3 cases reported so far.[37,38]

Multiple Endocrine Neoplasia Type 1

The syndrome of multiple endocrine neoplasia type 1 (MEN1) is an autosomal dominant condition characterized by the development of tumors in multiple endocrine and nonendocrine organs.[39] Primary hyperparathyroidism (the most constant feature of the syndrome), gastroenteropancreatic neuroendocrine tumors (GEP-NETs), and pituitary adenomas are the 3 main components or MEN1.[40] Eighty-five percent of the patients with MEN1 have familial presentation and penetrance that is age-specific and organ-specific, and almost complete by the fifth decade of life.[41] Ninety percent of the MEN1 cases bear loss-of-function germline mutations or deletions in the *MEN1* gene (on chromosome 11q13.1), encoding the tumor suppressor menin, a scaffolding protein that regulates the expression and function of proteins involved in transcriptional regulation, genome stability, and cell proliferation.[42–45] In mice, *Men1* full knockout is lethal in utero, but hypomorphic models develop a syndrome resembling the human phenotype.[40]

CS in the setting of MEN1 can be due to a corticotropinoma (79%), primary adrenal disease (21%), or very, rarely, ACTH secretion from a GEP-NET (a few case reports).[46] Approximately 30% to 40% of patients with MEN1 develop pituitary adenomas, and these tumors are the first disease manifestation in 17% to 29% of patients, usually arising at a young age.[47–49] Pituitary adenomas in patients with MEN1 are significantly larger and more invasive than those occurring in non-MEN1 sporadic patients (76%–85% are macroadenomas), but there is no increased prevalence of carcinomas.[47,50] Two-thirds of the patients with clinically evident pituitary disease have prolactinomas, whereas corticotropinomas represent only 3% to 10% of the MEN1-related pituitary adenomas.[47,49,50] Approximately 10% of patients with MEN1 develop adrenal tumors (most of them nonfunctioning), but the incidence of adrenal enlargement is much higher; the prevalence of adrenal cancer is 1%. Nevertheless, CS is relatively infrequent (5% of patients with MEN1 with adrenal tumors).[51]

Carney Complex

Carney complex (CNC) is a rare syndrome composed of multiple endocrine neoplasia and cardiocutaneous manifestations, with autosomal dominant inheritance.[52,53] Three-quarters of CNC cases are caused by loss-of-function mutations in the PRKAR1A gene (on chromosome 17q24.2), 6% are due to deletions in 17q24.2-q24.3, and a triplication of the PRKACB gene was identified as the cause of disease in a single patient, whereas other cases are linked to an uncharacterized defect in 2p16.[54–57] More than half of the cases display familial presentation, with almost full penetrance.[58] No germline or somatic PRKAR1A mutations have been identified in sporadic pituitary adenomas.[59–61] PRKAR1A loss-of-function causes unopposed activation of the cAMP/PKA pathway due to uncontrolled catalytic subunit activity.[53,62] One-quarter of CNC patients develop CS due to PPNAD, although histologic evidence of PPNAD has been detected in almost all CNC individuals at autopsy.[63] Patients develop hypercortisolism with insidious progression over the years that characteristically displays a paradoxical rise during the 6-day Liddle test.[64] Histologically, PPNAD consists of normal-sized or slightly enlarged adrenals with irregular contour, due to small subcapsular dark nodules and cortical atrophy.[65] So far, only 3 cases of CD have been reported among patients with CNC, all of them with frameshift PRKAR1A mutations, although the corticotropinoma was highly suspected but not fully proven in one of the patients.[66–68] Loss of heterozygosity (LOH) in the corticotropinoma tissue was demonstrated in 2 cases.[67,68] In the setting of CNC, CD represents a diagnostic challenge, due to the possible coexistence of CS of adrenal origin.[55,66]

GENETIC ALTERATIONS IN CUSHING'S DISEASE
Somatic Gain-of-Function USP8 Mutations

Mutations in the exon 14 of the USP8 gene (15q21.2), encoding the ubiquitin-specific protease 8, have been reported in 31% to 60% of corticotropinomas occurring in children and adults in tumor-extracted DNA, accounting for the most common somatic gene alteration in CD.[69–72] Such gene defects affect highly conserved residues localized in a hotspot within the 14-3-3 binding motif (residues 715–720). Under physiologic conditions, USP8 binds and deubiquitinates target ubiquitinated proteins to prevent their proteasomal degradation. Cleavage of USP8 at a site immediately upstream to the 14-3-3 binding motif by still unknown proteases results in enhanced deubiquitinase activity from a C-terminal 40-kDa protein fragment.[70] Phosphorylation and binding to 14-3-3 proteins regulates USP8 function by preventing cleavage, but loss of such interaction results in unrestricted protein function. A key target protein for USP8 in corticotroph cells is the epidermal growth factor receptor (EGFR), and USP8 gain-of-function mutations are translated into continuous EGFR recycling, and therefore increased EGFR signaling, resulting in increased POMC transcription.[70,71,73] Along these lines, corticotropinomas carrying USP8 mutations are usually microadenomas that strongly express POMC.[74]

Although EGFR overexpression is not a consistent finding in USP8 mutation-positive tumors, in vitro studies have proven that USP8 mutants inhibit the degradation of the ligand-bound EGFR in EGF-stimulated cells.[70,74] Expression of the somato-statin receptor type 5 (SSTR5) and O-6-methylguanine-DNA methyltransferase (MGMT) are increased in *USP8*-mutated tumors, suggesting that such tumors might be responsive to the pharmacologic treatment with pasireotide, but not with temozo-lomide.[74] The frequency of *USP8* mutations is higher in female individuals in all the cohorts reported so far, but there are discrepancies among studies regarding other clinical and biochemical features.[69–71,74] Interestingly, the frequency of *USP8* muta-tions in a recently reported cohort of patients with Nelson syndrome (45%), was not higher than what has been reported for CD, although such mutations were associated with lower frequency of ACTH normalization after surgery.[75]

Somatic RASD1 Mutation

Originally identified as a gene induced by dexamethasone treatment of AtT20 cells, *RASD1* encodes a glucocorticoid-inducible Ras guanosine triphospha-tase (RAS GTPase) that might have a physiologic role in the glucocorticoid negative feedback in corticotrophs, where it inhibits cAMP-stimulated secretion.[76,77] By inter-acting with G inhibitory proteins, RASD1 exerts a context-dependent activation or suppression of MAPK signaling.[78,79] *RASD1* also is expressed in other tissues, where it might mediate local responses to glucocorticoids; it displays a circadian rhythm of expression in the hypothalamus and has a role as a mediator of the photic response of the circadian clock.[76,80] A novel missense mutation in the *RASD1* gene was detected in a small allelic fraction by whole-exome sequencing in corticotropinoma tissue from a young adult CD female; a coexistent hotspot *USP8* mutation was identified in the same tumor.[81] It was hypothesized that, in this genetically heterogeneous tumor, the *RASD1* mutation could contribute to cell proliferation and ACTH secretion in a small subpopulation of cells.

Somatic TP53 Mutations

Only 3 CD cases have so far been associated with somatic inactivating missense *TP53* mutations, including 2 patients with ACTH-secreting pituitary carcinomas (1 heterozy-gous and 1 not specified) and 1 patient with an invasive corticotropinoma with high Ki-67 index and a homozygous mutation.[82,83] Immunostaining for TP53 was positive in the 3 cases, and particularly high for carcinomas (60% and 90% of positive cells). Interestingly, accumulation of TP53 protein has been observed in 50% of corticotro-pinomas, suggesting that alternative mechanisms should have a role in the over-expression of this tumor suppressor.[84]

Somatic and Germline N3CR1 Mutations

Mutations in the *N3CR1* gene, encoding the glucocorticoid receptor, have been iden-tified by direct sequencing in 2 cases of CD: a patient with a frameshift somatic mu-tation and Nelson syndrome, and a case of CD with generalized glucocorticoid resistance and a dominant-negative de novo germline mutation.[85,86] Whole-exome sequencing of 12 corticotropinomas demonstrated an additional case with a somatic nonsense mutation.[71] Loss-of-function of *N3CR1* in the corticotroph cells impairs the response to the negative adrenal feedback, rendering the cells resistant to the antipro-liferative and antisecretory effects of glucocorticoids. Other studies failed to identify further mutations, indicating that *N3CR1* gene defects are a rare cause of CD.[87,88]

Multiple Endocrine Neoplasia Type 2

Activating mutations in the rearranged during transfection proto-oncogene (*RET*, 10q.11.2) are associated with the syndrome of multiple endocrine neoplasia type 2

(MEN2), an autosomal dominant entity that includes 3 distinctive clinical presentations: familial medullary thyroid carcinoma (MTC), MEN2A (association of MTC, pheochromocytomas, and hyperparathyroidism), and MEN2B (MTC, pheochromocytomas, characteristic facies, marfanoid habitus, ocular abnormalities, musculoskeletal manifestations, and generalized ganglioneuromatosis).[89] RET encodes the tyrosine kinase membrane receptor for the glial-derived neurotrophic factor, expressed by the neural crest during embryogenesis. Activating mutations result in constitutive RET function and activation of pro-proliferative molecular pathways, including the RAS/RAF proto-oncogene serine/threonine-protein kinase (RAF)/mitogen-activated protein kinase (MAPK)/phosphoinositide 3-kinase (PI3K)/RAC-alpha serine/threonine-protein kinase (AKT) pathway.[89,90] Pituitary adenomas are not a classic component of MEN2, but an association between pituitary adenomas and RET mutations has been reported in 4 different patients. Three patients presented with an MEN2A-like phenotype; the fourth patient presented as MEN2B; among them, 2 CD cases have been associated with RET mutations.[91–94] Other patients with similar phenotypes have been described in the literature, although genetic testing was not available or was negative for RET mutations.[95] Although rarely, patients with MEN2 also can develop CS due to ectopic ACTH secretion from MTC.[89]

Multiple Endocrine Neoplasia Type 4

Human germline mutations in the cyclin-dependent kinase inhibitor 1B gene (CDKN1B, 12p13.1) cause approximately 2% of the cases of MEN1 mutation-negative multiple endocrine neoplasia.[96–98] These patients display a heterogeneous phenotype, referred to as MEN4, encompassing parathyroid and pituitary adenomas, neuroendocrine tumors, and various benign and malignant neoplasms.[96] MEN4 is an autosomal dominant disorder with incomplete penetrance, therefore it can present clinically as familial or sporadic cases.[99] The most common component of the syndrome is hyperparathyroidism, whereas renal angiomyolipoma, adrenal nonfunctional tumor, uterine fibroids, gastrinoma and gastric carcinoma, GEP-NETs, nonfunctioning pancreatic endocrine neoplasms, neuroendocrine cervical carcinoma, bronchial carcinoid, and papillary thyroid carcinoma also have been described as part of the syndrome.[96–98,100–105]

Pituitary tumors have been reported in 8 patients with MEN4 so far, only 1 of them with CD.[98,99,105] This female patient carried a frameshift CDKN1B mutation (p.K25fs) and was diagnosed with CD at the age of 46 years; loss of the normal allele was demonstrated in the tumor tissue. She also developed a small-cell neuroendocrine cervical carcinoma and hyperparathyroidism.[97] Although the association of CDKN1B mutations with human corticotropinomas is rare, CDKN1B plays a crucial role in the control of corticotroph proliferation. In addition, Cdkn1b knockout mice develop, among other phenotypic abnormalities, ACTH-secreting hyperplasia or adenomas of the pituitary pars intermedia with full penetrance.[106–108] Given that CDKN1B gene defects are infrequent, other gene regulatory mechanisms might play a role in the impaired CDKN1B function often observed in corticotropinomas.

Three P Association

The association of a pituitary adenoma with a pheochromocytoma or paraganglioma (pheo/PGL) in a single patient, recently defined as the "Three P Association" (3PAs), is a very infrequent phenotype, with only 82 cases identified in the literature.[95,109–119] Of the cases with a known genetic cause, 21 are due to germline loss-of-function mutations in genes that are known to be causative of pheo/PGL: SDHB, SDHD, SDHC and

SDHA genes (*SDHx* genes), in 9, 6, 2, 2, and 1 cases, respectively, whereas an *SDHAF2* and a *MAX* mutation were reported in 1 case each.[109–113,115,118,120–124] A few other cases presenting with this phenotype represent variants of classic syndromes of multiple endocrine neoplasia: 3 cases with *RET* mutations (MEN2A), 2 cases with *MEN1* mutations (MEN1), and 1 with a *VHL* mutation (Von Hippel-Lindau disease).[91,93,117,125] Four cases of CD presenting with 3PAs phenotype have been reported in the literature, one of them carrying a *RET* mutation (see "Multiple endocrine neoplasia type 2"). Genetic screening failed to identify causative mutations in 2 patients.[115,116] One patient was not genetically tested but had a family history compatible with MEN2A.[126] Although it is feasible that mutations in other pheo/PGL-related genes could lead to CD, this has not been demonstrated so far.

Familial Isolated Pituitary Adenoma

Familial isolated pituitary adenoma (FIPA) is defined by the presence of pituitary adenomas in 2 or more members of the same family in the absence of other clinical features, with autosomal dominant inheritance and incomplete penetrance, and accounts for approximately 2.5% of all pituitary adenomas.[127,128] One-fifth of the FIPA cases are due to germline loss-of-function mutations in the *AIP* gene (11q13.2).[129,130] *AIP* mutations are also detected in a subset of sporadic pituitary adenomas affecting young patients, and in one-third of cases of gigantism.[129,131] In the somatotroph cells, AIP has a complex effect as a negative regulator of the cAMP/PKA pathway and of the downstream effects of a G inhibitory protein–coupled receptor, probably an SSTR.[132,133] Ninety-three percent of the *AIP* mutation–positive patients have macroadenomas, and the clinical phenotype is growth hormone excess in 80% of the cases.[129,130] Only 3 cases of CD associated with *AIP* mutations have been described so far in 1 pediatric and 2 young adult patients with missense mutations (p.K103R in the pediatric case and p.R304Q in the adults), all of them with apparently sporadic presentation.[134,135] Nevertheless, the variants found in these patients have displayed inconsistent experimental results, therefore their pathogenic potential is uncertain (reviewed in Hernández-Ramírez and colleagues[136]).

FIPA with undetermined genetic cause represents a heterogeneous group of patients regarding pituitary tumor types, although half of these patients develop growth hormone excess.[137] Six percent of these patients have CD, and FIPA families with exclusively cases of CD have only been reported in the absence of *AIP* mutations.[129,138] X-linked acrogigantism, an infrequent form of gigantism with very young onset caused by *GPR101* (Xq26.3) gene amplification, occasionally has a familial presentation and is included by some, but not all investigators as part of FIPA. Nevertheless, *GPR101* gene defects have not been implicated in CD as yet.[139]

Cushing's Disease Associated with CABLES1 Mutations

The negative cell-cycle regulator *CABLES1* is a direct target gene for glucocorticoids in the corticotroph cells, therefore acting as a mediator of the regulatory adrenal-pituitary feedback loop.[140] CABLES1 stabilizes and prevents the degradation of cell-cycle regulators and interacts with TP53 and TP73 to trigger apoptosis; such tumor suppressor activity is inhibited by 14-3-3 or AKT-mediated phosphorylation.[141,142] CABLES1 expression is lost in a variety of human cancers, and *CABLES1* gene inactivation promotes cell proliferation and survival, as well as tumor formation in vitro, and replicates the human neoplasms in mouse models.[141] We have recently identified 4 patients with CD with loss-of-function *CABLES1* missense mutations, accounting for 2% of the patients tested.[143] The 4 patients had young-onset macroadenomas that were large and aggressive. The mutations were demonstrated at the germline level in 2 of the patients, whereas only tumor-derived DNA was available in the other 2 cases; 1 of the germline mutations was demonstrated in an apparently unaffected parent. These mutations displayed reduced ability to block corticotroph cell proliferation in response to dexamethasone stimulation in vitro. None of the patients had somatic *USP8* mutations, and immunohistochemistry revealed variable CABLES1 with very low nuclear CDKN1B staining. Given its function, *CABLES1* could provide a link between 2 of the main molecular mechanisms disrupted in corticotropinomas: dysfunction of the CDK/cyclin-dependent cell-cycle regulation and EGFR activation of the EGFR pathway, which uses AKT1 as one of its main effectors.[142,144,145]

DICER1 Syndrome

The DICER1 syndrome or pleuropulmonary blastoma (PPB) familial tumor and dysplasia syndrome consists of the association of PPB, ovarian sex cord-stromal tumors, cystic nephroma and thyroid gland tumors, such as multinodular goiter, adenomas, and differentiated thyroid cancer, together with other less common benign and malignant tumors.[146,147] This syndrome is caused by loss-of-function mutations in the *DICER1* gene (14q32.13), and has autosomal dominant presentation, with very low penetrance. Eighty percent of the mutations are inherited and 20% present de novo, and only one-third of the mutation carriers have a known familial history of *DICER1*-related tumors.[147] DICER1 is a multidomain enzyme with important functions in microRNA (miRNA) processing; the RNaseIIIa and RNaseIIIb domains, located at the C-terminal half, constitute the catalytic core of the enzyme. Somatic *DICER1* loss-of-function variants have been reported in *DICER1*-related tumors, most of them affecting the RNase IIIb catalytic domain, in the presence or absence of germline mutations.[148]

Pituitary blastoma is a rare and aggressive apparently congenital pituitary tumor presenting clinically as CD early in infancy.[149] A recent study reported 13 cases of DICER1 syndrome with pituitary blastoma, and 9 of 10 infants tested were positive for heterozygous *DICER1* mutations. Somatic *DICER1* mutations were detected in 7 cases, and 2 cases displayed LOH in the tumor, accounting for a total of 9 patients with somatic alterations; 7 of these cases were also positive for germline mutations.[149] This series, together with a recent case report, account for a total of 14 genetically screened cases of this neoplasm reported to date.[150] The first manifestation of disease appeared early in childhood, and in most cases (9/14) pituitary blastoma was the only manifestation of the syndrome; 5 of the patients died within 0 to 26 months of the first surgery.[149,150] At the histopathological examination, pituitary blastomas resemble the human fetal adenohypophysis at the age of 10 to 12 gestational weeks, when corticotrophs and somatotrophs are already differentiated, and the alpha-glycoprotein subunit starts to emerge, but other cell types are not yet evident.[151] Aside of pituitary blastoma, it remains uncertain whether *DICER1* could also play a role in CD due to pituitary adenomas.

Tuberous Sclerosis Complex

Tuberous sclerosis complex (TSC) is a syndrome characterized by multiple hamartomatous lesions affecting brain, skin, heart, lungs, and kidneys, associated with neurologic manifestations, such as seizures, autism, and cognitive disability. This syndrome is due to loss-of-function mutations in either the *TSC1* (9q34.13) or the *TSC2* (16p13.3) gene, whose protein products (hamartin and tuberin) act as negative regulators of the mammalian target of rapamycin complex 1, therefore inhibiting cell growth.[152] Pituitary adenomas are not a common feature of the TSC, but CD has been described in 2 of such patients so far: a pediatric patient with a *TSC2* mutation and a young adult who was not genetically tested; both patients presented with other coexistent manifestations of TSC.[61,153,154]

X-Linked Congenital Adrenal Hypoplasia

The clinical association of adrenal hypoplasia with glucocorticoid and mineralocorticoid deficiency and hypogonadotropic hypogonadism is due to loss-of-function mutations in the *DAX1* gene (Xp21.2), encoding an orphan nuclear receptor.[155] A single case of a corticotropinoma associated with a germline frameshift *DAX1* mutation has been described.[156] The patient had preexisting adrenal insufficiency, primary hypothyroidism, and hypogonadotrophic hypogonadism and was diagnosed with a CD at the age of 33 years, due to an invasive corticotropinoma. Maternal inheritance of the genetic defect was proven, but no other affected family members were identified.

SUMMARY

Great progress has been made in recent years to elucidate the genetic defects underlying CS of adrenal and pituitary origin. Frequent molecular abnormalities in adrenal lesions include cAMP/PKA and WNT/CTNNB1 signaling overactivation, whereas glucocorticoid resistance, abnormal expression of cell-cycle regulators, and overexpression of membrane receptors predominate in corticotropinomas. Although most of the patients present sporadically, CS is part of a growing number of syndromes of familial isolated CS or multiple endocrine and nonendocrine neoplasia. Moreover, it should be kept in mind that CS of adrenal and pituitary origin can coexist in the setting of some syndromic presentations, complicating the diagnosis. Further research efforts are required to unveil other molecular abnormalities in CS, which will hopefully lead to novel therapeutic targets.

REFERENCES

1. Lacroix A, Feelders RA, Stratakis CA, et al. Cushing's syndrome. Lancet 2015; 386(9996):913–27.
2. Berthon A, Stratakis CA. From beta-catenin to ARM-repeat proteins in adrenocortical disorders. Horm Metab Res 2014;46(12):889–96.
3. Gaujoux S, Tissier F, Groussin L, et al. Wnt/beta-catenin and 3′,5′-cyclic adenosine 5′-monophosphate/protein kinase A signaling pathways alterations and somatic beta-catenin gene mutations in the progression of adrenocortical tumors. J Clin Endocrinol Metab 2008;93(10):4135–40.
4. Tadjine M, Lampron A, Ouadi L, et al. Frequent mutations of beta-catenin gene in sporadic secreting adrenocortical adenomas. Clin Endocrinol (Oxf) 2008; 68(2):264–70.
5. Bonnet S, Gaujoux S, Launay P, et al. Wnt/beta-catenin pathway activation in adrenocortical adenomas is frequently due to somatic CTNNB1-activating mutations, which are associated with larger and nonsecreting tumors: a study in cortisol-secreting and -nonsecreting tumors. J Clin Endocrinol Metab 2011; 96(2):E419–26.
6. Tissier F, Cavard C, Groussin L, et al. Mutations of beta-catenin in adrenocortical tumors: activation of the Wnt signaling pathway is a frequent event in both benign and malignant adrenocortical tumors. Cancer Res 2005;65(17):7622–7.
7. Hsiao HP, Kirschner LS, Bourdeau I, et al. Clinical and genetic heterogeneity, overlap with other tumor syndromes, and atypical glucocorticoid hormone secretion in adrenocorticotropin-independent macronodular adrenal

hyperplasia compared with other adrenocortical tumors. J Clin Endocrinol Metab 2009;94(8):2930–7.

8. Gaujoux S, Pinson S, Gimenez-Roqueplo AP, et al. Inactivation of the APC gene is constant in adrenocortical tumors from patients with familial adenomatous polyposis but not frequent in sporadic adrenocortical cancers. Clin Cancer Res 2010;16(21):5133–41.

9. Beuschlein F, Fassnacht M, Assie G, et al. Constitutive activation of PKA catalytic subunit in adrenal Cushing's syndrome. N Engl J Med 2014;370(11): 1019–28.

10. Cao Y, He M, Gao Z, et al. Activating hotspot L205R mutation in PRKACA and adrenal Cushing's syndrome. Science 2014;344(6186):913–7.

11. Sato Y, Maekawa S, Ishii R, et al. Recurrent somatic mutations underlie corticotropin-independent Cushing's syndrome. Science 2014;344(6186): 917–20.

12. Goh G, Scholl UI, Healy JM, et al. Recurrent activating mutation in *PRKACA* in cortisol-producing adrenal tumors. Nat Genet 2014;46(6):613–7.

13. Lodish MB, Yuan B, Levy I, et al. Germline PRKACA amplification causes variable phenotypes that may depend on the extent of the genomic defect: molecular mechanisms and clinical presentations. Eur J Endocrinol 2015;172(6): 803–11.

14. Horvath A, Boikos S, Giatzakis C, et al. A genome-wide scan identifies mutations in the gene encoding phosphodiesterase 11A4 (PDE11A) in individuals with adrenocortical hyperplasia. Nat Genet 2006;38(7):794–800.

15. Horvath A, Mericq V, Stratakis CA. Mutation in PDE8B, a cyclic AMP-specific phosphodiesterase in adrenal hyperplasia. N Engl J Med 2008;358(7):750–2.

16. Horvath A, Giatzakis C, Tsang K, et al. A cAMP-specific phosphodiesterase (PDE8B) that is mutated in adrenal hyperplasia is expressed widely in human and mouse tissues: a novel PDE8B isoform in human adrenal cortex. Eur J Hum Genet 2008;16(10):1245–53.

17. Assie G, Libe R, Espiard S, et al. ARMC5 mutations in macronodular adrenal hyperplasia with Cushing's syndrome. N Engl J Med 2013;369(22):2105–14.

18. Faucz FR, Zilbermint M, Lodish MB, et al. Macronodular adrenal hyperplasia due to mutations in an armadillo repeat containing 5 (ARMC5) gene: a clinical and genetic investigation. J Clin Endocrinol Metab 2014;99(6):E1113–9.

19. Espiard S, Drougat L, Libe R, et al. ARMC5 mutations in a large cohort of primary macronodular adrenal hyperplasia: clinical and functional consequences. J Clin Endocrinol Metab 2015;100(6):E926–35.

20. Correa R, Zilbermint M, Berthon A, et al. The ARMC5 gene shows extensive genetic variance in primary macronodular adrenocortical hyperplasia. Eur J Endocrinol 2015;173(4):435–40.

21. Cavalcante IP, Nishi M, Zerbini MCN, et al. The role of ARMC5 in human cell cultures from nodules of primary macronodular adrenocortical hyperplasia (PMAH). Mol Cell Endocrinol 2018;460:36–46.

22. Berthon A, Faucz FR, Espiard S, et al. Age-dependent effects of Armc5 haploinsufficiency on adrenocortical function. Hum Mol Genet 2017;26(18):3495–507.

23. Gagliardi L, Schreiber AW, Hahn CN, et al. ARMC5 mutations are common in familial bilateral macronodular adrenal hyperplasia. J Clin Endocrinol Metab 2014; 99(9):E1784–92.

24. Alencar GA, Lerario AM, Nishi MY, et al. ARMC5 mutations are a frequent cause of primary macronodular adrenal hyperplasia. J Clin Endocrinol Metab 2014; 99(8):E1501–9.

25. Xekouki P, Stratakis CA. Succinate dehydrogenase (*SDHx*) mutations in pituitary tumors: could this be a new role for mitochondrial complex II and/or Krebs cycle defects? Endocr Relat Cancer 2012;19(6):C33–40.
26. Fragoso MC, Alencar GA, Lerario AM, et al. Genetics of primary macronodular adrenal hyperplasia. J Endocrinol 2015;224(1):R31–43.
27. Matyakhina L, Freedman RJ, Bourdeau I, et al. Hereditary leiomyomatosis associated with bilateral, massive, macronodular adrenocortical disease and atypical cushing syndrome: a clinical and molecular genetic investigation. J Clin Endocrinol Metab 2005;90(6):3773–9.
28. Shuch B, Ricketts CJ, Vocke CD, et al. Adrenal nodular hyperplasia in hereditary leiomyomatosis and renal cell cancer. J Urol 2013;189(2):430–5.
29. Louiset E, Duparc C, Young J, et al. Intraadrenal corticotropin in bilateral macronodular adrenal hyperplasia. N Engl J Med 2013;369(22):2115–25.
30. Lecoq AL, Stratakis CA, Viengchareun S, et al. Adrenal GIPR expression and chromosome 19q13 microduplications in GIP-dependent Cushing's syndrome. JCI Insight 2017;2(18) [pii:92184].
31. Swords FM, Baig A, Malchoff DM, et al. Impaired desensitization of a mutant adrenocorticotropin receptor associated with apparent constitutive activity. Mol Endocrinol 2002;16(12):2746–53.
32. Swords FM, Noon LA, King PJ, et al. Constitutive activation of the human ACTH receptor resulting from a synergistic interaction between two naturally occurring missense mutations in the MC2R gene. Mol Cell Endocrinol 2004;213(2): 149–54.
33. Collins MT, Singer FR, Eugster E. McCune-Albright syndrome and the extraskeletal manifestations of fibrous dysplasia. Orphanet J Rare Dis 2012;7(Suppl 1):S4.
34. Landis CA, Masters SB, Spada A, et al. GTPase inhibiting mutations activate the alpha chain of Gs and stimulate adenylyl cyclase in human pituitary tumours. Nature 1989;340(6236):692–6.
35. Brown RJ, Kelly MH, Collins MT. Cushing syndrome in the McCune-Albright syndrome. J Clin Endocrinol Metab 2010;95(4):1508–15.
36. Carney JA, Young WF, Stratakis CA. Primary bimorphic adrenocortical disease: cause of hypercortisolism in McCune-Albright syndrome. Am J Surg Pathol 2011;35(9):1311–26.
37. Williamson EA, Ince PG, Harrison D, et al. G-protein mutations in human pituitary adrenocorticotrophic hormone-secreting adenomas. Eur J Clin Invest 1995; 25(2):128–31.
38. Riminucci M, Collins MT, Lala R, et al. An R201H activating mutation of the GNAS1 (Gsalpha) gene in a corticotroph pituitary adenoma. Mol Pathol 2002; 55(1):58–60.
39. Wermer P. Genetic aspects of adenomatosis of endocrine glands. Am J Med 1954;16(3):363–71.
40. Thakker RV. Multiple endocrine neoplasia type 1 (MEN1) and type 4 (MEN4). Mol Cell Endocrinol 2014;386(1–2):2–15.
41. Thakker RV, Newey PJ, Walls GV, et al. Clinical practice guidelines for multiple endocrine neoplasia type 1 (MEN1). J Clin Endocrinol Metab 2012;97(9): 2990–3011.
42. Lemmens I, Van de Ven WJ, Kas K, et al. Identification of the multiple endocrine neoplasia type 1 (MEN1) gene. The European Consortium on MEN1. Hum Mol Genet 1997;6(7):1177–83.
43. Chandrasekharappa SC, Guru SC, Manickam P, et al. Positional cloning of the gene for multiple endocrine neoplasia-type 1. Science 1997;276(5311):404–7.

44. Lemos MC, Thakker RV. Multiple endocrine neoplasia type 1 (*MEN1*): analysis of 1336 mutations reported in the first decade following identification of the gene. Hum Mutat 2008;29(1):22–32.

45. Concolino P, Costella A, Capoluongo E. Multiple endocrine neoplasia type 1 (MEN1): An update of 208 new germline variants reported in the last nine years. Cancer Genet 2016;209(1–2):36–41.

46. Simonds WF, Varghese S, Marx SJ, et al. Cushing's syndrome in multiple endocrine neoplasia type 1. Clin Endocrinol (Oxf) 2012;76(3):379–86.

47. Verges B, Boureille F, Goudet P, et al. Pituitary disease in MEN type 1 (MEN1): data from the France-Belgium MEN1 multicenter study. J Clin Endocrinol Metab 2002;87(2):457–65.

48. Farrell WE, Azevedo MF, Batista DL, et al. Unique gene expression profile associated with an early-onset multiple endocrine neoplasia (MEN1)-associated pituitary adenoma. J Clin Endocrinol Metab 2011;96(11):E1905–14.

49. de Laat JM, Dekkers OM, Pieterman CR, et al. Long-term natural course of pituitary tumors in patients with MEN1: results from the DutchMEN1 Study Group (DMSG). J Clin Endocrinol Metab 2015;100(9):3288–96.

50. Trouillas J, Labat-Moleur F, Sturm N, et al. Pituitary tumors and hyperplasia in multiple endocrine neoplasia type 1 syndrome (MEN1): a case-control study in a series of 77 patients versus 2509 non-MEN1 patients. Am J Surg Pathol 2008;32(4):534–43.

51. Gatta-Cherifi B, Chabre O, Murat A, et al. Adrenal involvement in MEN1. Analysis of 715 cases from the Groupe d'etude des Tumeurs Endocrines database. Eur J Endocrinol 2012;166(2):269–79.

52. Carney JA, Gordon H, Carpenter PC, et al. The complex of myxomas, spotty pigmentation, and endocrine overactivity. Medicine (Baltimore) 1985;64(4):270–83.

53. Correa R, Salpea P, Stratakis CA. Carney complex: an update. Eur J Endocrinol 2015;173(4):M85–97.

54. Stratakis CA, Carney JA, Lin JP, et al. Carney complex, a familial multiple neoplasia and lentiginosis syndrome. Analysis of 11 kindreds and linkage to the short arm of chromosome 2. J Clin Invest 1996;97(3):699–705.

55. Kirschner LS, Carney JA, Pack SD, et al. Mutations of the gene encoding the protein kinase A type I-alpha regulatory subunit in patients with the Carney complex. Nat Genet 2000;26(1):89–92.

56. Forlino A, Vetro A, Garavelli L, et al. PRKACB and carney complex. N Engl J Med 2014;370(11):1065–7.

57. Salpea P, Horvath A, London E, et al. Deletions of the PRKAR1A Locus at 17q24.2-q24.3 in carney complex: genotype-phenotype correlations and implications for genetic testing. J Clin Endocrinol Metab 2014;99(1):E183–8.

58. Horvath A, Bertherat J, Groussin L, et al. Mutations and polymorphisms in the gene encoding regulatory subunit type 1-alpha of protein kinase A (PRKAR1A): an update. Hum Mutat 2010;31(4):369–79.

59. Kaltsas GA, Kola B, Borboli N, et al. Sequence analysis of the *PRKAR1A* gene in sporadic somatotroph and other pituitary tumours. Clin Endocrinol (Oxf) 2002;57(4):443–8.

60. Sandrini F, Kirschner LS, Bei T, et al. PRKAR1A, one of the Carney complex genes, and its locus (17q22-24) are rarely altered in pituitary tumours outside the Carney complex. J Med Genet 2002;39(12):e78.

61. Stratakis CA, Tichomirowa MA, Boikos S, et al. The role of germline AIP, MEN1, PRKAR1A, CDKN1B and CDKN2C mutations in causing pituitary adenomas in a

large cohort of children, adolescents, and patients with genetic syndromes. Clin Genet 2010;78(5):457–63.

62. Meoli E, Bossis I, Cazabat L, et al. Protein kinase A effects of an expressed PRKAR1A mutation associated with aggressive tumors. Cancer Res 2008; 68(9):3133–41.

63. Stratakis CA, Kirschner LS, Carney JA. Clinical and molecular features of the Carney complex: diagnostic criteria and recommendations for patient evaluation. J Clin Endocrinol Metab 2001;86(9):4041–6.

64. Stratakis CA, Sarlis N, Kirschner LS, et al. Paradoxical response to dexamethasone in the diagnosis of primary pigmented nodular adrenocortical disease. Ann Intern Med 1999;131(8):585–91.

65. Stratakis CA, Kirschner LS. Clinical and genetic analysis of primary bilateral adrenal diseases (micro- and macronodular disease) leading to Cushing syndrome. Horm Metab Res 1998;30(6–7):456–63.

66. Basson CT, Aretz HT. Case records of the Massachusetts General Hospital. Weekly clinicopathological exercises. Case 11-2002. A 27-year-old woman with two intracardiac masses and a history of endocrinopathy. N Engl J Med 2002;346(15):1152–8.

67. Hernández-Ramírez LC, Tatsi C, Lodish MB, et al. Corticotropinoma as a Component of Carney Complex. J Endocr Soc 2017;1(7):918–25.

68. Kiefer FW, Winhofer Y, Iacovazzo D, et al. PRKAR1A mutation causing pituitary-dependent Cushing disease in a patient with Carney complex. Eur J Endocrinol 2017;177(2):K7–12.

69. Pérez-Rivas LG, Theodoropoulou M, Ferrau F, et al. The gene of the ubiquitin-specific protease 8 is frequently mutated in adenomas causing Cushing's disease. J Clin Endocrinol Metab 2015;100(7):E997–1004.

70. Reincke M, Sbiera S, Hayakawa A, et al. Mutations in the deubiquitinase gene USP8 cause Cushing's disease. Nat Genet 2015;47(1):31–8.

71. Ma ZY, Song ZJ, Chen JH, et al. Recurrent gain-of-function USP8 mutations in Cushing's disease. Cell Res 2015;25(3):306–17.

72. Faucz FR, Tirosh A, Tatsi C, et al. Somatic USP8 gene mutations are a common cause of pediatric Cushing disease. J Clin Endocrinol Metab 2017;102(8): 2836–43.

73. Mizuno E, Iura T, Mukai A, et al. Regulation of epidermal growth factor receptor down-regulation by UBPY-mediated deubiquitination at endosomes. Mol Biol Cell 2005;16(11):5163–74.

74. Hayashi K, Inoshita N, Kawaguchi K, et al. The USP8 mutational status may predict drug susceptibility in corticotroph adenomas of Cushing's disease. Eur J Endocrinol 2016;174(2):213–26.

75. Pérez-Rivas LG, Theodoropoulou M, Puar TH, et al. Somatic USP8 mutations are frequent events in corticotroph tumor progression causing Nelson's tumor. Eur J Endocrinol 2018;178(1):59–65.

76. Kemppainen RJ, Behrend EN. Dexamethasone rapidly induces a novel ras superfamily member-related gene in AtT-20 cells. J Biol Chem 1998;273(6): 3129–31.

77. Graham TE, Key TA, Kilpatrick K, et al. Dexras1/AGS-1, a steroid hormone-induced guanosine triphosphate-binding protein, inhibits 3′,5′-cyclic adenosine monophosphate-stimulated secretion in AtT-20 corticotroph cells. Endocrinology 2001;142(6):2631–40.

78. Cismowski MJ, Takesono A, Ma C, et al. Genetic screens in yeast to identify mammalian nonreceptor modulators of G-protein signaling. Nat Biotechnol 1999;17(9):878–83.
79. Graham TE, Prossnitz ER, Dorin RI. Dexras1/AGS-1 inhibits signal transduction from the Gi-coupled formyl peptide receptor to Erk-1/2 MAP kinases. J Biol Chem 2002;277(13):10876–82.
80. Cheng HY, Obrietan K, Cain SW, et al. Dexras1 potentiates photic and suppresses nonphotic responses of the circadian clock. Neuron 2004;43(5): 715–28.
81. Uzilov AV, Cheesman KC, Fink MY, et al. Identification of a novel RASD1 somatic mutation in a USP8-mutated corticotroph adenoma. Cold Spring Harb Mol Case Stud 2017;3(3):a001602.
82. Tanizaki Y, Jin L, Scheithauer BW, et al. P53 gene mutations in pituitary carcinomas. Endocr Pathol 2007;18(4):217–22.
83. Kawashima ST, Usui T, Sano T, et al. P53 gene mutation in an atypical corticotroph adenoma with Cushing's disease. Clin Endocrinol (Oxf) 2009;70(4):656–7.
84. Buckley N, Bates AS, Broome JC, et al. P53 protein accumulates in Cushing's adenomas and invasive non-functional adenomas. J Clin Endocrinol Metab 1994;79(5):1513–6.
85. Karl M, Lamberts SW, Koper JW, et al. Cushing's disease preceded by generalized glucocorticoid resistance: clinical consequences of a novel, dominant-negative glucocorticoid receptor mutation. Proc Assoc Am Physicians 1996; 108(4):296–307.
86. Karl M, Von Wichert G, Kempter E, et al. Nelson's syndrome associated with a somatic frame shift mutation in the glucocorticoid receptor gene. J Clin Endocrinol Metab 1996;81(1):124–9.
87. Dahia PL, Honegger J, Reincke M, et al. Expression of glucocorticoid receptor gene isoforms in corticotropin-secreting tumors. J Clin Endocrinol Metab 1997; 82(4):1088–93.
88. Antonini SR, Latronico AC, Elias LL, et al. Glucocorticoid receptor gene polymorphisms in ACTH-secreting pituitary tumours. Clin Endocrinol (Oxf) 2002; 57(5):657–62.
89. Wells SA Jr, Pacini F, Robinson BG, et al. Multiple endocrine neoplasia type 2 and familial medullary thyroid carcinoma: an update. J Clin Endocrinol Metab 2013;98(8):3149–64.
90. Machens A, Dralle H. Multiple endocrine neoplasia type 2 and the RET protooncogene: from bedside to bench to bedside. Mol Cell Endocrinol 2006;247(1–2): 34–40.
91. Saito T, Miura D, Taguchi M, et al. Coincidence of multiple endocrine neoplasia type 2A with acromegaly. Am J Med Sci 2010;340(4):329–31.
92. Heinlen JE, Buethe DD, Culkin DJ, et al. Multiple endocrine neoplasia 2a presenting with pheochromocytoma and pituitary macroadenoma. ISRN Oncol 2011;2011:732452.
93. Naziat A, Karavitaki N, Thakker R, et al. Confusing genes: a patient with MEN2A and Cushing's disease. Clin Endocrinol (Oxf) 2013;78(6):966–8.
94. Kasturi K, Fernandes L, Quezado M, et al. Cushing disease in a patient with multiple endocrine neoplasia type 2B. J Clin Transl Endocrinol Case Rep 2017;4: 1–4.
95. O'Toole SM, Denes J, Robledo M, et al. 15 years of paraganglioma: the association of pituitary adenomas and phaeochromocytomas or paragangliomas. Endocr Relat Cancer 2015;22(4):T105–22.

96. Pellegata NS, Quintanilla-Martinez L, Siggelkow H, et al. Germ-line mutations in *p27Kip1* cause a multiple endocrine neoplasia syndrome in rats and humans. Proc Natl Acad Sci U S A 2006;103(42):15558–63.
97. Georgitsi M, Raitila A, Karhu A, et al. Germline *CDKN1B/p27Kip1* mutation in multiple endocrine neoplasia. J Clin Endocrinol Metab 2007;92(8):3321–5.
98. Agarwal SK, Mateo CM, Marx SJ. Rare germline mutations in cyclin-dependent kinase inhibitor genes in multiple endocrine neoplasia type 1 and related states. J Clin Endocrinol Metab 2009;94(5):1826–34.
99. Lee M, Pellegata NS. Multiple endocrine neoplasia syndromes associated with mutation of *p27*. J Endocrinol Invest 2013;36(9):781–7.
100. Molatore S, Marinoni I, Lee M, et al. A novel germline *CDKN1B* mutation causing multiple endocrine tumors: clinical, genetic and functional characterization. Hum Mutat 2010;31(11):E1825–35.
101. Belar O, De la Hoz C, Perez-Nanclares G, et al. Novel mutations in *MEN1, CDKN1B* and *AIP* genes in patients with multiple endocrine neoplasia type 1 syndrome in Spain. Clin Endocrinol (Oxf) 2012;76(5):719–24.
102. Malanga D, De GS, Riccardi M, et al. Functional characterization of a rare germ-line mutation in the gene encoding the cyclin-dependent kinase inhibitor *p27Kip1 (CDKN1B)* in a Spanish patient with multiple endocrine neoplasia (MEN)-like phenotype. Eur J Endocrinol 2012;166(3):551–60.
103. Occhi G, Regazzo D, Trivellin G, et al. A novel mutation in the upstream open reading frame of the *CDKN1B* gene causes a MEN4 phenotype. PLoS Genet 2013;9(3):e1003350.
104. Pardi E, Mariotti S, Pellegata NS, et al. Functional characterization of a *CDKN1B* mutation in a Sardinian kindred with multiple endocrine neoplasia type 4 (MEN4). Endocr Connect 2015;4(1):1–8.
105. Sambugaro S, Di RM, Ambrosio MR, et al. Early onset acromegaly associated with a novel deletion in *CDKN1B* 5'UTR region. Endocrine 2015;49(1):58–64.
106. Fero ML, Rivkin M, Tasch M, et al. A syndrome of multiorgan hyperplasia with features of gigantism, tumorigenesis, and female sterility in p27(Kip1)-deficient mice. Cell 1996;85(5):733–44.
107. Kiyokawa H, Kineman RD, Manova-Todorova KO, et al. Enhanced growth of mice lacking the cyclin-dependent kinase inhibitor function of p27(Kip1). Cell 1996;85(5):721–32.
108. Nakayama K, Ishida N, Shirane M, et al. Mice lacking p27(Kip1) display increased body size, multiple organ hyperplasia, retinal dysplasia, and pituitary tumors. Cell 1996;85(5):707–20.
109. Lopez-Jimenez E, de Campos JM, Kusak EM, et al. *SDHC* mutation in an elderly patient without familial antecedents. Clin Endocrinol (Oxf) 2008;69(6):906–10.
110. Xekouki P, Pacak K, Almeida M, et al. Succinate dehydrogenase (SDH) D sub-unit (SDHD) inactivation in a growth-hormone-producing pituitary tumor: a new association for SDH? J Clin Endocrinol Metab 2012;97(3):E357–66.
111. Varsavsky M, Sebastian-Ochoa A, Torres VE. Coexistence of a pituitary macro-adenoma and multicentric paraganglioma: a strange coincidence. Endocrinol Nutr 2013;60(3):154–6.
112. Dematti S, Branz G, Casagranda G, et al. Pituitary tumors in SDH mutation carriers. 12th ENSAT Meeting. 2013. p. 29.
113. Dwight T, Mann K, Benn DE, et al. Familial *SDHA* mutation associated with pituitary adenoma and pheochromocytoma/paraganglioma. J Clin Endocrinol Metab 2013;98(6):E1103–8.

114. Niemeijer ND, Papathomas TG, Korpershoek E, et al. Succinate dehydrogenase (SDH)-deficient pancreatic neuroendocrine tumor expands the SDH-related tumor spectrum. J Clin Endocrinol Metab 2015;100(10):E1386–93.
115. Xekouki P, Szarek E, Bullova P, et al. Pituitary adenoma with paraganglioma/ pheochromocytoma (3PAs) and succinate dehydrogenase defects in humans and mice. J Clin Endocrinol Metab 2015;100(5):E710–9.
116. Johnston PC, Kennedy L, Recinos PF, et al. Cushing's disease and co-existing phaeochromocytoma. Pituitary 2016;19(6):654–6.
117. Okada R, Shimura T, Tsukida S, et al. Concomitant existence of pheochromocytoma in a patient with multiple endocrine neoplasia type 1. Surg Case Rep 2016; 2(1):84.
118. Guerrero Perez F, Lisbona Gil A, Robledo M, et al. Pituitary adenoma associated with pheochromocytoma/paraganglioma: a new form of multiple endocrine neoplasia. Endocrinol Nutr 2016;63(9):506–8.
119. Niemeijer ND, Rijken JA, Eijkelenkamp K, et al. The phenotype of SDHB germline mutation carriers: a nationwide study. Eur J Endocrinol 2017;177(2):115–25.
120. Benn DE, Richardson AL, Marsh DJ, et al. Genetic testing in pheochromocytoma- and paraganglioma-associated syndromes. Ann N Y Acad Sci 2006; 1073:104–11.
121. Majumdar S, Friedrich CA, Koch CA, et al. Compound heterozygous mutation with a novel splice donor region DNA sequence variant in the succinate dehydrogenase subunit B gene in malignant paraganglioma. Pediatr Blood Cancer 2010;54(3):473–5.
122. Papathomas TG, Gaal J, Corssmit EP, et al. Non-pheochromocytoma (PCC)/paraganglioma (PGL) tumors in patients with succinate dehydrogenase-related PCC-PGL syndromes: a clinicopathological and molecular analysis. Eur J Endocrinol 2014;170(1):1–12.
123. Denes J, Swords F, Rattenberry E, et al. Heterogeneous genetic background of the association of pheochromocytoma/paraganglioma and pituitary adenoma: results from a large patient cohort. J Clin Endocrinol Metab 2015;100(3): E531–41.
124. Roszko KL, Blouch E, Blake M, et al. Case report of a prolactinoma in a patient with a novel MAX mutation and bilateral pheochromocytomas. J Endocr Soc 2017;1(11):1401–7.
125. Denes J, Swords FM, Xekouki P, et al. Familial pituitary adenoma and paraganglioma syndrome - a novel type of multiple endocrine neoplasia. Endocr Rev 2012;33:OR41–2, 04_MeetingAbstracts.
126. Steiner AL, Goodman AD, Powers SR. Study of a kindred with pheochromocytoma, medullary thyroid carcinoma, hyperparathyroidism and Cushing's disease: multiple endocrine neoplasia, type 2. Medicine (Baltimore) 1968;47(5): 371–409.
127. Vierimaa O, Georgitsi M, Lehtonen R, et al. Pituitary adenoma predisposition caused by germline mutations in the AIP gene. Science 2006;312(5777): 1228–30.
128. Daly AF, Jaffrain-Rea ML, Ciccarelli A, et al. Clinical characterization of familial isolated pituitary adenomas. J Clin Endocrinol Metab 2006;91(9):3316–23.
129. Hernandez-Ramirez LC, Gabrovska P, Denes J, et al. Landscape of familial isolated and young-onset pituitary adenomas: prospective diagnosis in AIP mutation carriers. J Clin Endocrinol Metab 2015;100(9):E1242–54.
130. Daly AF, Tichomirowa MA, Petrossians P, et al. Clinical characteristics and therapeutic responses in patients with germ-line AIP mutations and pituitary

adenomas: an international collaborative study. J Clin Endocrinol Metab 2010; 95(11):E373–83.

131. Rostomyan L, Daly AF, Petrossians P, et al. Clinical and genetic characterization of pituitary gigantism: an international collaborative study in 208 patients. Endocr Relat Cancer 2015;22(5):745–57.

132. Chahal HS, Trivellin G, Leontiou CA, et al. Somatostatin analogs modulate AIP in somatotroph adenomas: the role of the ZAC1 pathway. J Clin Endocrinol Metab 2012;97(8):E1411–20.

133. Tuominen I, Heliovaara E, Raitila A, et al. AIP inactivation leads to pituitary tumorigenesis through defective Galphai-cAMP signaling. Oncogene 2015;34(9): 1174–84.

134. Georgitsi M, Raitila A, Karhu A, et al. Molecular diagnosis of pituitary adenoma predisposition caused by aryl hydrocarbon receptor-interacting protein gene mutations. Proc Natl Acad Sci U S A 2007;104(10):4101–5.

135. Cazabat L, Bouligand J, Salenave S, et al. Germline AIP mutations in apparently sporadic pituitary adenomas: prevalence in a prospective single-center cohort of 443 patients. J Clin Endocrinol Metab 2012;97(4):E663–70.

136. Hernández-Ramírez LC, Trivellin G, Stratakis CA. Role of phosphodiesterases on the function of aryl hydrocarbon receptor-interacting protein (AIP) in the pituitary gland and on the evaluation of AIP gene variants. Horm Metab Res 2017; 49(4):286–95.

137. Beckers A, Daly AF. The clinical, pathological, and genetic features of familial isolated pituitary adenomas. Eur J Endocrinol 2007;157(4):371–82.

138. Beckers A, Aaltonen LA, Daly AF, et al. Familial isolated pituitary adenomas (FIPA) and the pituitary adenoma predisposition due to mutations in the aryl hydrocarbon receptor interacting protein (AIP) gene. Endocr Rev 2013;34(2): 239–77.

139. Trivellin G, Correa RR, Batsis M, et al. Screening for GPR101 defects in pediatric pituitary corticotropinomas. Endocr Relat Cancer 2016;23(5):357–65.

140. Roussel-Gervais A, Couture C, Langlais D, et al. The Cables1 gene in glucocorticoid regulation of pituitary corticotrope growth and Cushing disease. J Clin Endocrinol Metab 2016;101(2):513–22.

141. Huang JR, Tan GM, Li Y, et al. The emerging role of cables1 in cancer and other diseases. Mol Pharmacol 2017;92(3):240–5.

142. Shi Z, Park HR, Du Y, et al. Cables1 complex couples survival signaling to the cell death machinery. Cancer Res 2015;75(1):147–58.

143. Hernández-Ramírez LC, Gam R, Valdés N, et al. Loss-of-function mutations in the CABLES1 gene are a novel cause of Cushing's disease. Endocr Relat Cancer 2017;24(8):379–92.

144. Fukuoka H, Cooper O, Ben-Shlomo A, et al. EGFR as a therapeutic target for human, canine, and mouse ACTH-secreting pituitary adenomas. J Clin Invest 2011;121(12):4712–21.

145. Liu NA, Jiang H, Ben-Shlomo A, et al. Targeting zebrafish and murine pituitary corticotroph tumors with a cyclin-dependent kinase (CDK) inhibitor. Proc Natl Acad Sci U S A 2011;108(20):8414–9.

146. Slade I, Bacchelli C, Davies H, et al. DICER1 syndrome: clarifying the diagnosis, clinical features and management implications of a pleiotropic tumour predisposition syndrome. J Med Genet 2011;48(4):273–8.

147. Doros L, Schultz KA, Stewart DR, et al. DICER1-Related Disorders. In: Adam MP, Ardinger HH, Pagon RA, et al, editors. GeneReviews. Seattle (WA): University of Washington, Seattle; 1993-2018.

148. Foulkes WD, Priest JR, Duchaine TF. *DICER1*: mutations, microRNAs and mechanisms. Nat Rev Cancer 2014;14(10):662–72.
149. de Kock L, Sabbaghian N, Plourde F, et al. Pituitary blastoma: a pathognomonic feature of germ-line *DICER1* mutations. Acta Neuropathol 2014;128(1):111–22.
150. Sahakitrungruang T, Srichomthong C, Pornkunwilai S, et al. Germline and somatic *DICER1* mutations in a pituitary blastoma causing infantile-onset Cushing's disease. J Clin Endocrinol Metab 2014;99(8):E1487–92.
151. Scheithauer BW, Kovacs K, Horvath E, et al. Pituitary blastoma. Acta Neuropathol 2008;116(6):657–66.
152. Lam HC, Nijmeh J, Henske EP. New developments in the genetics and pathogenesis of tumours in tuberous sclerosis complex. J Pathol 2017;241(2):219–25.
153. Tigas S, Carroll PV, Jones R, et al. Simultaneous Cushing's disease and tuberous sclerosis; a potential role for TSC in pituitary ontogeny. Clin Endocrinol (Oxf) 2005;63(6):694–5.
154. Nandagopal R, Vortmeyer A, Oldfield EH, et al. Cushing's syndrome due to a pituitary corticotropinoma in a child with tuberous sclerosis: an association or a coincidence? Clin Endocrinol (Oxf) 2007;67(4):639–41.
155. McCabe ER. DAX1: increasing complexity in the roles of this novel nuclear receptor. Mol Cell Endocrinol 2007;265-266:179–82.
156. De Menis E, Roncaroli F, Calvari V, et al. Corticotroph adenoma of the pituitary in a patient with X-linked adrenal hypoplasia congenita due to a novel mutation of the DAX-1 gene. Eur J Endocrinol 2005;153(2):211–5.

Morbidity of Cushing's Syndrome and Impact of Treatment

Susan M. Webb, MD, PhD[a,b], Elena Valassi, MD, PhD[a,b,*]

KEYWORDS

- Cushing's syndrome • Morbidity • Remission • Quality of life

KEY POINTS

- Endogenous glucocorticoid excess determines many deleterious effects in patients with Cushing's syndrome, leading to increased morbidity.
- Patients with active Cushing's syndrome present cardiovascular and metabolic complications, musculoskeletal alterations, and neuropsychiatric disorders.
- Many abnormalities associated with hypercortisolism do not completely revert despite successful treatment in patients with Cushing's syndrome, leading to sustained impaired health-related quality of life.

INTRODUCTION

Chronic exposure to endogenous glucocorticoid (GC) excess in patients with Cushing's syndrome (CS) is associated with a cluster of complications, which negatively impact morbidity and mortality, including the metabolic syndrome, cardiovascular events, muscle weakness, bone fractures, neurocognitive impairment, and psychiatric disorders.[1] Resolution of hypercortisolism after successful treatment does not lead to complete clinical remission, owing to the irreversible effects of previous hormone excess on many GC-sensitive tissues.[2] Residual psychophysical morbidity in "cured" CS makes their recovery slow and incomplete, and severely affects health-related quality of life (HRQoL) even in the long term after control of cortisol excess.[3]

The authors have nothing to disclose.

[a] Department of Endocrinology, Hospital Sant Pau, Universitat Autònoma de Barcelona, Centro de Investigación Biomédica en Red de Enfermedades Raras (CIBER-ER, Unidad 747), IIB-Sant Pau, ISCIII, c/Sant Antoni Maria Claret 167, Barcelona 08025, Spain; [b] Department of Medicine, Hospital Sant Pau, Universitat Autònoma de Barcelona, Centro de Investigación Biomédica en Red de Enfermedades Raras (CIBER-ER, Unidad 747), IIB-Sant Pau, ISCIII, c/Sant Antoni Maria Claret 167, Barcelona 08025, Spain

* Corresponding author. Department of Endocrinology, Research Center for Pituitary Diseases, Hospital Sant Pau, c/Sant Antoni Maria Claret 167, Barcelona 08025, Spain.
E-mail address: EValassi@santpau.cat

Endocrinol Metab Clin N Am 47 (2018) 299–311
https://doi.org/10.1016/j.ecl.2018.01.001
0889-8529/18/© 2018 Elsevier Inc. All rights reserved.

METABOLISM AND THE CARDIOVASCULAR SYSTEM

CS is a fat-partitioning disorder, characterized by decreased total subcutaneous fat and increased total adipose fat, visceral fat, and trunk subcutaneous fat, leading to impaired adipokine production and related metabolic consequences.[4] Indeed, chronic GC excess in CS is commonly associated with cardiovascular risk factors[5] (**Table 1**).

Impaired glucose tolerance and overt diabetes have been described in 64% and 47% of patients with CS, respectively, owing to the effects of cortisol excess on glucose homeostasis[6] (**Box 1**). Although after remission insulin levels decrease compared with active disease, insulin resistance persists after correcting hypercortisolism and cured patients with CS have higher insulin than controls.[6]

Both soluble tumor necrosis factor-α receptor 1 and interleukin-6 remain higher in patients surgically cured of hypercortisolism for 11 years as compared with controls, suggesting persistent proinflammatory signaling alteration, even in the long term after achieving eucortisolism.[7] In this study, remitted patients also had greater total and trunk fat mass than controls, as assessed by dual-energy x-ray absorptiometry (DXA).[7] A polymorphism of a gene related to GC sensitivity and ongoing GC replacement, are associated with persistent abdominal obesity in cured CS.[8] Remission of hypercortisolism is associated with fat reduction and improvement of fat distribution, consistent with a more favorable cardiovascular risk profile.[9] However, 20 months after remission lipid profiles remain altered, with low adiponectin.[9]

Persistently increased cardiovascular risk in patients with Cushing's disease (CD) 5 years after cure is related to maintenance of increased waist/hip ratio, diastolic blood pressure, total/high-density lipoprotein cholesterol ratio, and plasma fibrinogen, compared with controls.[10] After long-term remission, a greater prevalence of coronary calcifications and noncalcified atheroma plaques, as quantified by cardiac multidetector computed tomography angiogram scan, were described in patients with cured CS compared with controls.[11,12]

Hypertension is a prevalent cardiovascular risk factor, reported in up to 85% of patients with CS, and associated with duration of hypercortisolism[13] (see **Box 1**). Moderate hypertension, with absent nocturnal blood pressure dipping, persists despite effective treatment of hypercortisolism in up to 56% of cured patients, depending on age, duration of GC exposure, and duration of hypertension before surgery.[13,14] Compared with hypertensive controls, hypertensive patients with CS presented

---

Table 1
Summary of cardiometabolic complications associated with cortisol excess in Cushing's syndrome

Cardiovascular Features	Metabolic Features
Left ventricle hypertrophy	Increased total adipose fat, visceral fat, and trunk subcutaneous fat
Concentric remodeling	
Decreased midwall systolic performance with diastolic dysfunction	Decreased total subcutaneous fat
Myocardial fibrosis	Alteration of adipokine secretory pattern (elevated leptin, resistin, tumor necrosis factor-alpha and interleukin-6, reduced adiponectin)
Reduced heart rate variability	
Prolonged QTc dispersion	
Hypertension; absent nocturnal blood pressure dipping	Insulin resistance
Atherosclerosis	Impaired glucose tolerance
Hypercoagulability, increased risk of venous thromboembolism	Dyslipidemia

Data from Refs.[9,13,17,22]

Box 1
Pathophysiology of impaired glucose tolerance and hypertension in patients with Cushing's syndrome

Impaired Glucose Tolerance	Hypertension
Increased gluconeogenesis	Inhibition of the vasodilating system
Disruption of insulin receptor signaling	Activation of the renin–angiotensin–aldosterone system
Reduced insulin sensitivity in liver and skeletal muscle	Inhibition of peripheral catecholamine catabolism
Altered adipokine profile	Increased cardiac output
	Increased total peripheral and renovascular resistance
	Enhanced cortisol binding to the mineralocorticoid receptor

Data from Ferraú F, Korbonits M. Metabolic comorbidities in Cushing's syndrome. Eur J Endocrinol 2015;173:311–9; and Isidori A, Graziadio C, Paragliola RM, et al. The hypertension of Cushing's syndrome: controversies in the pathophysiology and focus on cardiovascular complications. J Hypertens 2015;33:44–60.

---

more severe cardiac structural and functional changes, including left ventricular (LV) hypertrophy with concentric remodeling, and reduced midwall systolic performance with diastolic dysfunction, suggesting that the detrimental effects of hypertension on the heart are worsened by cortisol excess.[15]

Some echocardiographic parameters (interventricular septum thickness, posterior wall thickness, and LV mass index), were still altered in patients with CS in remission for 1 year compared with controls.[16] Moreover, although parameters of systolic function, including ejection fraction and midwall fractional shortening, were within the normal range in cured patients, mean values were still lower than controls.[16] Yet, using cardiac MRI, subclinical systolic biventricular dysfunction and increased LV mass were found in patients with CS.[17] After remission, biventricular improvement of systolic performance and reduced LV mass were observed, together with regression of concentric LV remodeling pattern, independent of body mass index and glucose metabolism.[17] Myocardial fibrosis, frequently found in active CS, regresses after correction of cortisol excess, independent of LV hypertrophy and hypertension.[18]

Prolonged QTcd (QTc dispersion) and reduced heart rate variability (an abnormality of cardiovascular autonomic regulation) are also found in CS.[19,20]

Active CS presents a procoagulative phenotype, and increased incidence of venous thromboembolism in CS compared with the general population (2.5–3.1 per 1000 persons/year vs 1.0–2.0 per 1000 persons/year, respectively; **Box 2**).[21] Patients who undergo surgery for CD have greater risk of thromboembolism than those with a nonfunctional pituitary adenoma, highlighting the role of cortisol (or adrenocorticotrophic

---

Box 2
Procoagulative phenotype of patients with Cushing's syndrome

- Elevation of procoagulant factors (factors VIII and IX, and von Willebrand factor)
- Impaired fibrinolytic capacity owing to increased plasminogen activator inhibitor type 1
- Shortening of activated partial thromboplastin time
- Increased thrombin generation

Data from van der Pas R, Leebeck FWG, Hofland LJ, et al. Hypercoagulability in Cushing's syndrome: prevalence, pathogenesis and treatment. Clin Endocrinol (Oxf) 2013;78:481–8.

hormone) in impairing hemostatic and fibrinolytic factors.[22] After remission, these parameters partially ameliorate, but von Willebrand factor, and factors VII and IX might remain increased at 1 year after cure.[23]

Medications used to treat hypercortisolism might also have metabolic effects in patients with CS. The steroidogenesis inhibitor metyrapone may cause hirsutism and hypertension owing to the accumulation of androgens and desoxycorticosterone in the cortisol synthetic pathway, which could limit long-term treatment with this agent.[24] Pasireotide, a multireceptor-targeted somatostatin analog with a high binding affinity for somatostatin receptor type 5, induces hyperglycemia-related adverse effects in up to 73% of patients, especially in those with preexisting diabetes or impaired glucose tolerance, owing to inhibition of insulin and incretin secretion.[24] Assessment of glucose levels and optimization of glucose-lowering therapy is recommended before and during treatment with pasireotide. It may also reduce weight and blood pressure.[25] Mifepristone, a nonselective GC receptor antagonist, is associated with a favorable metabolic profile, namely, a decrease in body weight, waist circumference, and fat mass, and increased insulin sensitivity in up to 87% of patients treated for 6 months.[25] Sustained weight loss was reported at 2 years of follow-up.[25] More than one-half of patients with impaired glucose tolerance had an improved glucose profile after therapy with this medication.[25] However, mifepristone may also cause severe hypertension owing to mineralocorticoid receptor activation.[25] Osilodrostat, a novel inhibitor of 11 beta-hydroxylase under experimentation, was reported to decrease body mass index after 19 months of treatment.[25]

Abnormal growth hormone secretion, found in up to 65% of CD patients in long-term remission, may contribute to metabolic derangements.[26]

In conclusion, CS is associated with an unfavorable cardiometabolic profile, which may persist in the long term after remission, so that specific management strategies should be contemplated to normalize cardiovascular risk factors and prevent morbidity in these patients.

MUSCULOSKELETAL SYSTEM

GC excess enhances muscle protein catabolism and inhibits anabolic signaling, leading to atrophy, especially in type IIa muscle fibers, which are involved in fast power contraction.[27] Consequently, myopathy and muscle weakness, mainly of the lower limb proximal musculature, are reported in 70% of active CS, especially in females[28] (**Table 2**). A DXA study demonstrated a 15% reduction of limb lean mass in active patients with CS compared with obese controls with the same total body fat mass, and an MRI study showed that muscle mass is reduced in CS compared with controls match

Table 2	
Summary of musculoskeletal alterations associated with cortisol excess in Cushing's syndrome	
Muscle	**Bone**
Muscle atrophy, especially of the lower limbs	Vertebral fractures
Muscle weakness	Low bone mineral density and bone mineral content
Reduced performance on chair rising test	Low osteocalcin levels
Reduced hand grip strength	Spine abnormalities

Data from Berr CM, Stieg MR, Deutschbein T, et al. Persistence of myopathy in Cushing's syndrome: evaluation of the German Cushing's registry. Eur J Endocrinol 2017;176:737–46.

for body mass index.[4,29] An MRI body composition assessment 20 months after remission showed a reduced total and limb skeletal muscle mass in successfully treated CD patients compared with baseline, inversely related to the duration of GC replacement.[9]

Muscle performance was also impaired in active CS, with decreased hand grip strength and performance on chair rising test compared with controls.[27] Patients with CS still have lower limb skeletal muscle mass than controls, as shown on DXA,[8] 13 years after achieving remission, which is associated with muscle weakness and altered muscle function compared with healthy subjects.[27] Hand grip strength was even more decreased than in active patients, unrelated to muscle loss, suggesting that altered quality of muscle (eg, fatty infiltration) may contribute to sustained functional muscle limitations in previously hypercortisolemic patients.[30]

Bone is also severely affected in CS, owing to the inhibitory effects of GC on replication and differentiation of osteoblasts, and intestinal and renal calcium reabsorption. One-half of active patients with CS have osteoporosis, and 30% to 50% experience fractures, especially of the vertebrae.[31] Consistently, patients with endogenous hypercortisolism have reduced DXA-derived trabecular bone score, a marker of bone microarchitecture, along with decreased volumetric bone density and impaired cortical microstructure, as assessed by high-resolution peripheral quantitative computed tomography.[32,33] Secondary hypogonadism and/or concomitant growth hormone deficiency further contribute to bone loss in endogenous cortisol excess[31] (see **Table 2**).

Whether biochemical control of hypercortisolism reverses bone impairment remains controversial, probably owing to the heterogeneity of the studies published. Whereas some authors showed full recovery of bone mineral density 6 to 8 years after remission, paralleled by restoration of coupled remodeling and increased osteocalcin, a marker of bone formation, others demonstrated that estrogen-sufficient women with cured CS after 11 years had persistently lower bone mineral density and osteocalcin than controls, suggesting that the protective effect of estrogens on bone mass is lost in hypercortisolism.[34,35] The duration of postoperative GC replacement and endogenous cortisol excess predict abnormal BMC and bone mineral density.[35] Accordingly, Ragnarsson and colleagues[8] demonstrated that cured patients with ongoing GC replacement presented reduced lumbar spine bone mineral density, and a polymorphism of a gene related to GC sensitivity was associated with reduced femoral bone mineral density.

Interestingly, Faggiano and colleagues[36] demonstrated an increased prevalence of spine abnormalities in CS compared with controls 4 years after the resolution of hypercortisolism. Thus, like in other types of secondary osteoporosis, geometric and mechanical bone properties might be impaired persistently if previously exposed to GC excess, regardless of DXA-measured bone mineral density, and this may severely affect long-term fracture risk.

In conclusion, the detrimental effects of hypercortisolism on the musculoskeletal system, leading to muscle weakness, low muscle performance, osteoporosis, and bone fractures, might not be fully reversible after remission of CS, by mechanisms not yet clearly established.

RENAL FUNCTION

Nephrolithiasis is described in one-half of the patients with active CS, owing to hypercalciuria, hyperuricosuria, and hyperoxalaturia.[37] Although the lithogenic pattern of metabolites and electrolytes ameliorate after remission, the prevalence of silent nephrolithiasis remains higher in cured CS than in controls. Obesity, hypertension, and diabetes mellitus might contribute to kidney stones in CS.[37]

IMMUNE SYSTEM

Cortisol excess inhibits the immune system, causing increased susceptibility to infections and improvement of autoimmune diseases during the active phase of CS. After hypercortisolism correction, new onset of autoimmune diseases or exacerbation of previous ones may occur, as immune activity improves, after longstanding suppression.[38] Autoimmune thyroiditis is the most frequent disorder in patients with cured CS, especially with preexisting goiter or positive antithyroid antibodies.[38] Thus, strict monitoring of patients with CS to identify and treat early immune disorders after achievement of eucortisolism is recommended.

COGNITIVE FUNCTION AND MOOD

Chronic hypercortisolism is associated with cognitive and psychiatric dysfunctions[39,40] (**Table 3**), a consequence of the structural and functional changes induced by hypercortisolism in brain areas rich in GC receptors, mainly the hippocampus,

Table 3
Summary of brain alterations and neuropsychiatric disorders associated with cortisol excess in Cushing's syndrome

Brain Structural Abnormalities	Brain Functional and Biochemical Abnormalities	Deficits in Cognitive Function	Psychopathology
Brain atrophy (mainly hippocampus, amygdala and anterior cingulate cortex)	Reduced functional response of prefrontal cortex during memory testing and emotional processing	Memory	Depression
Decreased cortical thickness	Altered connectivity between the prefrontal cortex and the posterior cingulate cortex	Verbal learning	Anxiety
Reduced gray matter volumes of the cerebellum and anterior cingulate cortex	Alteration of the cholinergic system	Language	Mania
Widespread reduction of white matter integrity	Low levels of N-acetyl-aspartate (marker of neuronal integrity), and high levels of glutamate (excitatory neurotransmitter causing cell damage) in the hippocampus	Spatial information	Maladaptive personality
		Working memory Executive function Mental fatigue	Panic Suicidal ideation

Data from Andela CD, van Haalen FM, Ragnarsson O, et al. Mechanisms in endocrinology: Cushing's syndrome causes irreversible effects on the human brain: a systematic review of structural and functional magnetic resonance imaging studies. Eur J Endocrinol 2015;173:R1–14; and Pivonello R, Simeoli C, De Martino MC, et al. Neuropsychiatric disorders in Cushing's syndrome. Front Neurosci 2015;9:129.

amygdala, and anterior cingulated cortex, which constitute the neurocircuitry of stress[41,42] (**Box 3**). In active CS, decreased hippocampal volumes were associated with impaired verbal learning and recall, and increased activation of the left middle frontal gyrus was related to accuracy of emotion identification.[42,43]

Neuropsychiatric improvement may be delayed and incomplete after resolution of cortisol excess.[40] Long-lasting alterations are reported in several cognitive domains and executive functions.[44–46] Hypopituitarism and hydrocortisone dependency are associated with poor performance on some cognitive tests.[44] Impaired decision making along with decreased cortical thickness in selective frontal areas, irrespective of disease activity, have also been observed in CS compared with controls, suggesting that chronic hypercortisolemia promotes brain changes that are not reversible after endocrine remission.[47] Accordingly, patients in long-term remission showed more severe depression and negative affect, with an increased prevalence of maladaptive personality and psychopathology, as compared with both matched controls and patients with nonfunctioning pituitary macroadenomas.[48] Mental fatigue, characterized by mental exhaustion and long recovery time after mentally strenuous tasks, is more common in remitted CS than controls.[49] Recent structural and functional MRI studies in patients with long-term cured CS versus controls identified several abnormalities in the patients with CS (see **Table 3**).[42,50,51] A decrease in white matter integrity in the left uncinate fasciculus was associated negatively with depression[52] in CS after long-term remission, whereas reduced functional brain responses, mainly in the prefrontal cortex, were detected during memory testing in CS women 7 years after treatment.[53]

A recent genetic study demonstrated that common genetic variants in the GC receptor and the *11β-HSD1* gene influence cognitive impairment in the patient with CS in long-term remission.[54] Reduced methylation of FKBP5 (a protein regulating intracellular GC receptor sensitivity) and retinoic acid receptor related genes are also associated with psychopathology in patients with cured CS.[55]

Although remission achieved after irradiation improved affectivity, the effects of radiation therapy on cognitive function remain controversial, owing to the scarcity and heterogeneity of published studies.[43] Either a decrease in cortisol production induced by steroidogenesis inhibitors (ketoconazole and metyrapone) or blockade of the GC receptor by mifepristone has improved psychopathology in CS.[43] Treatment with mifepristone has been associated with global clinical improvement, including psychiatric and cognitive symptoms and quality of life, in 88% of patients after 24 weeks.[25]

In conclusion, exposure to excess cortisol may have irreversible functional and structural effects on brain areas controlling cognitive function and mood. Consequently, neuropsychiatric disorders may persist in patients with cured CS, despite long-lasting eucortisolism.

Box 3
Pathophysiology of brain damage in patients with Cushing's syndrome

- Reduced synthesis of neurotrophic factors leading to impaired memory and learning process
- Suppression of neurogenesis in the dentate gyrus, leading to hippocampal volume loss
- Increased excitatory amino acids causing neural toxicity and dendritic atrophy
- Reduced glucose uptake in the brain leading to cerebral atrophy

Data from Pivonello R, Simeoli C, De Martino MC, et al. Neuropsychiatric disorders in Cushing's syndrome. Front Neurosci 2015;9:129.

HEALTH-RELATED QUALITY OF LIFE

Poorer HRQoL, as measured with generic or specific questionnaires, has invariably been described in patients with patients with active CS compared with normal population and patients with other pituitary neoplasms.[56,57] Patients with CS report bodily pain, weakness or fatigability, sleep disturbances, worries related to physical appearance, depression/anxiety, troubles with their family life and partner relations, and decreased work or school performance.[58]

Interestingly, obese patients with CS scored worse on physical functional assessment of HRQoL than obese controls without CS, regardless of body mass index, suggesting that specific factors associated with active hypercortisolism determine HRQoL in the obese patients with CS.[59] Most systemic and psychological dysfunctions observed in CS contribute to impair patients' well-being, including neurocognitive dysfunctions, emotional distress, and depression.[28,43]

HRQoL scoring in remitted patients improves compared with baseline, but remains worse than in healthy controls, years after correction of hypercortisolism.[60–63] Patients with cured CS complain of sustained fatigue, anxiety/depression, and poor psychosocial functioning,[64] consistent with the long-lasting negative effects of previous hypercortisolism on cognitive function and behavior.[65] The improvement of physical alterations and emotional distress, characteristic of the active phase, is not immediate after treatment; some physical complaints, like fatigability, take up to 4 years to recover.[66] The first weeks after surgery can be very disheartening owing to a sort of cortisol deprivation phase, with worsening of pain, fatigability, and a sense of helplessness. Moreover, cured patients typically show impairment of coping strategy and persistently negative illness perception, the latter influencing HRQoL after more than 10 years of remission.[67,68]

Although the impact of gender, age, and radiotherapy on HRQoL is controversial, duration of remission and coexistence of depressive symptomatology are positive and negative predictors of HRQoL, respectively.[63,67,69,70] Additionally, the duration of adrenal insufficiency and hydrocortisone use are inversely associated with HRQoL in treated CS, irrespective of etiology[57,62,64] (**Fig. 1**). Pasireotide treatment is

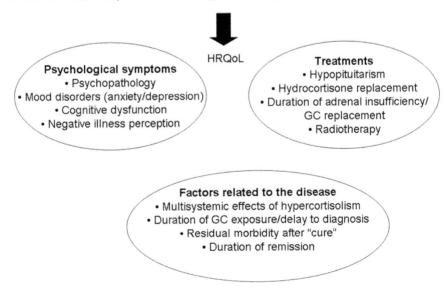

Fig. 1. Factors potentially influencing health-related quality of life (HRQoL) in patients with Cushing's syndrome. GC, glucocorticoids.

associated with improvement of HRQoL at 12 months, especially in patients reaching biochemical control.[24]

In conclusion, HRQoL is severely affected in CS in the active phase, consistent with the deleterious, systemic effects of cortisol excess, and after long-term hormone control, owing to persistently impaired physical and psychological features, including cognitive changes, depression, less self-confidence, and altered illness perception.

SUMMARY

Cortisol excess is associated with metabolic, cardiovascular, and neuropsychological alterations that are only partially reversible after resolution of hypercortisolism. Early detection of hypercortisolism and effective treatment aimed at achieving persistent remission is mandatory in patients with CS. Life-long evaluation is also highly recommended, even long term after remission, to control complications of previous hypercortisolism and improve HRQoL. Periodic laboratory and clinical assessment, and appropriate management of comorbidities (diabetes, hypertension, dyslipidemia) should be carried out according to current guidelines. New diagnostic tools and therapeutic options to reduce the delay to diagnosis and improve long-term prognosis are highly desired. Controlled, prospective studies are also needed to evaluate the impact of radiation and pharmacologic therapy on long-term morbidity.

REFERENCES

1. Newell-Price J, Bertagna X, Grossman AB, et al. Cushing's syndrome. Lancet 2006;367:1605–17.
2. Valassi E, Crespo I, Santos A, et al. Clinical consequences of Cushing's syndrome. Pituitary 2012;15:319–29.
3. Webb SM, Crespo I, Santos A, et al. Quality of life tools for the management of pituitary disease. Eur J Endocrinol 2017;177:R13–26.
4. Geer EB, Shen W, Gallagher D, et al. MRI assessment of lean and adipose tissue distribution in female patients with Cushing's disease. Clin Endocrinol (Oxf) 2010; 73:469–75.
5. Valassi E, Biller BM, Klibanski A, et al. Adipokines and cardiovascular risk in Cushing's syndrome. Neuroendocrinology 2012;95:187–206.
6. Ferraú F, Korbonits M. Metabolic comorbidities in Cushing's syndrome. Eur J Endocrinol 2015;173:311–9.
7. Barahoma MJ, Sucunza N, Resmini E, et al. Persistent body fat mass and inflammatory markers increase after long-term cure of Cushing's syndrome. J Clin Endocrinol Metab 2009;94:3365–71.
8. Ragnarsson O, Glad CA, Bergthorsdottir R, et al. Body composition and bone mineral density in women with Cushing's syndrome in remission and the association with common genetic variants influencing glucocorticoid sensitivity. Eur J Endocrinol 2015;172:1–10.
9. Geer EB, Shen W, Stromayer E, et al. Body composition and cardiovascular risk markers after remission of Cushing's disease: a prospective study using whole-body MRI. J Clin Endocrinol Metab 2012;97:1702–11.
10. Colao A, Pivonello R, Spiezia R, et al. Persistence of increased cardiovascular risk in patients with Cushing's disease after five years of successful cure. J Clin Endocrinol Metab 1999;84:3991–9.
11. Barahona MJ, Resmini E, Vilades D, et al. Coronary artery disease detected by multislice computed tomography in patients after long-term cure of Cushing's syndrome. J Clin Endocrinol Metab 2013;98:1093–9.

12. Neary NM, Booker OJ, Abel BS, et al. Hypercortisolism is associated with increased coronary arterial atherosclerosis: analysis of noninvasive coronary angiography using multidetector computerized tomography. J Clin Endocrinol Metab 2013;98:2045–52.

13. Isidori A, Graziadio C, Paragliola RM, et al. The hypertension of Cushing's syndrome: controversies in the pathophysiology and focus on cardiovascular complications. J Hypertens 2015;33:44–60.

14. Giraldi FP, Toja PM, De Martin M, et al. Circadian blood pressure profile in patients with Cushing's syndrome before and after cure. Horm Metab Res 2007; 39:908–14.

15. Muiesan ML, Lupia M, Salvetti M, et al. Left ventricular structural and functional characteristics in Cushing's syndrome. J Am Coll Cardiol 2003;41:2275–9.

16. Toja PM, Branzi G, Ciambellotti F, et al. Clinical relevance of cardiac structure and function abnormalities in patients with Cushing's syndrome before and after cure. Clin Endocrinol (Oxf) 2012;76:332–8.

17. Kamenicky P, Redheuil A, Roux C, et al. Cardiac structure and function in Cushing's syndrome: a cardiac magnetic resonance imaging study. J Clin Endocrinol Metab 2014;99:E2144–53.

18. Yiu KH, Marsan NA, Delgado V, et al. Increased myocardial fibrosis and Leith ventricular dysfunction in Cushing's syndrome. Eur J Endocrinol 2012;166:27–34.

19. Alexandraki KI, Kaltsas GA, Vouliotis AI, et al. Specific electrocardiographic features associated with Cushing's disease. Clin Endocrinol (Oxf) 2011;74:558–64.

20. Chandran DS, Ali N, Jaryal AK, et al. Decreased autonomic modulation of heart rate and altered cardiac sympathovagal balance in patients with Cushing's syndrome: role of endogenous hypercortisolism. Neuroendocrinology 2013;97:309–17.

21. van der Pas R, Leebeck FWG, Hofland LJ, et al. Hypercoagulability in Cushing's syndrome: prevalence, pathogenesis and treatment. Clin Endocrinol (Oxf) 2013; 78:481–8.

22. Stujiver DJF, van Zaane B, Feelders RA, et al. Incidence of venous thromboembolism in patients with Cushing's syndrome: a multicenter cohort study. J Clin Endocrinol Metab 2011;96:3525–32.

23. Manetti L, Bogazzi F, Giovannetti C, et al. Changes in coagulation indexes and occurrence of venous thromboembolism in patients with Cushing's syndrome: results from a prospective study before and after surgery. Eur J Endocrinol 2010; 23:145–50.

24. Pivonello R, De Leo M, Cozzolino A, et al. The treatment of Cushing's disease. Endocr Rev 2015;36:386–486.

25. Cuevas-Ramos D, Lim DST, Fleseriu M. Update on medical treatment for Cushing's disease. Clin Diabetes Endocrinol 2016;2:16.

26. Webb SM, Mo D, Lamberts SWJ, et al. Metabolic, cardiovascular and cerebrovascular outcomes in GH deficient subjects with previous Cushing's disease or non-functioning pituitary adenoma: a Hypopituitary Control and Complications Study (HypoCCS) analysis. J Clin Endocrinol Metab 2010;95:630–8.

27. Berr CM, Stieg MR, Deutschbein T, et al. Persistence of myopathy in Cushing's syndrome: evaluation of the German Cushing's registry. Eur J Endocrinol 2017; 176:737–46.

28. Valassi E, Santos A, Yaneva M, et al. The European registry on Cushing's syndrome: 2-year experience. Baseline demographic and clinical characteristics. Eur J Endocrinol 2011;165:383–92.

29. Wajchenberg BL, Bosco A, Marrone MM, et al. Estimation of body fat and lean tissue distribution by dual energy X-ray absorptiometry and abdominal body

fat evaluation by computed tomography in Cushing's disease. J Clin Endocrinol Metab 1995;80:2791–4.

30. Drey M, Berr CM, Reincke M, et al. Cushing's syndrome: a model for sarcopenic obesity. Endocrine 2017;57:481–5.
31. Mancini T, Doga M, Mazziotti G, et al. Cushing's syndrome and bone. Pituitary 2004;7:249–52.
32. Belaya ZE, Hans D, Rozhinskaya LY, et al. The risk factors for fractures and trabecular bone-score value in patients with endogenous Cushing's syndrome. Arch Osteoporos 2015;10:44.
33. Dos Santos CV, Vieira Neto L, Madeira M, et al. Bone density and microarchitecture in endogenous hypercortisolism. Clin Endocrinol (Oxf) 2015;83:468–74.
34. Manning PJ, Evans MC, Reid IR. Normal bone density following cure of Cushing's syndrome. Clin Endocrinol 1992;36:229–34.
35. Barahona MJ, Sucunza N, Resmini E, et al. Deleterious effects of glucocorticoid replacement on bone in women after long-term remission of Cushing's syndrome. J Bone Miner Res 2009;24:1841–6.
36. Faggiano A, Pivonello R, Filippella M, et al. Spine abnormalities and damage in patients cured from Cushing's disease. Pituitary 2001;4:153–61.
37. Faggiano A, Pivonello R, Melis D, et al. Nephrolithiasis in Cushing's disease: prevalence, etiopathogenesis, and modification after disease cure. J Clin Endocrinol Metab 2003;88:2076–80.
38. da Mota F, Murray C, Ezzat S. Overt immune dysfunction after Cushing's syndrome remission: a consecutive case series and review of the literature. J Clin Endocrinol Metab 2011;96:E1670–4.
39. Forget H, Lacroix A, Somma M, et al. Cognitive decline in patients with Cushing's syndrome. J Int Neuropsychol Soc 2000;6:20–9.
40. Sonino N, Fava GA, Raffi AR, et al. Clinical correlates of major depression in Cushing's disease. Psychopathology 1998;31:302–6.
41. Starkman MN, Gebarski SS, Berent S, et al. Hippocampal formation volume, memory dysfunctions, and cortisol levels in patients with Cushing's syndrome. Biol Psychiatry 1992;32:756–65.
42. Andela CD, van Haalen FM, Ragnarsson O, et al. Mechanisms in endocrinology: Cushing's syndrome causes irreversible effects on the human brain: a systematic review of structural and functional magnetic resonance imaging studies. Eur J Endocrinol 2015;173:R1–14.
43. Pivonello R, Simeoli C, De Martino MC, et al. Neuropsychiatric disorders in Cushing's syndrome. Front Neurosci 2015;9:129.
44. Tiemensma J, Kokshoorn NE, Biermasz NR, et al. Subtle cognitive impairments in in patients with long-term cure of Cushing's disease. J Clin Endocrinol Metab 2010;95:2699–714.
45. Resmini E, Santos A, Gómez-Anson B, et al. Verbal and visual memory performance and hippocampal volumes, measured by 3-Tesla magnetic resonance imaging, in patients with Cushing's syndrome. J Clin Endocrinol Metab 2012;97: 663–71.
46. Ragnarsson O, Berglund P, Eder DN, et al. Long-term cognitive impairments and attentional deficits in patients with Cushing's disease and cortisol-producing adrenal adenoma in remission. J Clin Endocrinol Metab 2012;97:E1640–8.
47. Crespo I, Granell-Moreno E, Santos A, et al. Impaired decision-making and selective cortical frontal thinning in Cushing's syndrome. Clin Endocrinol (Oxf) 2014;81: 826–33.

48. Tiemensma J, Biermasz MR, Middelkoop HA, et al. Increased prevalence of psychopathology and maladaptive personality traits after long-term cure of Cushing's disease. J Clin Endocrinol Metab 2010;95:E129–41.

49. Papakokkinou E, Johansson B, Berglund P, et al. Mental fatigue and executive dysfunctions in patients with Cushing's syndrome in remission. Behav Neurol 2015;2015:173653.

50. Bas-Hoogendam JM, Andela CD, van der Werff SJA, et al. Altered neural processing of emotional faces in remitted Cushing's disease. Psychoneuroendocrinology 2015;59:134–6.

51. Resmini E, Santos A, Gómez-Anson B, et al. Hippocampal dysfunction in cured Cushing's syndrome patients, detected by 1H-MR-spectroscopy. Clin Endocrinol 2013;79:700–7.

52. Van der Werff SJ, Andela CD, Pannekoek JN, et al. Widespread reductions of white matter integrity in patients with long-term remission of Cushing's disease. Neuroimage Clin 2014;4:659–67.

53. Ragnarsson O, Stomby A, Dahlqvist P, et al. Decreased prefrontal functional brain response during memory testing in women with Cushing's syndrome in remission. Psychoneuroendocrinology 2017;82:117–25.

54. Ragnarsson O, Glad CA, Berglund P, et al. Common genetic variants in the glucocorticoid receptor and the 11β-hydroxysteroid dehydrogenase type 1 genes influence long-term cognitive impairments in patients with Cushing's syndrome in remission. J Clin Endocrinol Metab 2014;99:1803–7.

55. Glad CA, Andersson-Assarsson JC, Berglund P, et al. Reduced DNA methylation and psychopathology following endogenous hypercortisolism – a genome-wide study. Sci Rep 2017;7:44445.

56. Sonino N, Fava GA. Psychological aspects of endocrine disease. Clin Endocrinol (Oxf) 1998;49:1–7.

57. Webb SM, Badia X, Barahona MJ, et al. Evaluation of Health-Related Quality of Life in patients with Cushing's syndrome with a new questionnaire (CushingQoL). Eur J Endocrinol 2008;158:623–30.

58. Gotch PM. Cushing's syndrome from the patient's perspective. Endocrinol Metab Clin North Am 1994;23:607–17.

59. Abraham SB, Abel BS, Rubino D, et al. A direct comparison of quality of life in obese and Cushing's syndrome patients. Eur J Endocrinol 2013;168:787–93.

60. Lindsay JR, Nansel T, Baid S, et al. Long-term impaired quality of life in Cushing's syndrome despite initial improvement after surgical remission. J Clin Endocrinol Metab 2006;91:447–53.

61. van Aken MO, Pereira AM, Biermasz NR, et al. Quality of life in patients after long-term biochemical cure of Cushing's disease. J Clin Endocrinol Metab 2005;90:3279–86.

62. Wagenmakers MAEM, Neta-Meier RT, Prins JB, et al. Impaired quality of life in patients in long-term remission of Cushing's syndrome of both adrenal and pituitary origin: a remaining effect of longstanding hypercortisolism? Eur J Endocrinol 2012;167:687–95.

63. Milian M, Kreitschmann-Andermahr I, Siegel S, et al. Validation of the Tuebingen CD-25 inventory as a measure of postoperative health-related quality of life in patients treated for Cushing's disease. Neuroendocrinology 2015;102:60–7.

64. Tiemensma J, Depaoli S, Felt MJ. Using subscales when scoring the Cushing's quality of life questionnaire. Eur J Endocrinol 2016;174:33–40.

65. Andela CD, Scharloo M, Pereira AM, et al. Quality of life (QoL) impairments in patients with a pituitary adenoma a systematic review of QoL studies. Pituitary 2015;18:752–76.
66. Sippel RS, Elaraj DM, Kebebew E, et al. Waiting for change: symptom resolution after adrenalectomy for Cushing's syndrome. Surgery 2008;144:1054–61.
67. Tiemensma J, Kaptein AA, Pereira AM, et al. Negative illness perceptions are associated with impaired quality of life in patients after long-term remission of Cushing's syndrome. Eur J Endocrinol 2011;165:527–35.
68. Tiemensma J, Kaptein AA, Pereira AM, et al. Coping strategies in patients after treatment for functioning or non-functioning pituitary adenomas. J Clin Endocrinol Metab 2011;96:964–71.
69. Santos A, Resmini E, Martinez-Momblan MA, et al. Psychometric performance of the CushingQoL questionnaire in conditions of real clinical practice. Eur J Endocrinol 2012;167:337–42.
70. Valassi E, Crespo I, Keevil BG, et al. Affective alterations in patients with Cushing's syndrome in remission are associated with decreased BDNF and cortisone levels. Eur J Endocrinol 2017;176:221–31.

Mortality in Patients with Endogenous Cushing's Syndrome

Pedram Javanmard, MD[a], Daisy Duan, MD[a], Eliza B. Geer, MD[b],*

KEYWORDS

- Mortality • Cushing's syndrome • Cushing's disease • Ectopic Cushing's
- Adrenal Cushing's • Subclinical Cushing's

KEY POINTS

- Cushing's syndrome, chronic endogenous cortisol hypersecretion, is associated with an overall increased mortality risk.
- The leading causes of mortality in Cushing's are cardiovascular events, infection, sepsis, and thromboembolism.
- Patients with Cushing's due to a pituitary tumor or a benign adrenal adenoma seem to have the best survival outcomes; persistent or recurrent disease confers high mortality risk.
- Overall, patients with Cushing's due to an ectopic adrenocorticotrophic hormone-secreting tumor or adrenocortical carcinoma have the worst survival rate.
- Prompt diagnosis and treatment of Cushing's and specific monitoring and treatment of comorbidities are paramount to decreasing the burden of mortality.

INTRODUCTION

Endogenous hypercortisolism, known as Cushing's syndrome (CS), is a chronic endocrine disorder caused by excessive adrenal cortisol secretion, with an estimated incidence of 0.7 to 2.4 cases per million population per year.[1–4] The majority (70%) of endogenous CS cases are caused by excess adrenocorticotrophic hormone (ACTH) production from pituitary corticotroph tumors, known as Cushing's disease (CD). ACTH-independent adrenal cortisol production due to an adrenal tumor or hyperplasia is responsible for 20% of CS cases. The remaining 10% of CS cases are due to ectopic ACTH (or very rarely corticotropin-releasing hormone) production.[1–3]

The authors have no relevant disclosures.

[a] Department of Medicine, Division of Endocrinology, Diabetes, and Bone Disease, Icahn School of Medicine, The Mount Sinai Hospital, 1 Gustave L Levy Place, Box 1055, New York, NY 10029, USA; [b] Division of Endocrinology, Department of Medicine, Multidisciplinary Pituitary and Skull Base Tumor Center, Memorial Sloan Kettering Cancer Center, 1275 York Avenue, Box 419, New York, NY 10065, USA
* Corresponding author.
E-mail address: geere@mskcc.org

Endocrinol Metab Clin N Am 47 (2018) 313–333
https://doi.org/10.1016/j.ecl.2018.02.005
0889-8529/18/© 2018 Elsevier Inc. All rights reserved.

CS can occur at any age. It is, however, more frequent during the fourth to sixth decades of life and more common in women: 79% of pituitary CS, 81% of adrenocortical adenomas, and 60% to 70% of adrenocortical carcinoma (ACC) cases are female, whereas among patients with ectopic CS (ECS), males have an equal or even higher predominance.[5–7]

With regard to the overall predictors for mortality in CS, male gender, older age at diagnosis, overall disease activity duration, disease status (persistent or recurrent disease vs remission), persistent hypercortisolism after initial surgery, and hypertension at last follow-up have been associated with higher mortality risk.[6,8–10] This article reviews the predictors of mortality in patients with endogenous CS. The majority of available mortality data are on patients with CD, and therefore CD is the focus of the review.

ADRENOCORTICOTROPHIC HORMONE-DEPENDENT CUSHING'S DISEASE

CD, due to an ACTH-secreting pituitary corticotroph adenoma, is the most common form of endogenous CS and accounts for 70% of all cases of CS.[3,8,9] In the original series published by Harvey Cushing's in 1932,[11] the median survival in untreated CD was 4.6 years. This finding was validated in a later study[12] that reported a 5-year survival rate of 50%. The main causes of mortality in CD are cardiovascular complications including strokes and myocardial infarctions (**Table 1**).[13,14]

In the past 2 decades, there have been 12 retrospective nationwide or single-center cohort studies that have reported standardized mortality ratios (SMRs) in CD, with 5 of these studies also reporting mortality data on other causes of CS (**Table 2**). Most studies have been conducted in Europe, the United States, or New Zealand, and had median follow-up periods from 6 to 20 years since the onset of treatment. The overall SMR for all-cause mortality in CD ranges from 0.98 to 9.30, indicating that mortality risk in patients with CD is similar to or higher than that of the general population. The majority of these studies further stratify mortality risk based on disease activity status (ie, remission vs recurrent or persistent disease). In addition, several of these studies identify independent mortality risk factors in patients with CD. A limitation of these studies are the small sample sizes, thus, with even smaller numbers of deaths. As several meta-analyses have pointed out, there is also considerable heterogeneity with respect to the definitions of remission, persistence, and recurrence of disease, the timing of the assessment after initial treatment, methods of treatment, and the duration of follow-up periods (**Table 3**). Despite these challenges, there is consistent evidence that persistent CD after pituitary surgery confers the highest risk of mortality, although there are conflicting data regarding mortality risk in patients with disease remission after treatment.

Predictors of Mortality and Risk Factors for Increased Mortality in Patients with Cushing's Disease Overall

Cardiovascular disease results in a 4-fold increase in mortality among patients with persistent CD compared with control populations.[9,15,16] More recent studies suggest a more pronounced mortality risk, with a reported SMR of 13.8 for vascular disease.[17] Some mortality risk may also be present in patients with CD who have been in remission for more than 10 years.[18] In addition, given that the cause of mortality in patients with CD is largely attributed to cardiovascular diseases, certain cardiovascular risk factors have been identified as independent predictors of mortality. The presence of diabetes, but not hypertension, was an independent risk factor for mortality (hazard ratio [HR], 2.82; 95% confidence interval [CI], 1.29–6.17) in 1 study[18]; in other studies,[7,9,17] however, the persistence of both diabetes or glucose metabolism

Table 1
Causes of death reported in patients with CS

References	Mortality Rate	Causes of Death
Clayton et al,[18] 2016	CD: 16%	CD CV[a] 62.7%; malignancy 17.6%; PE 7.8%; sepsis 3.9%; others or unknown 19.6%
Ntali et al,[24] 2013	CS overall: 9.6%; CD: 9%; AC: 3%; ECS 30%	CD CV 50%; malignancy 25%; infection/sepsis 21.4%; multiple organ failure 3.6%; perioperative 3.6%; unknown 3.6% AC CV 100% ECS Metastatic carcinomatosis 40%; Sepsis 30%; postoperative 20%; unknown 10%
Yaneva et al,[6] 2013	CS overall: 30.3%; CD: 27.5%; ECS: 58.3%; AA: 14.3%; ACC: 89.7%; BAH: 18.2%; unproven: 40%	CD CV 32%; CVA 15%; infections/sepsis 9%; other neoplasms 7.7%; DM 6.4%; CS 5.1%; thromboembolism 1.3%; ARF 1.3%; hepatic failure 1.3%; others 1.3%; unknown 16.7% ECS CV 43%; infection/sepsis 29%; osteoporosis 14%; unknown 14% AA Thromboembolism 19%; infections/sepsis 12.5%; CVA 12.5%; other neoplasms 12.5%; unknown 31% ACC CS 45%; CV 24%; infections/sepsis 21%; CVA 3.4%; unknown 7% BAH NR
Hassan-smith et al,[26] 2012	CD: 16.3%	CD CV 61.5%; malignancy 23.1%; infection 7.7%; CD 7.7%
Bolland et al,[7] 2011	CS overall: 14%	CS (including CD, ECS, AA, BAH) CV 19%; carcinoma 22%; CVA 17%; sepsis 17%; PE 17%; suspected adrenal insufficiency 2.8%
Clayton et al,[17] 2011	CD: 22%	CD CV 53.8%; CVA 23.1%; malignancy 15.4%; GI bleed 7.7%
Dekker et al,[21] 2007	CD: 16.2%	CD CV 33.3%; CVA 8.3%; malignancy 8.3%; infection 8.3%; persistent disease 8.3%; unknown 16.7%; other 16.7%
Hammer et al,[10] 2004	CD: 10%	CD NR
Lindholm et al,[8] 2001	CS overall 28.9%; CD 18.2%; AA 10.8%; ACC 100%	CS (including CD, AA, ACC)[b] Malignancy 40%; CV[c] 20%; CVA 20%; sepsis 10%; surgical complication 10%

(continued on next page)

Table 1 (continued)		
References	**Mortality Rate**	**Causes of Death**
Swearingen et al,[23] 1999	CD: 3.8%	CD CV 33.3%; CVA 33.3%; lymphoma 16.7%; trauma 16.7%
Pikkarainen et al,[49] 1999	CS overall: 13.5%	CS (including CD, AA) CV 20%; PE 20%; aspiration pneumonia 10%; mitral valve insufficiency and CHF 10%; lung cancer 10%; pancreatitis 10%; intracerebral hemorrhage 10%; morbus Parkinson 10%

Abbreviations: AA, adrenal adenoma; AC, adrenal Cushing's; ACC, adrenocortical carcinoma; ARF, acute renal failure; BAH, bilateral adrenal hyperplasia; CD, Cushing's disease; CHF, congestive heart failure; CS, Cushing's syndrome; CV, cardiovascular; CVA, cerebrovascular accident; DM, diabetes mellitus; ECS, ectopic Cushing's syndrome; GI, gastrointestinal; NR, not reported; PE, pulmonary embolism.

[a] Includes CVA-related deaths and ruptured aortic aneurysms.
[b] Causes of death were reported for 90 patients with CS who had long-term follow-up data. Only 10 deaths were reported in this cohort.
[c] CV included ruptured aortic aneurysm and myocardial infarction.

dysfunction and hypertension after treatment were found to increase mortality. Moreover, cardiovascular risk in patients with CD who had been in remission for 5 years remained higher when compared with an age- and gender-matched population.[15] In a small prospective trial on patients with CS,[19] there was significant decrease in glucose impairment, hyperlipidemia, and hypertension only in adrenal but not pituitary Cushing's 1 year after biochemical remission, a finding that could explain the persistent mortality risk some studies have shown in patients with CD despite treatment.

Lambert and colleagues[20] examined mortality data from 346 patients with CD over a span of 31 years of follow-up. This study demonstrated that longer exposure to excess glucocorticoids, defined here by a duration of symptoms before diagnosis until remission, was associated with increased risk of death. This observation supports the hypothesis that poor outcomes in CD is a consequence of hypercortisolism, as suggested by studies demonstrating that patients with CD have increased mortality compared with patients with nonfunctioning and growth hormone-secreting pituitary adenomas.[21,22]

Other factors associated with increased mortality found in Lambert and colleagues[20] include older age at diagnosis and preoperative plasma ACTH concentrations. Among patients with CD who achieved overall and immediate remission, depression at presentation and male sex also increased the risk of death. Older age at diagnosis has been frequently associated with increased mortality in both CD and CS.[6,7,9,17,23,24] Male gender has also been identified in additional studies as a mortality risk factor in both CD and CS.[6,10]

Mortality in Patients with Persistent or Recurrent Cushing's Disease

Multiple cohort studies and meta-analyses have consistently demonstrated that patients with CD with persistent or recurrent disease have significantly elevated SMR when compared with the general population. Of note, in all but 1 cohort study,[7] a combined SMR was calculated for patients with persistent disease and those with recurrent disease, even if these were distinctly defined groups during data collection. In addition, recurrence rates vary among studies, ranging between 10% and 20% at

Table 2
Summary of studies reporting Standardized Mortality Ratio (SMR) in Cushing's syndrome and/or Cushing's disease[a]

References	Study Design	CS vs. CD	Study Participants	Study Period	# of Pts	Median Followup (y)	SMR for All Cause Mortality	SMR for Remission	SMR for Persistent Disease	Indep. Risk Factors of Mortality
Clayton et al,[18] 2016	Retrospective multi-center cohort	CD	• UK, Denmark, Netherlands, New Zealand tertiary referral centers • Pts cured of hypercortisolism for minimum of 10 y[b]	1948–2014[c]	320	11.8[d]	1.61	NR	NR	DM; higher number of treatments
Ntali et al,[24] 2013	Retrospective multi-center cohort[e]	CS (CD, ECS, AA, BAH)[f]	• 1 tertiary referral centers in Oxford, UK[e]	1967–2009	209 CS; 182 CD; 16 AC; 11 ECS	CD 12; AC 5; ECS 4.5	CD 9.3; AC 5.3; ECS 68.5	CD 8.3; ECS 83.3	CD 9.9; ECS 66.7	Older age at diagnosis
Yaneva et al,[6] 2013	Retrospective single-center cohort	CS (CD, ECS, AA, ACC, BAH)	• 1 tertiary referral center in Sofia, Bulgaria	1965–2010	386 CS; 240 CD; 12 ECS; 84 AA; 11 BAH; 10 etiology unproven	7.0	CS 4.05; CD 1.88; ECS 13.33; AA 1.67; ACC 48; BAH 1.14; unproven 4	CS 1.67	CS 2.4	Older age at diagnosis; male; CD pts without initial remission after TSS; duration of activity of symptoms
Hassan-Smith et al,[26] 2012	Retrospective single-center cohort	CD	• 1 center in the UK • Pts who underwent TSS with 1 surgeon	1988–2009	80[g]	10.9[h]	3.17	2.47	4.12[i]	NR
Bolland et al,[7] 2011	Retrospective nationwide cohort	CS (CD, ECS, AA, BAH)	• 4 endocrinology services in New Zealand[j]	1960–2005	253 CS; 188 CD; AA 37; BAH 9; occult ECS 10; probable ECS 9	6.4	CS 4.1; CD macroadenoma 3.5; CD microadenoma 3.2; AA 7.5; BAH 14; occult ECS 27; probable ECS 3.1	CD macroadenoma 2.5; CD microadenoma 3.2	CD macroadenoma 5.7; CD microadenoma 2.4	CD only – older age at diagnosis; BDX; pituitary irradiation; CD and CS – HTN, DM at final follow-up
Clayton et al,[17] 2011	Retrospective single-center study cohort	CD	• 1 UK center	1958–2010	60	15	4.8	3.3	16.0	HTN; DM; disease persistence
Dekker et al,[21] 2007	Retrospective single-center cohort	CD	• 1 center in the Netherlands • Patients who underwent TSS for NFMA and CD	1977–2005	Total 248; CD 74; NFMA 174	10.1 (mean)	2.39	1.8	4.38	Disease persistence
Hammer et al,[10] 2004	Retrospective single-center cohort	CD	• 1 tertiary referral center in the US • Pts who underwent TSS with 1 surgeon[k]	1975–1998	189	11.1	1.42	1.18	2.8	Male; higher tumor stage

(continued on next page)

Table 2
(continued)

References	Study Design	CS vs. CD	Study Participants	Study Period	# of Pts	Median Followup (y)	SMR for All Cause Mortality	SMR for Remission	SMR for Persistent Disease	Indep. Risk Factors of Mortality
Lindholm et al,[8] 2001	Retrospective national registry cohort	CS (CD, AA, ACC)	• National Patient Register of the Danish National Board of Health	1985–1995	166 CS; 99 CD total[l]; 48 adrenal tumors; 11 ACC; 16 cancer-associated; 3 others	8.1	CS 3.68; proven CD 1.7; unproven CD 11.5; AA 3.48; ACC 11/11 died-no SMR	CD 0.31	CS 5.06	Disease persistence
Swearingen et al,[23] 1999	Retrospective single-center cohort	CD	• 1 tertiary referral center in the US • Pts who underwent TSS with 1 surgeon	1978–1996	161	8.0	0.98	NR	NR	Older age at diagnosis
Pikkarainen et al,[49] 1999	Retrospective single-center cohort	CS (CD, AA, ECS, ACC, BAH)	• 1 tertiary referral center in Finland	1981–1994	74 CS; 43 CD; ECS 4; unclear ACTH dep 1; AA 20; ACC 4; BAH 2	7.4 (mean)	CS: 1.68; CD: 2.67; AA 1.35; benign pituitary or adrenal disease 2.02; not reported for ECS or ACC	NR	NR	NR
Etxabe et al,[9] 1994	Retrospective national registry cohort	CD	• National Health Service Records in Vizcaya, Spain	1975–1992	49	4.7	3.8	NR	NR	Older age at diagnosis; persistent HTN; persistent abnormalities of glucose metabolism

Abbreviations: AA, adrenal adenoma; AC, adrenal Cushing's; ACC, adrenocortical carcinoma; BAH, bilateral adrenal hyperplasia; BDX, bilateral adrenalectomy; HTN, hypertension; indep, independent; NFMA, non-functioning pituitary macroadenoma; NR, not reported; pts, patients; SMR, standardized mortality ratio; TSS, transsphenoidal surgery.

a Studies were included if they are: 1. A cohort study of patients with Cushing's syndrome and/or Cushing's disease; and 2. Mortality risk expressed as SMR.

b Patient had continued cure with no relapse until database was frozen or until death.

c Frozen data dates ranged 2009–2014.

d 11.8 years from study entry + 10 years in remission.

e Study also included a second cohort from Athens, Greece but data for this table only included Oxford cohort as SMR was only calculated for this cohort.

f Patients with ACC were excluded.

g 72 patients with clinical follow-up data.

h 10.9 yrs median follow-up for mortality; 4.6 yrs median for clinical follow-up.

i Recurrent and persistent disease were combined.

j Patients with ACC or malignant ECS were excluded.

k Excluded patients who had undergone previous pituitary or adrenal surgery or had Nelson's syndrome.

l 73 CD proven; 26 CD unproven.

Table 3

Definitions of remission/cure and recurrent/persistent disease in mortality studies on Cushing's syndrome

References	Definition of Remission and/or Cure	Definition of Recurrent or Persistent Disease
Clayton et al,[18] 2016	Variable depending on the center	NR
Ntali et al,[24] 2013	• Undetectable 9-h serum cortisol after pituitary surgery, adrenalectomy or removal of an ectopic ACTH-producing tumor • After pituitary radiotherapy, normal 24 h UFC or mean serum cortisol 150–300 nmol/l on a 5-point cortisol day curve or had developed ACTH deficiency and during medical treatment, if the patient had achieved a mean serum cortisol 150–300 nmol/l on a 5-point day curve	Recurrence: clinical and biochemical (elevated 24 h UFC and lack of suppression on overnight or low dose DST)
Yaneva et al,[6] 2013	Remission – resolution of clinical symptoms after treatment, adrenal insufficiency with need for GC replacement therapy, normalization of UFC Cure– absence of clinical and biochemical hypercortisolism (normal/low UFC or 17-OH and ketosteroids in earlier cases and normal DST at last clinical visit)	NR
Hassan-Smith et al,[26] 2012	Initial remission: morning post-op cortisol <1.8 ug/dL measured between day 4 and week 6) Cure: initial remission and continued biochemical cure during follow-up	Recurrence: biochemical (raised UFC or failure of cortisol suppression on DST) and clinical after initial remission Persistence: biochemically by post-op cortisol >1.8 ug/dL
Bolland et al,[7] 2011	Adrenal insufficiency and required GC replacement or normal 24-h UFC or normal overnight 1 mg DST	Recurrence: recurrence of CS following initial biochemical cure
Clayton et al,[17] 2011	Clinically - resolution of symptoms and signs Biochemically - normal UFC and low-dose DST, normal mean plasma cortisol day curve for those on metyrapone; achieved within 3 y after treatment	Persistence: failure to achieve remission targets within 3 y despite treatment

(continued on next page)

Table 3
(continued)

References	Definition of Remission and/or Cure	Definition of Recurrent or Persistent Disease
Dekker et al,[21] 2007	Normal 1 mg DST and 24-h UFC in 2 consecutive samples	Persistence: failure to meet biochemical criteria for remission 3–6 mo after 1st operation; Recurrence: recurrence of hypercortisolism (increased 24-h UFC, abnormal 1 mg DST, and normal or exaggerated response of serum ACTH and cortisol to IV CRH stimulation
Hammer et al,[10] 2004	Initial remission: within 1 wk post-op, basal or 1 mg DST plasma cortisol <5 ug/dL; or within 6 mo post-op, low or normal plasma or urinary cortisol, resolution of clinical features, and no additional therapy Long-term remission: at 6 mo post-op, continued clinical remission, plasma cortisol after 1 mg DST cortisol of <5 ug/dL or normal 24-h UFC at last follow-up and had not undergone additional therapy	Recurrence: initial remission followed by recurrent hypercortisolism or additional therapy 6 mo or more post-op
Lindholm et al,[8] 2001	• Plasma cortisol <18 ug/dL at 30 min after IV 250 ug of corticotropin and/or UFC <18 ug/24 h measured 12–180 d after operation • If the results were ambiguous postop, panhypopituitarism or if UFC <90 ug/24 h at >5 y after first operation	Recurrence: after cure is initially achieved, UFC >90 ug/24 h at any time during follow-up
Swearingen et al,[23] 1999	Fasting serum cortisol <138 nmol/l and UFC <55 nmol/d at 10-d post-op	Recurrence: based on questionnaire response and results of routine endocrine reevaluation, without independent repeated assay
Pikkarainen et al,[49] 1999	Normal UFC, disappearance of symptoms, no relapse	NR
Etxabe et al,[9] 1994	Normalization of UFC and normal DST	NR

Abbreviations: CRH, corticotropin-releasing hormone; DST, dexamethasone suppression test; GC, glucocorticoid; NR, not reported; UFC, urinary free cortisol.

10 years in patients with a microadenoma and between 12% and 45% in patients with a macroadenoma.[25] Aside from individual differences in disease severity and tumor size and characteristics, the variation in reported recurrence rates could reflect differences in treatment outcomes between centers as well as inconsistency in definitions used for establishing recurrent and persistent disease. Given these discrepancies, mortality data for persistent and recurrent CD are presented together.

In the 4 cohort studies[10,17,21,26] that focus on patients with CD only, the SMR for patients with persistent or recurrent disease ranged from 2.8 to 16.0, and was significantly increased compared with SMR for patients with disease in remission, which ranged from 1.18 to 4.12. Most recently, a meta-analysis of 8 studies that reported mortality rates in CD[27] calculated a pooled SMR of 4.6 (95% CI, 2.9–7.3) for patients with persistent or recurrent disease, compared with an SMR of 2.5 (95% CI, 1.4–4.2) for patients with remitted disease, as defined in each study. Given the overwhelming evidence of poor outcomes for patients with persistent or recurrent disease, early diagnosis and aggressive intervention are imperative.

Mortality in Patients with Cushing's Disease in Remission

In contrast with studies describing mortality in patients with persistent disease, studies that focus on patients with disease remission have yielded conflicting results. Several studies report an SMR (ranging from 1.18 to 1.67) for patients with disease remission similar to that of the general population,[6,10,21] but some data suggest treatment type may play a role in mortality risk.[8,18] A recent study by Clayton and colleagues[18] analyzed census data from multiple tertiary referral centers in the UK, Denmark, the Netherlands, and New Zealand on 320 patients with CD in remission, as defined by each center's criteria for normalization of hypercortisolism without recurrence for at least 10 years. A strength of this study was its long follow-up (median of 11.8 years from study entry), totaling more than 20 years of survival data. All-cause mortality in patients with disease remission from any treatment for at least 10 years remained increased, with an SMR of 1.61 (95% CI, 1.23–2.12). However, patients who achieved remission after transsphenoidal surgery (TSS) alone had long-term survival comparable to that of the general population (SMR ,0.95; CI, 0.58–1.55). Similarly, a previous study by Lindholm and colleagues[8] reported that the mortality risk for patients with CD cured by initial TSS was no different from that of the general population (SMR, 0.31; 95% CI, 0.01–1.72).

Other studies, however, report a significantly increased SMR (range, 2.47–8.30) in patients with CD who achieve remission versus the general population.[7,17,24,26,28] Moreover, in Bolland and colleagues series,[7] SMR remained elevated even in patients who were cured after first TSS, although the confidence intervals were wide (the SMR was 2.3 for pituitary macroadenoma with a 95% CI of 0.4–7.5, and 3.1 for pituitary microadenoma with a 95% CI of 1.8–4.9). A more recent meta-analysis by van Haalen and colleagues,[27] which extracted data from 8 cohort studies totaling 766 patients,[6–8,17,21,24,26] reported a pooled SMR for patients with disease remission of 2.5 (95% CI, 1.4–4.2), suggesting irreversible effects of long-term excess glucocorticoid exposure. It can be concluded that, although there is some evidence that mortality risk for patients with CD in remissions remain elevated, survival outcomes are still significantly improved compared with patients with CD with persistent or recurrent disease. Moreover, patients with CD cured by TSS alone seem to have the best survival outcomes, possibly no different from that of the general population. The use of consistent definitions of CD remission, persistence, and recurrence between investigators would improve the ability to clearly define mortality risk for each of these groups.

The pathophysiology behind the persistently elevated mortality risk despite biochemical remission in CD is not well-characterized. It has been hypothesized that perhaps, due to the difficulty in diagnosis and cure, the prolonged cortisol excess before remission results in irreversible or long-lasting adverse effects that predispose to increased mortality. In support of this hypothesis, Dekkers and colleagues[21] reported that the SMR for patients with CD was significantly higher than SMR for patients with nonfunctioning pituitary macroadenomas (2.39 vs 1.24), and mortality in CD was increased compared with acromegaly after adjustment for sex and age (HR, 2.4; 95% CI, 1.13–4.91), suggesting that hypercortisolism is responsible for the increased mortality. In addition, a study by Colao and colleagues[15] found that atherosclerosis and cardiovascular risk factors remained elevated in patients who had CD despite being in remission for an average of 5 years. In addition, although whole-body MRI showed that CD remission resulted in favorable changes in body fat distribution and decrease in some cardiovascular risk factors, other markers such as adiponectin and C-reactive protein did not change after remission.[29] Proinflammatory cytokines also remained increased after CD remission, likely contributing to increased cardiovascular mortality.[30] Similarly, Hassan-Smith and colleagues[26] showed that although weight loss and improvement in blood pressure were evident with treatment, a significant proportion of patients with CD in remission demonstrated end-organ cardiovascular damage that was likely irreversible, including evidence of left ventricular hypertrophy and myocardial ischemia. Aside from cardiovascular complications, other comorbidities such as bone impairment and neuropsychiatric dysfunction have been shown to persist despite biochemical cure.[31,32]

Effect of Treatment Type on Mortality in Cushing's Disease

Surgical resection, when feasible and performed by an experienced surgeon, remains first-line treatment for CD. As discussed, some data show that patients who were able to achieve remission with pituitary surgery alone had mortality risk similar to that of the general population. However, immediate remission rates with pituitary surgery range from 65% to 90% for microadenomas and are less than 65% for macroadenomas,[25] and pituitary surgery is associated with long-term failure with an average recurrence rate of 32%.[4] Perioperative mortality rate range between 0% and 7.1% with a mean of 0.6%.[4] In the event of persistent or recurrent disease despite initial pituitary surgery, treatment options include repeat pituitary surgery, pituitary radiotherapy, medical therapy, and bilateral adrenalectomy (BLA). However, there are several drawbacks to these second- and third-line therapies. The disadvantages of pituitary radiotherapy include the delay in effect, potential cerebrovascular complications, and risk for developing hypopituitarism. Limitations of BLA include the development of permanent adrenal insufficiency and the risk of corticotroph tumor progression and development of Nelson syndrome.

Although several cohort studies report an association between mortality risk and treatment modality, this must be interpreted with caution because these are all retrospective studies.[6,7,17,18] Furthermore, differences in availability and indications for treatment over time and factors contributing to the individual patient's surgical candidacy can confound these findings. Thus, the observed effects of treatment modality on mortality may not accurately reflect the direct effects of the treatment but rather the inherent mortality risks of patients who received these treatments. In a CD cohort followed for a median of 106 months (range, 0–494 months) studied within the larger CS study by Yaneva and colleagues,[6] survival outcome at the end of study differed significantly according to the first-line treatment modality received by the patients (P = .012). Only 29% of patients who received radiotherapy alone were alive at the end of the study, compared with 58% of patients who received medical therapy alone, 46% treated with BLA alone, and 50% who underwent unilateral adrenalectomy alone or in combination with other treatment. The survival rate for patients who underwent TSS alone or in combination with other therapy was not directly reported, but 79% of these patients were in remission at last follow-up, implying a high survival rate. However, it was not reported why some patients did not have TSS as part of their treatment course and it is possible that these patients may have been poor surgical candidates (ie, more frail or had inoperable tumors) and thus had increased mortality risk even before treatment. In the study by Bolland and colleagues,[7] BLA alone and pituitary irradiation alone or in combination with any treatment modality were independently associated with increased mortality (OR, 3.1 and 3.0, respectively), whereas treatment with pituitary surgery had improved mortality (OR, 0.2). In addition, Clayton and colleagues[17] noted that the majority of deaths in the study occurred in patients treated with pituitary radiotherapy alone or in combination with metyrapone, raising the possibility that pituitary radiotherapy itself may be a risk factor for mortality, as it is linked to excess mortality in patients with acromegaly and nonfunctioning pituitary tumors.[33] However, as indicated in the study, patients who received radiotherapy and later died were diagnosed with CD before TSS was routinely offered as first-line treatment. In contrast, Dekkers and colleagues[21] reported that radiotherapy in addition to TSS was not associated with increased mortality in CD.

In the disease remission cohort studied by Clayton and colleagues,[18] higher mortality was noted with higher number of treatments. The HR was 1.77 for 2 versus 1 treatment, and 2.6 for 3 versus 1 treatment. The median survival time from study entry for 1 treatment was 33 years, for 2 was 27 years, and for 3 treatments was 21 years. This is not a surprising finding, because the more complex cases often require multimodal treatment.

ECTOPIC ADRENOCORTICOTROPHIC HORMONE-DEPENDENT CUSHING'S SYNDROME

ECS was first recognized in 1962 in a case series by Meador and colleagues.[34] Nearly one-half of reported cases are due to small cell lung cancer, which is often associated with rapid tumor progression and disseminated disease.[5,35] ECS can also be caused by carcinoid tumors (commonly bronchial or thymic), islet cell tumors, medullary thyroid carcinomas, and pheochromocytomas, with very rare causes including non–small cell lung cancers and cancers of the prostate, breast, ovary, gallbladder, and colon.[5,36,37]

Treatment modalities for ECS generally consist of one or a combination of primary tumor resection, medical management/chemotherapy, BLA, and radiotherapy. Series providing survival data are relatively limited given the rarity of this disease. Nonetheless, almost all published studies indicate significantly increased mortality compared with the general population, with neoplastic progression, infection/sepsis, cardiovascular disease, and thromboembolic disease the primary causes of mortality in most cases.[14]

Regarding predictors of mortality, age at diagnosis, gender, remission status, and the presence of lymph node metastases have not been shown to be independent predictors of survival.[24] However, Isidori and colleagues[38] reported that the presence of distant metastases and tumor histology were important predictors of overall survival. Furthermore, among patients with ECS, patients with small cell carcinoma overall had the worst prognosis, whereas patients with other tumors, especially bronchial carcinoid tumors, showed relatively prolonged survival. Of note, improved overall survival has been described in patients with an occult ectopic source, particularly with adequate control of hypercortisolemia, compared with patients who have apparent malignant sources of ACTH, including small cell lung cancer and medullary thyroid carcinoma.[37–40]

A retrospective review of 43 patients with ECS diagnosed between 1979 and 2009 reported deaths in 27 patients (62.8%) and a median overall survival of 32.2 months, with no significant differences in median overall survival durations between men (32.2 months) and women (32.4 months). Progression of primary malignancies and systemic infections at the time of death were the leading causes of mortality, and 2 patients died from pulmonary embolism.[41]

Yaneva and colleagues[6] described 12 patients with ECS followed for a median of 55 months (range, 1-256 months). The SMR was significant at 13.3 with the most common etiologies of mortality being cardiovascular diseases (43%), infections/sepsis (29%), and osteoporosis-related fracture and its complications (14%).

In a retrospective cohort study of 33 patients with ECS followed for a median of 4 years (range, 0–18 years), Ntali and colleagues[24] reported 10 deaths and the highest SMR described in the literature, namely, an overall SMR of 68.5. The main causes of death in this population were progression of the primary malignancy and infection/sepsis. Sepsis was again highlighted as a leading cause of mortality in a retrospective review of 21 patients with ECS in southern India who were followed for a mean 20.1 months, with 3 of 5 reported deaths (60%) attributed to sepsis and the remainder owing to metastatic disease and postoperative pulmonary embolism.[42]

When possible, surgical removal of the ectopic ACTH tumor is the first-line treatment. However, when the tumor cannot be located or is unresectable (as seen in widespread metastatic disease), and medical therapy is ineffective, BLA is effective in alleviating symptoms and comorbidities owing to excess cortisol production.[35] The advantage of BLA is immediate control of hypercortisolism, although lifelong glucocorticoid and mineralocorticoid replacement is necessary. However, with severe hypercortisolemia, surgical morbidity and mortality is not trivial in the setting of immunosuppression, myopathy, metabolic derangements, and hypercoagulability.[42]

O'Riordain and colleagues[43] reported survival outcomes in 18 patients with ECS who underwent BLA, with 1-, 2-, and 5-year survival rates of 67%, 44%, and 39%, respectively. Among these patients, 73% of deaths were directly related to metastatic malignant disease, with the remaining 27% attributed to cardiovascular and cardiopulmonary disease. A higher 5-year survival rate of 51% among 35 patients with ECS after BLA was reported in a retrospective chart review conducted from 1996 to 2005.[5] Furthermore, complete primary tumor resection, if feasible, was highlighted as the ideal treatment for ECS with no patient deaths reported among 5 patients cured by complete tumor resection in a retrospective review of 38 patients from 1990 to 2011 diagnosed and treated for ECS in a tertiary referral center.[35] Additionally, a high mortality rate and often inadequate response to medical therapy was illustrated with all 9 patients treated medically, dying at a median of 1.5 months, and 15 of 24 patients (62%) treated with BLA dying with median survival time of 14.5 months.[35]

In a nationwide retrospective survey of 253 patients with CS between 1960 and 2005 in New Zealand, 10 patients with a localized etiology of ECS had a significant SMR of 27 (95% CI, 8.5–65.20). Notably, the 9 patients classified as 'probable' ECS (no tumor source identified) did not show a significant increase in mortality compared with the matched general New Zealand population, however, with an SMR of 3.1 (95% CI, 0.5–10.0) and a P-value of .16.[7] This is the only known study with a nonsignificant SMR for patients with ECS, albeit in patients with unconfirmed and 'probable' ECS. Given the rarity and tumor heterogeneity among patients with ECS, additional data with larger series will be essential to better characterize mortality risk for these patients.

ADRENOCORTICOTROPHIC HORMONE-INDEPENDENT ADRENAL CUSHING'S SYNDROME

ACTH-independent adrenal Cushing's accounts for approximately 20% of endogenous CS in adults.[44] Unilateral adrenal tumors account for approximately 90% of these cases, 80% of which are benign adenomas with much fewer cases due to ACC; additional adrenal causes that are rare include micronodular/macronodular adrenal hyperplasia and primary pigmented nodular adrenal disease.[44] Patients with adrenal adenomas as compared with carcinomas are younger (39.6 ± 14.4 years vs 51.5 ± 16.6 years) and generally present with smaller tumors (3.3 ± 1.0 cm vs 8.6 ± 4.5 cm).[45] Overall, among patients with adrenal CS, a female predominance has been noted.[45] The First-line treatment for patients with adrenal CS is surgical resection, either unilateral or BLA, depending on the etiology. Perioperative complications and morbidity have dramatically decreased in recent decades with advancements in surgical techniques, including the introduction of minimally invasive laparoscopic adrenalectomy.[5,46]

Cushing's Syndrome Due to Adrenal Adenoma

The incidence of CS due to an adrenal adenoma is approximately 0.6 per million per year.[8] Numerous studies have been published on this patient population, and overall, mortality seems to be less pronounced as compared with CS of other etiologies. A systematic review and meta-analysis of mortality studies demonstrated that mortality for treated patients with a benign cortisol-producing adrenal adenoma did not differ significantly from the general population with an SMR of 1.90 (95% CI, 0.93–3.91).[47] Of note, age at diagnosis, sex, and observation time do not seem to impact mortality in patients with CS due to a benign adrenal adenoma.[24,47] Furthermore, biochemical cure rates of up to 100%, after surgical removal of benign adrenal adenomas, with a long-term mortality similar to the general population, has been reported by Iacobone and colleagues.[48]

In a retrospective study analyzing 45 years of data, the SMR was not significantly increased among patients with CS due to adrenal adenomas at 1.67 (95% CI, 0.20–6.02).[6] In this group, thromboembolic complications were the most frequent cause of death (19%), followed by infections (12.5%), cerebrovascular diseases (12.5%), and other neoplasms (12.5%). All but 2 of 84 patients with cortisol-secreting adenomas underwent surgery, and the remaining 2 patients died with severe active disease that prevented them from undergoing major surgery.[6] Similarly, Pikkarainen and colleagues[49] described a normal SMR of 1.35 (95% CI, 0.16–4.89) among patients with CS due to an adrenal adenoma. The efficacy of adrenalectomy among this patient population was highlighted in a study showing no recurrences among 27 patients with adrenal adenoma causing CS treated with adrenalectomy followed for 5.0 ± 5.5 years, with 1 death (perioperative hypoglycemia presumably due to adrenal insufficiency).[45]

In another large series, Ntali and colleagues[24] analyzed mortality in 74 patients with adrenal CS, of which 57 of 74 patients (77%) had unilateral adrenal adenomas. Two 2 patients (3%) with adrenal Cushing's died, neither of whom was in remission, both due to cardiovascular events. Overall, the 10-year probability of survival was 95.5% and the SMR was similar to that of the general population at 5.3 (95% CI, 0.3–26.0) with a *P*-value of .2. Similarly, a cohort of 54 patients with cortisol-secreting adenomas had an excellent 5-year survival rate (all causes) of 90%.[5]

Other studies, however, report an increased mortality risk in patients with benign adrenal CS. Among 37 patients with CS due to an adrenal adenoma, 4 (10.8%) died during a median period of 7.1 years (range, 3.1–13.8 years) yielding an SMR of 3.48 (95% CI, 0.95–8.90).[8] Of note, pretreatment 24-hour urinary free cortisol levels did not differ significantly between survivors and nonsurvivors. In this study, excess mortality was noted within the first year after the initial admission for hypercortisolism. However, the mortality rate was subsequently not significantly higher than that of the general population.[8]

Dekkers and colleagues[50] reported an increased mortality risk in 132 patients with adrenal CS (excluding ACC, and not differentiating adenoma vs bilateral hyperplasia) compared with the control population (HR, 2.4; 95% CI, 1.6–3.5). Of note, given that data were obtained from population-based registries without access to individual records, the authors comment that some patients with pituitary CD treated with adrenalectomy without concomitant pituitary surgery could have been misclassified as adrenal CS, hence skewing their results.

Bolland and colleagues[7] also noted an elevated SMR of 7.5 (95% CI, 1.9–20.0) among 37 patients with adrenal adenomas. Notably, however, 2 of the total 3 deaths occurred in untreated patients preoperatively due to pulmonary embolism and sepsis, with only 1 death occurring after treatment, albeit in the immediate postoperative period due to ischemic heart disease. Therefore, although the SMR for adrenal adenoma was increased in this cohort, untreated patients were included, and there were no deaths outside of the immediate postoperative follow-up period.[7] Overall, the mortality risk was most prevalent in the early stages after diagnosis and perioperatively. These studies highlight the importance of timely treatment, perioperative thromboembolic prophylaxis, optimization of cardiovascular status, and prompt identification and treatment of adrenal insufficiency in patients with adrenal CS.

Cushing's Syndrome Due to Adrenocortical Carcinoma

The incidence of Cushing's due to ACC is approximately 0.2 per million per year.[8] Complete surgical resection is the only potentially curative treatment for ACC.[51] As opposed to benign adrenal pathology, where laparoscopic surgery is preferable, open surgery is often required for patients with ACC, thus increasing risk for potential perioperative complications.[52,53] Furthermore, surgical remission is uncommon due to a high prevalence of tumor invasiveness and metastasis and, therefore, adjuvant therapy, including mitotane and other cytotoxic agents are often needed.[54] Data on mortality in patients with ACC are limited, but most cases are associated with a poor prognosis and a high mortality rate.

One cohort of 29 patients with ACC had an SMR of 48.0 (95% CI, 30.75–71.42) with a mean survival from the time of diagnosis of 18 months, the most common causes of death being cardiovascular and infectious/sepsis.[6] In total, 24 of 29 patients with ACC underwent adrenalectomy and the remaining 5 (all whom subsequently died) had severe active, metastatic disease that precluded them from undergoing surgery.[6] All 11 patients in another cohort with ACC died soon after admission (median survival time was 7 months; range, 0.9–46.7 months).[8]

Another study reported that, among 13 patients with ACC undergoing adrenalectomy, 76.9% had recurrences at a mean follow-up of 33 months with the 3- and 5-year survival rates being 41.5% and 31.2%, respectively.[45] Porterfield and colleagues[5] also described a grim 5-year survival rate (all causes) of 23% among 10 patients with ACC.

Bilateral Adrenal Hyperplasia

Given the rarity of this disease, only a few studies have commented specifically on mortality among patients with ACTH-independent CS due to bilateral adrenal hyperplasia. In 1 study of 9 patients with bilateral adrenal hyperplasia followed for a mean of 5.7 years, 3 deaths were reported yielding an SMR of 14 (95% CI, 3.7–40.0).[7] In contrast, another study did not identify increased mortality among 11 patients with bilateral adrenal hyperplasia causing CS compared with the general population, with an SMR of 1.14 (95% CI, 0.21–6.34).[6] BLA is the treatment of choice among this population. A systematic review of patients treated with BLA, including 45 patients with CS due to bilateral adrenal hyperplasia, showed a median mortality rate of 0% (95% CI, 0–100), with a total of 4 deaths over the median follow-up time of 36 months (range, 23–294 months).[55] More studies are needed to clarify risk factors and etiologies of mortality in this population.

MORTALITY IN SUBCLINICAL OR MILD ADRENAL CUSHING'S SYNDROME

With the increase in use of radiology and advanced imaging technology, adrenal incidentalomas are being discovered with increasing frequency. Incidental adrenal masses are found in 4.5% of computed tomography imaging done for an unrelated cause, with an incidence of up to 10% in patients older than 70 years.[56,57] Adrenal lesions are more commonly seen in the elderly population, in women, and in the left adrenal gland.[58,59] Among patients with adrenal incidentalomas, up to 30% may exhibit evidence of autonomous cortisol production.[60,61] However, the overwhelming majority of these patients do not demonstrate classical features of CS and, therefore, this diagnosis has been termed subclinical CS or mild hypercortisolism.[62] There is no consensus regarding the biochemical definition of subclinical CS. Most studies define adrenal CS by autonomous cortisol production, with lack of complete serum cortisol suppression after the low dose (1 mg) overnight dexamethasone suppression test (DST); however, serum cortisol cutoffs range from 1.8 to 5 µg/dL, with 1.8 µg/dL being the most sensitive test for defining mild hypercortisolemia, but also yielding a higher false-positive rate.[63]

The term subclinical may not accurately define this condition, however, given that even low-grade cortisol excess has been linked with morbidities, including hypertension, diabetes, dyslipidemia, cardiovascular events, obesity, metabolic bone disease, and a potentially a higher mortality risk (**Table 4**).[57,62,64–67] Di Dalmazi and colleagues[64] described 198 patients with adrenal incidentalomas who were followed for a mean of 7.5 years. Compared with patients with nonfunctioning adenomas, all-cause mortality (91% vs 57%) and cardiovascular-specific mortality (98% vs 78%) were worse in patients with subclinical CS, defined as cortisol levels of greater than 5 µg/dL after a 1-mg overnight DST. Notably, factors significantly associated with mortality in this study were age and mean concentrations of serum cortisol after DST.

These findings were echoed in a retrospective, longitudinal cohort study by Debono and colleagues[57] of 206 patients with benign adrenocortical adenomas. Survival rates decreased with increasing serum cortisol levels after a 1-mg overnight DST: compared with patients with post-DST serum cortisol levels of less than 1.8 µg/dL, the HR of death was 12.0 (95% CI, 1.6–92.6) and 22.0 (95% CI, 2.6–188.3) in patients with serum cortisol values of 1.8 to 5.0 µg/dL, and greater than 5 µg/dL, respectively. In fact, among the 18 patient deaths in this cohort, 94% had post-DST serum cortisol of greater than 1.8 µg/dL, with cardiovascular (50%) and respiratory/infectious (33%) causes being the major causes of death.

Likewise, in a recent retrospective study spanning 13 years, Patrova and colleagues[68] showed increased mortality in patients with adrenal incidentalomas with autonomous cortisol secretion compared with nonfunctioning adrenal incidentalomas. 365 patients with adrenal incidentalomas were classified as having normal post-DST

Table 4
Summary of cohort studies assessing mortality in subclinical Cushing's syndrome

References	Study Design	Study Participants	Study Period	Definitions (Cortisol Level After 1 mg DST)	# of Pts	Mean Follow-up (y)	Mortality or Survival Rates (%)	Signif Predictors of Mortality	Causes of Death
Patrova et al,[68] 2017	Retrospective single-center cohort	Single center in Sweden	2003–2010	• Normal (<1.8 mcg/dL) • Possible autonomous (1.8–5 mcg/dL) • Autonomous cortisol secretion (>5 mcg/dL)	365 total; NS 204; possible autonomous 128; autonomous 33	5.2 ± 2.3	Mortality Rates: NS 7.8% Possible autonomous 11.7% Autonomous 18.2%	Cortisol levels post-DST as a continuous variable; age; tumor size	• NS: malignancy[a] 3.9%; CV 2%; pulm 1%; unknown 2.5% • Possible autonomous: cancer 3.9%; CV 3.1%; pulm 0.8%; unknown 3.9% • Autonomous: malignancy[a] 18.2%
Debono et al,[57] 2014	Retrospective single-center cohort	Single center in the UK	2005–2013	• Normal (<1.8 mcg/dL) • Group 1 (1.8–5 mcg/dL) • Group 2 (>5 mcg/dL)	206 total; • Cortisol <1.8: n = 95 • Cortisol 1.8–5: n = 92 • Cortisol >5: n = 19	4.2 ± 2.3	Mortality Rates: Overall 9% • Cortisol <1.8: 1% • Cortisol 1.8–5: 13% • Cortisol >5: 26%[b]	Cortisol levels post-DST	CV 50%; respiratory/infectious 33%; malignancy[a] 6%
Di dalmazi et al,[64] 2014	Retrospective single-center cohort	Single center in Italy	1995–2010	• NS (<1.8 mcg/dL) • Intermediate (1.8–5 mcg/dL) • Subclinical CS (>5 mcg/dL)	198 total; NS 129; intermediate 59; subclinical CS 10	7.5 ± 3.2	Survival Rates: • Intermediate or subclinical CS 57% • NS 91.2%	Age; mean concentrations of cortisol post DST	CV 48%; malignancy 43%; hip fracture complications 10%

Abbreviations: CS, Cushing's syndrome; CV, cardiovascular; DST, dexamethasone suppression test; NS, non-secreting.
[a] Excluding adrenocortical carcinoma.
[b] Mortality HR compared with DST cortisol <1.8 mcg/dL vs 1.8–5 mcg/dL is 12.0 (95% CI 1.6–92.6); DST cortisol <1.8 mcg/dL vs >5 mcg/dL is 22.0 (95% CI 2.6–188.3).

cortisol secretion (<1.8 µg/dL), possible autonomous (1.8–5 µg/dL), and autonomous (>5 µg/dL) cortisol secretion. 37 patients (10.1%) died during the follow-up period (5.2 ± 2.3 years), 7.8% of whom were in the nonsecreting group, 11.7% in the possible autonomous, and 18.2% in the autonomous cortisol secreting group (P = .019). Interestingly, all deaths in the autonomous group were attributed to cancer (excluding ACC), whereas in the possible autonomous group cardiovascular, followed by cancer, and pulmonary etiologies were the leading causes of death, respectively.[68] Taken together, patients with subclinical CS may be at risk for increased mortality, and the risk may correlate with the degree of cortisol autonomy.

Unilateral adrenalectomy in patients with subclinical CS has been shown in a number of studies to improve multiple long-term cardiovascular and metabolic outcomes, including blood pressure, fasting blood glucose, obesity, dyslipidemia, and even vertebral fractures.[69–72] However, the effect on mortality is less clear. There is currently is no definitive evidence showing a mortality benefit from adrenalectomy among patients with subclinical CS.

With regard to the effect of medical therapy in subclinical CS, there are very few data. Only 1 small study evaluating medical therapy in the setting of mild hypercortisolism has been reported in the literature to date. DeBono and colleagues[73] showed that HOMA-IR (an index of insulin resistance) improved significantly in all 6 patients treated for 4 weeks with the glucocorticoid receptor antagonist mifepristone. Further studies are needed to clarify which patients with subclinical CS may benefit from surgery versus medical therapy or even serial monitoring, and how these management modalities affect long-term mortality risk.

SUMMARY

With improved biochemical and imaging diagnostics, surgical techniques, as well as medical and radiation therapies, survival for patients with CS has improved since the data of Plotz in the 1950s and particularly since the time of Harvey Cushing's when the mean survival period was only 4.7 years.[11,12] Nonetheless, CS is still associated with several comorbidities as well as increased mortality. Prompt and effective treatment resulting in normalization of cortisol levels improves both comorbidities and mortality, in some series mirroring that of the general population. It is imperative that patients with persistent disease receive prophylaxis and active surveillance for infections and cardiovascular and thromboembolic events to mitigate the burden of these comorbidities. Finally, there is a need for studies with high-quality data involving larger cohorts of all subtypes of CS, thus, better characterizing morbidity and mortality and informing treatment guidelines for patients with CS.

REFERENCES

1. Pivonello R, De Martino MC, De Leo M, et al. Cushing's syndrome. Endocrinol Metab Clin North Am 2008;37(1):135–49, ix.
2. Newell-Price J, Bertagna X, Grossman AB, et al. Cushing's syndrome. Lancet 2006;367(9522):1605–17.
3. Steffensen C, Bak AM, Rubeck KZ, et al. Epidemiology of Cushing's syndrome. Neuroendocrinology 2010;92(Suppl 1):1–5.
4. Pivonello R, De Leo M, Cozzolino A, et al. The treatment of Cushing's disease. Endocr Rev 2015;36(4):385–486.
5. Porterfield JR, Thompson GB, Young WF, et al. Surgery for Cushing's syndrome: an historical review and recent ten-year experience. World J Surg 2008;32(5): 659–77.

6. Yaneva M, Kalinov K, Zacharieva S. Mortality in Cushing's syndrome: data from 386 patients from a single tertiary referral center. Eur J Endocrinol 2013;169(5): 621–7.

7. Bolland MJ, Holdaway IM, Berkeley JE, et al. Mortality and morbidity in Cushing's syndrome in New Zealand. Clin Endocrinol 2011;75(4):436–42.

8. Lindholm J, Juul S, Jørgensen JO, et al. Incidence and late prognosis of Cushing's syndrome: a population-based study. J Clin Endocrinol Metab 2001;86(1): 117–23.

9. Etxabe J, Vazquez JA. Morbidity and mortality in Cushing's disease: an epidemiological approach. Clin Endocrinol 1994;40(4):479–84.

10. Hammer GD, Tyrrell JB, Lamborn KR, et al. Transsphenoidal microsurgery for Cushing's disease: initial outcome and long-term results. J Clin Endocrinol Metab 2004;89(12):6348–57.

11. Cushing H. The basophil adenomas of the pituitary body and their clinical manifestations (pituitary basophilism). 1932. Obes Res 1994;2(5):486–508.

12. Plotz CM, Knowlton AI, Ragan C. The natural history of Cushing's syndrome. Am J Med 1952;13(5):597–614.

13. Clayton RN. Mortality in Cushing's disease. Neuroendocrinology 2010;92(Suppl 1):71–6.

14. Pivonello R, Isidori AM, De Martino MC, et al. Complications of Cushing's syndrome: state of the art. Lancet Diabetes Endocrinol 2016;4(7):611–29.

15. Colao A, Pivonello R, Spiezia S, et al. Persistence of increased cardiovascular risk in patients with Cushing's disease after five years of successful cure. J Clin Endocrinol Metab 1999;84(8):2664–72.

16. Pivonello R, Faggiano A, Lombardi G, et al. The metabolic syndrome and cardiovascular risk in Cushing's syndrome. Endocrinol Metab Clin North Am 2005;34(2): 327–39, viii.

17. Clayton RN, Raskauskiene D, Reulen RC, et al. Mortality and morbidity in Cushing's disease over 50 years in Stoke-on-Trent, UK: audit and meta-analysis of literature. J Clin Endocrinol Metab 2011;96(3):632–42.

18. Clayton RN, Jones PW, Reulen RC, et al. Mortality in patients with Cushing's disease more than 10 years after remission: a multicentre, multinational, retrospective cohort study. Lancet Diabetes Endocrinol 2016;4(7):569–76.

19. Giordano R, Picu A, Marinazzo E, et al. Metabolic and cardiovascular outcomes in patients with Cushing's syndrome of different aetiologies during active disease and 1 year after remission. Clin Endocrinol 2011;75(3):354–60.

20. Lambert JK, Goldberg L, Fayngold S, et al. Predictors of mortality and long-term outcomes in treated Cushing's disease: a study of 346 patients. J Clin Endocrinol Metab 2013;98(3):1022–30.

21. Dekkers OM, Biermasz NR, Pereira AM, et al. Mortality in patients treated for Cushing's disease is increased, compared with patients treated for nonfunctioning pituitary macroadenoma. J Clin Endocrinol Metab 2007;92(3):976–81.

22. Biermasz NR, Dekker FW, Pereira AM, et al. Determinants of survival in treated acromegaly in a single center: predictive value of serial insulin-like growth factor I measurements. J Clin Endocrinol Metab 2004;89(6):2789–96.

23. Swearingen B, Biller BM, Barker FG, et al. Long-term mortality after transsphenoidal surgery for Cushing disease. Ann Intern Med 1999;130(10):821–4.

24. Ntali G, Asimakopoulou A, Siamatras T, et al. Mortality in Cushing's syndrome: systematic analysis of a large series with prolonged follow-up. Eur J Endocrinol 2013;169(5):715–23.

25. Biller BMK, Grossman AB, Stewart PM, et al. Treatment of adrenocorticotropin-dependent Cushing's syndrome: a consensus statement. J Clin Endocrinol Metab 2008;93(7):2454–62.

26. Hassan-Smith ZK, Sherlock M, Reulen RC, et al. Outcome of Cushing's disease following transsphenoidal surgery in a single center over 20 years. J Clin Endocrinol Metab 2012;97(4):1194–201.

27. van Haalen FM, Broersen LHA, Jorgensen JO, et al. Management of endocrine disease: mortality remains increased in Cushing's disease despite biochemical remission: a systematic review and meta-analysis. Eur J Endocrinol 2015; 172(4):R143–9.

28. Pivonello R, Vitale P, Mantovani L, et al. MISSION STUDY. A worldwide epidemiological study on the mortality associated with Cushing's syndrome performed in nearly 5000 patients. 2013. Available at: http://www.endocrine.org/meetings/endo-annual-meetings/abstract-details?ID=9808. Accessed October 27, 2017.

29. Geer EB, Shen W, Strohmayer E, et al. Body composition and cardiovascular risk markers after remission of Cushing's disease: a prospective study using whole-body MRI. J Clin Endocrinol Metab 2012;97(5):1702–11.

30. Shah N, Ruiz HH, Zafar U, et al. Proinflammatory cytokines remain elevated despite long-term remission in Cushing's disease: a prospective study. Clin Endocrinol 2017;86(1):68–74.

31. Tiemensma J, Biermasz NR, Middelkoop HAM, et al. Increased prevalence of psychopathology and maladaptive personality traits after long-term cure of Cushing's disease. J Clin Endocrinol Metab 2010;95(10):E129–41.

32. Pivonello R, De Martino MC, De Leo M, et al. Cushing's disease: the burden of illness. Endocrine 2017;56(1):10–8.

33. Ayuk J, Stewart PM. Mortality following pituitary radiotherapy. Pituitary 2009; 12(1):35–9.

34. Meador CK, Liddle GW, Island DP, et al. Cause of Cushing's syndrome in patients with tumors arising from "nonendocrine" tissue. J Clin Endocrinol Metab 1962; 22(7):693–703.

35. Alberda WJ, van Eijck CHJ, Feelders RA, et al. Endoscopic bilateral adrenalectomy in patients with ectopic Cushing's syndrome. Surg Endosc 2012;26(4): 1140–5.

36. Hernández I, Espinosa-de-los-Monteros AL, Mendoza V, et al. Ectopic ACTH-secreting syndrome: a single center experience report with a high prevalence of occult tumor. Arch Med Res 2006;37(8):976–80.

37. Aniszewski JP, Young WF Jr, Thompson GB, et al. Cushing syndrome due to ectopic adrenocorticotropic hormone secretion. World J Surg 2001;25(7):934–40.

38. Isidori AM, Kaltsas GA, Pozza C, et al. The ectopic adrenocorticotropin syndrome: clinical features, diagnosis, management, and long-term follow-up. J Clin Endocrinol Metab 2006;91(2):371–7.

39. Howlett TA, Drury PL, Perry L, et al. Diagnosis and management of ACTH-dependent Cushing's syndrome: comparison of the features in ectopic and pituitary ACTH production. Clin Endocrinol 1986;24(6):699–713.

40. Ilias I, Torpy DJ, Pacak K, et al. Cushing's syndrome due to ectopic corticotropin secretion: twenty years' experience at the National Institutes of Health. J Clin Endocrinol Metab 2005;90(8):4955–62.

41. Ejaz S, Vassilopoulou-Sellin R, Busaidy NL, et al. Cushing syndrome secondary to ectopic adrenocorticotropic hormone secretion: the University of Texas MD Anderson Cancer Center Experience. Cancer 2011;117(19):4381–9.

42. Sathyakumar S, Paul TV, Asha HS, et al. Ectopic Cushing syndrome: a 10-year experience from a tertiary care center in Southern India. Endocr Pract 2017; 23(8):907–14.

43. O'Riordain DS, Farley DR, Young WF Jr, et al. Long-term outcome of bilateral adrenalectomy in patients with Cushing's syndrome. Surgery 1994;116(6): 1088–93 [discussion: 1093–4].

44. Sharma ST, Nieman LK, Feelders RA. Cushing's syndrome: epidemiology and developments in disease management. Clin Epidemiol 2015;7:281–93.

45. Daitch JA, Goldfarb DA, Novick AC. Cleveland clinic experience with adrenal Cushing's syndrome. J Urol 1997;158(6):2051–5 [quiz: 2275].

46. Young WF Jr, Thompson GB. Role for laparoscopic adrenalectomy in patients with Cushing's syndrome. Arq Bras Endocrinol Metabol 2007;51(8):1349–54.

47. Graversen D, Vestergaard P, Stochholm K, et al. Mortality in Cushing's syndrome: a systematic review and meta-analysis. Eur J Intern Med 2012;23(3):278–82.

48. Iacobone M, Mantero F, Basso SM, et al. Results and long-term follow-up after unilateral adrenalectomy for ACTH-independent hypercortisolism in a series of fifty patients. J Endocrinol Invest 2005;28(4):327–32.

49. Pikkarainen L, Sane T, Reunanen A. The survival and well-being of patients treated for Cushing's syndrome. J Intern Med 1999;245(5):463–8.

50. Dekkers OM, Horváth-Puhó E, Jørgensen JOL, et al. Multisystem morbidity and mortality in Cushing's syndrome: a cohort study. J Clin Endocrinol Metab 2013; 98(6):2277–84.

51. Allolio B, Hahner S, Weismann D, et al. Management of adrenocortical carcinoma. Clin Endocrinol 2004;60(3):273–87.

52. Miller BS, Ammori JB, Gauger PG, et al. Laparoscopic resection is inappropriate in patients with known or suspected adrenocortical carcinoma. World J Surg 2010;34(6):1380–5.

53. Else T, Kim AC, Sabolch A, et al. Adrenocortical carcinoma. Endocr Rev 2014; 35(2):282–326.

54. Terzolo M, Angeli A, Fassnacht M, et al. Adjuvant mitotane treatment for adrenocortical carcinoma. N Engl J Med 2007;356(23):2372–80.

55. Ritzel K, Beuschlein F, Mickisch A, et al. Clinical review: outcome of bilateral adrenalectomy in Cushing's syndrome: a systematic review. J Clin Endocrinol Metab 2013;98(10):3939–48.

56. Bovio S, Cataldi A, Reimondo G, et al. Prevalence of adrenal incidentaloma in a contemporary computerized tomography series. J Endocrinol Invest 2006;29(4): 298–302.

57. Debono M, Bradburn M, Bull M, et al. Cortisol as a marker for increased mortality in patients with incidental adrenocortical adenomas. J Clin Endocrinol Metab 2014;99(12):4462–70.

58. Kloos RT, Gross MD, Francis IR, et al. Incidentally discovered adrenal masses. Endocr Rev 1995;16(4):460–84.

59. Kim J, Bae KH, Choi YK, et al. Clinical characteristics for 348 patients with adrenal incidentaloma. Endocrinol Metab (Seoul) 2013;28(1):20–5.

60. Sippel RS, Chen H. Subclinical Cushing's syndrome in adrenal incidentalomas. Surg Clin North Am 2004;84(3):875–85.

61. Terzolo M, Bovio S, Reimondo G, et al. Subclinical Cushing's syndrome in adrenal incidentalomas. Endocrinol Metab Clin North Am 2005;34(2):423–39.

62. Chiodini I. Clinical review: diagnosis and treatment of subclinical hypercortisolism. J Clin Endocrinol Metab 2011;96(5):1223–36.

63. Chiodini I, Albani A, Ambrogio AG, et al, on behalf of the ABC Group. Six controversial issues on subclinical Cushing's syndrome. Endocrine 2016;56(2):262–6.
64. Di Dalmazi G, Vicennati V, Garelli S, et al. Cardiovascular events and mortality in patients with adrenal incidentalomas that are either non-secreting or associated with intermediate phenotype or subclinical Cushing's syndrome: a 15-year retrospective study. Lancet Diabetes Endocrinol 2014;2(5):396–405.
65. Di Dalmazi G, Vicennati V, Rinaldi E, et al. Progressively increased patterns of subclinical cortisol hypersecretion in adrenal incidentalomas differently predict major metabolic and cardiovascular outcomes: a large cross-sectional study. Eur J Endocrinol 2012;166(4):669–77.
66. Tauchmanovà L, Rossi R, Biondi B, et al. Patients with subclinical Cushing's syndrome due to adrenal adenoma have increased cardiovascular risk. J Clin Endocrinol Metab 2002;87(11):4872–8.
67. Debono M, Prema A, Hughes TJB, et al. Visceral fat accumulation and postdexamethasone serum cortisol levels in patients with adrenal incidentaloma. J Clin Endocrinol Metab 2013;98(6):2383–91.
68. Patrova J, Kjellman M, Wahrenberg H, et al. Increased mortality in patients with adrenal incidentalomas and autonomous cortisol secretion: a 13-year retrospective study from one center. Endocrine 2017;58(2):267–75.
69. Chiodini I, Morelli V, Salcuni AS, et al. Beneficial metabolic effects of prompt surgical treatment in patients with an adrenal incidentaloma causing biochemical hypercortisolism. J Clin Endocrinol Metab 2010;95(6):2736–45.
70. Akaza I, Yoshimoto T, Iwashima F, et al. Clinical outcome of subclinical Cushing's syndrome after surgical and conservative treatment. Hypertens Res 2011;34(10):1111–5.
71. Salcuni AS, Morelli V, Eller Vainicher C, et al. Adrenalectomy reduces the risk of vertebral fractures in patients with monolateral adrenal incidentalomas and subclinical hypercortisolism. Eur J Endocrinol 2016;174(3):261–9.
72. Toniato A, Merante-Boschin I, Opocher G, et al. Surgical versus conservative management for subclinical Cushing syndrome in adrenal incidentalomas: a prospective randomized study. Ann Surg 2009;249(3):388–91.
73. Debono M, Chadarevian R, Eastell R, et al. Mifepristone reduces insulin resistance in patient volunteers with adrenal incidentalomas that secrete low levels of cortisol: a pilot study. PLoS One 2013;8(4):e60984.

Prognostic Factors of Long-Term Remission After Surgical Treatment of Cushing's Disease

Adriana G. Ioachimescu, MD, PhD

KEYWORDS

- Cushing's disease • ACTH-secreting pituitary adenoma • Transsphenoidal surgery
- Recurrence • Outcomes • Cortisol • ACTH

KEY POINTS

- Biochemical remission rates after transsphenoidal surgery for Cushing's disease vary between 59% and 94%.
- Predictors of remission include low cortisol levels measured immediately postoperatively, visualization of a microadenoma on preoperative imaging, and histologic identification of an adrenocorticotropic hormone–secreting adenoma.
- Recurrence of hypercortisolism occurs in 8% to 66% cases, more frequently in the first 5 years postoperatively.
- Although patients with low immediate postoperative cortisol levels are less likely to experience recurrence, this cannot reliably be excluded by any cortisol threshold.
- A systematic assessment of clinical, biochemical, histologic, and radiological parameters is useful to evaluate the individual risk of recurrence.

INTRODUCTION

Cushing's disease is a state of chronic hypercortisolism caused by an adrenocorticotropic hormone (ACTH)–secreting pituitary adenoma and represents the most frequent cause of endogenous Cushing's syndrome. Cushing's disease predominantly affects young adults, causing significant morbidity and increased mortality.[1] Treatment goals are reversal of clinical manifestations of hypercortisolism, normalization of biochemical abnormalities with minimal morbidity, and long-term control without recurrence.[2]

Disclosure Statement: The author has received institution-directed research support from Chiasma (NCT03252353), Novartis (NCT02180217), and Pfizer and has done occasional consulting for Pfizer.
Department of Medicine (Endocrinology) and Neurosurgery, Emory University School of Medicine, 1365 B Clifton Road Northeast, B6209, Atlanta, GA 30322, USA
E-mail address: aioachi@emory.edu

Endocrinol Metab Clin N Am 47 (2018) 335–347
https://doi.org/10.1016/j.ecl.2018.02.002
0889-8529/18/© 2018 Elsevier Inc. All rights reserved.

Transsphenoidal surgery (TSS) by an experienced neurosurgeon is the treatment of choice for patients with Cushing's disease. Long-term survival of patients achieving remission after TSS as a single treatment is similar with that of the general population.[3] Patients who do not attain biochemical remission commonly undergo a reoperation, usually within few weeks of the initial TSS. Several studies published after 1993 suggested that very low serum cortisol (s-cortisol) levels measured in the first 10 to 14 days postoperatively may indicate surgical cure. Therefore, this parameter became decisive for the recommendation of a repeat TSS. With subsequent data accumulation, caveats and fine-tuning of this approach have emerged. First, some patients become eucortisolemic without experiencing a low cortisol phase. Second, despite initially very low (even undetectable) postoperative s-cortisol levels, some patients experience recurrence of hypercortisolism during subsequent years. Third, other factors other than the s-cortisol level may contribute to the stratification of the risk for recurrence. The author reviews the clinical, biochemical, radiological, and histologic parameters that have been evaluated in relation with the biochemical outcomes of TSS.

For the purposes of this review, the author defines biochemical remission as resolution of hypercortisolism after surgery used as single treatment of Cushing's disease and defines recurrence as return of hypercortisolism after the initial remission.

TRANSSPHENOIDAL SURGERY RESULTS AND CAVEATS REGARDING INTERPRETATION

Remission rates after TSS vary between 59% and 94% in different studies that examined outcomes of surgery in different institutions.[4–8] A recent meta-analysis calculated a remission rate of 76% (95% confidence interval [CI], 72%–79%).[9] Failure to achieve remission can occur in several circumstances: incomplete resection of a large and/or invasive adenoma, inability to find a small adenoma during exploration of the pituitary gland, removal of an incidental non–ACTH-secreting lesion or incorrect diagnosis of Cushing's disease. Lack of remission is usually followed by a second early reoperation, which consists of another attempt to identify the adenoma or a more radical procedure, that is, partial or total hypophysectomy. Reoperation is usually performed within a few weeks from the initial TSA (often during the same hospitalization) to avoid later scarring. The data on outcomes of early reoperation are scarce; some studies indicate similar short-term remission rates with the first procedure.[5,10] Given the more extensive procedure that is often required, the risk of hypopituitarism is higher for the early reoperation.[10–12]

Although the technical aspects of TSS are beyond the scope of this review,[4] several aspects are important to mention. TSS can be performed by microscopic or endoscopic approach, depending on neurosurgeon's preference. The microscopic approach offers a binocular stereoscopic view. The endoscopic approach allows a wider field of view of the pituitary region, including lateral edges of the sella and cavernous sinuses. In recent years, some centers have used 3-dimensional endoscopic technology to improve the endoscopic depth perception.[13] The data on direct comparison between the two techniques in patients with Cushing's disease at the same institution are sparse and suggest similar biochemical outcomes.[14,15] Historical comparisons of remission rates by endoscopic versus microscopic technique yielded the same results.[11,15,16] A technical factor that may contribute to surgical success entails using the pseudocapsule formed by the compressed normal pituitary gland as a surgical capsule.[17]

Finding an experienced neurosurgeon is essential to achieve biochemical remission, complete tumor resection, and avoid complications. Particularly, TSS in Cushing's cases with adenomas too small to be visualized on preoperative imaging requires excellent surgical skills. The number of patients needed to operate to achieve the desired outcomes is not known. Most studies report postoperative remission rates greater than 70% and originate from reputable centers that perform a high number of TSS.[6,18–21] Only a few studies evaluated biochemical outcomes in relation to the number of years of neurosurgical experience. Yap and colleagues[22] found that the first decade of neurosurgery practice was associated with lower Cushing's remission rates compared with the second and third decade. In contrast, a study by Hofmann and Fahlbusch[23] found that remission rates did not increase over the years. A meta-analysis published in 2016 identified a signal regarding the possible association of neurosurgeons' experience with rates of biochemical remission.[9]

Interpretation of surgical results is confounded by the lack of standardization of remission criteria (**Box 1**). Over the years, different centers have used different criteria, including low immediate postoperative serum cortisol (in-house s-cortisol),[12,24,25] low immediate 24-hour urine free cortisol (u-cortisol),[20] need for glucocorticoid (GC) replacement,[26] suppression to low-dose dexamethasone,[26–28] or a combination of these criteria.[29] In addition, testing was done at variable intervals postoperatively. Immediate postoperative cortisol levels may be influenced by routine empirical postoperative administration of GC, which is required by the protocol in some centers.[20,22,28] Other centers only administer GC in case of hypocortisolism.[11,29–33] Another caveat to consider when interpreting surgical results is the preoperative medical treatment of hypercortisolism. Patients taking cortisol-lowering or cortisol receptor blocking medications may not experience a precipitous decrease of cortisol levels despite successful removal of the adenoma.

Long-term recurrence of hypercortisolism has been reported with significant variability of 8% and 66%.[6,8,11,18,22,26,28,34,35] The meta-analysis published in 2016 reported a relatively low recurrence rate of 10% (95% CI, 6%–16%).[9] In general, studies with extended follow-up found higher recurrence rates. The risk is higher in the first 5 years postoperatively[7] but can occur several decades after surgery.[36–38] In addition, the tests used to detect recurrence have evolved, with recent studies favoring late-night salivary cortisol over the u-cortisol or low-dose dexamethasone suppression test.[39,40] The duration of postoperative corticoadrenal insufficiency is inversely correlated with the risk of recurrence. One study found that more than 50% of patients who overcame this phase in the first 2 years postoperatively experienced recurrence of the hypercortisolism.[18] Patients with recurrence undergo one or several additional treatments, including pituitary reoperation, radiation, medical treatment, and bilateral adrenalectomy. The second TSS for recurrent Cushing's disease has been shown to have lower remission rates compared with the first procedure.[11,41]

Box 1
Caveats regarding interpretation of studies evaluating surgical remission

- How was remission defined: need for glucocorticoid replacement, serum cortisol, urine cortisol, or low-dose dexamethasone suppression test?

- When was testing done in relation with surgery?

- Were empirical glucocorticoids administered in the first few days postoperatively?

- Were cortisol-lowering medications used before surgery?

- How long were patients followed postoperatively?

PREOPERATIVE PARAMETERS' IMPACT ON SURGICAL REMISSION RATES

Cushing's disease affects both children and adults, particularly young women in the third and fourth decades of life. Most studies agree that sex and age at surgery do not have prognostic significance with regard to biochemical outcomes.[11] A study by Aranda and colleagues[35] suggested that older age at diagnosis was associated with a lower likelihood for durable remission, but statistical significance was borderline. Although not extensively studied, clinical presentation does not seem to influence the biochemical outcomes.[11]

The biochemical severity of hypercortisolism has not been consistently studied in relation to postoperative outcomes. However, higher preoperative ACTH levels have been associated with lower biochemical remission rates.[20,42,43]

Preoperative radiological characteristics of pituitary adenomas are important prognostic factors of surgical outcomes. Cavernous sinus invasion has been identified as the single most important factor associated with subtotal resection in patients with growth-hormone–secreting and nonfunctioning pituitary adenomas.[44,45] Approximately 20% patients with Cushing's disease present with macroadenomas. In these patients, cavernous sinus invasion has been shown to reduce the likelihood of biochemical remission.[43] Tumor diameter is also important for surgical outcomes in all types of pituitary adenomas. Some studies in patients with Cushing's disease have implicated an inverse correlation between tumor diameter and remission rates,[20,26,46,47] whereas others did not confirm these findings.[11,18,22] A meta-analysis of 87 articles on 8113 patients found patients with microadenomas have higher remission rates than patients with macroadenomas.[9] In addition, Blevins and colleagues'[33] study demonstrated patients with macroadenomas were more likely to recur (36% at 16 months) than patients with microadenomas, who also experienced recurrence later (12% at 49 months). The same study indicated that cavernous sinus disease and a diameter greater than 2.0 cm were associated with lower postoperative remission rates. On the other hand, patients with microadenomas visualized preoperatively had a higher likelihood of remission than patients in whom adenoma was not identified.[48–51]

HISTOLOGIC PARAMETERS INFLUENCE ON SURGICAL REMISSION RATES

Up to 25% of patients with Cushing's disease have small microadenomas that are not detected by preoperative MRI scan. Confirmation of an adenoma that stains positive for ACTH by pathology becomes very important in these cases. The ACTH-positive adenomas have been identified in 48% to 77% cases in different surgical series.[11,22,35,52] Some studies found an association between the identification of the ACTH-adenoma by immunohistochemistry and surgical remission,[18,20,26,51] whereas other did not.[11,22] The lack of concordance between the identification of the adenoma and biochemical remission is explained by the loss of pathologic material in the operative suction apparatus and its small size, sometimes insufficient to perform immunohistochemistry. In addition, even if the adenoma is not entirely removed, vascular changes may occur postoperatively, which can lead to necrosis and temporary loss of hormonal secretion of the ACTH-secreting adenoma. On the other hand, failure to identify the adenoma during surgery and by pathology is an important signal of unsuccessful outcome.

Dural invasion by the adenomas is a risk factor for incomplete resection and recurrence of hypercortisolism. Some centers perform histologic examination of the dura to guide the extent of surgical removal. Lonser and colleagues[53] prospectively studied 87 consecutive patients undergoing TSS along with histologic analysis of the anterior sella dura and other sites of dural invasion that were evident at surgery. There were 30 (34%) cases with histologic evidence of dural invasion, and the MRI scan indicated invasion in only 4 (22%). The most frequent site of invasion was the wall of the cavernous sinus followed by the sella dura. The size of the adenomas correlated with the risk of dural invasion.[53]

To augment the pathologic diagnosis, Erfe and colleagues[54] proposed the use of real-time quantitation of ACTH in resected pituitary specimens with a novel double-antibody sandwich assay. This method warrants further study and validation in larger cohorts.

IMMEDIATE POSTOPERATIVE CORTISOL LEVELS AND SURGICAL OUTCOMES

Three possibilities exist with regard to cortisol levels measured in the first 2 weeks postoperatively: low, normal, and persistently high. Preoperatively, the ACTH secretion from the nontumoral corticotroph adenohypophysis is suppressed by the chronic hypercortisolism. Postoperatively, complete tumor resection leads to the prompt cessation of tumoral ACTH production, whereas ACTH secretion from the normal pituitary gland remains suppressed. The result is a temporary phase of corticoadrenal insufficiency. Alternatively, normal or high cortisol levels measured in the first few days postoperatively would imply the presence of a tumor residual. This interpretation has several caveats: near-total resection of the tumor may also result in a marked drop of ACTH hypersecretion and brief corticoadrenal insufficiency. On the other hand, delayed remission can also occur, and several mechanisms have been implicated. First, prolonged ACTH stimulation induces adrenal glands hypertrophy with possible partial autonomy from the ACTH-secreting pituitary adenoma. This scenario would imply restoring eucortisolism postoperatively while ACTH levels become suppressed. Second, postoperatively, the residual adenoma may undergo necrosis in the first few weeks postoperatively. This scenario may be accompanied by a lack of identification of the ACTH-secreting tumor by pathology. Third, transient lack of hypocortisolism immediately postoperatively may reflect a nontumoral corticotroph response to surgical stress, which is supported by lower s-cortisol levels at 2 weeks compared with the first few days postoperatively.[55] Finally, the rare circumstance of cyclic Cushing's with surgery done in a phase of disease inactivity entails with the lack of postoperative hypocortisolism.

After the initial studies in the 1990s suggested that s-cortisol levels measured immediately after surgery correlate with long-term remission, this measure has been widely used in clinical practice. The study by McCance and colleagues,[25] in 10 patients with Cushing's disease, demonstrated that all patients with 8 AM s-cortisol lower than 10 mcg/dL on postoperative day 14 remained in remission after a mean follow-up of 59 months. Trainer and colleagues'[12] study of 48 patients reported remission at a median of 40 months for patients who achieved an s-cortisol of 1.8 mcg/dL or less in the first 10 days postoperatively. Additional studies confirmed the relationship between low early postoperative s-cortisol levels and durable remission at various thresholds: 1.8 mcg/dL,[22] 3.0 mcg/dL,[35,52] 3.2 mcg/dL,[29] 3.6 mcg/dL,[51] 5.0 mcg/dL,[31,56] 5.7 mcg/dL,[11] 8.0 mcg/dL,[57] and 10 mcg/dL.[32,34] A study by Patil and colleagues[58] demonstrated patients with an s-cortisol nadir of 2 mcg/dL or less were 2.5 times less likely to recur than those with s-cortisol greater than 2 mcg/dL.[58] On the other hand, several studies pointed out some patients recurred despite initially achieving undetectable s-cortisol levels.[22,34,59] **Table 1** illustrates one of the author's cases that recurred twice (after 2 different TSS procedures) despite achieving a nadir s-cortisol level of 0.6 and 1.2 mcg/dL, respectively. A large study by Lindsay and colleagues[28]

Table 1
Case illustrating that very low postoperative serum cortisol levels do not preclude recurrence of Cushing's disease

Date Measurement	June 2011	July 2011 (s/p TSS#1)	April 2012	February 2013	May 2013 (s/p TSS#2)	July 2013	July 2014	September 2015
Morning s-cortisol (6.7–22.6 µg/dL)	10.2	0.6[a]	5.2	—	1.2[a]	3.3	28.7	9.1
Plasma ACTH (6–58 pg/mL)	31	—	6	—	—	14	134	24
UFC (≤45 µg/d)	725	9.0	—	877	—	—	800	—
Bedtime salivary cortisol (nmol/L)	—	—	—	15 ×UNL	—	—	25 ×UNL	Normal
Morning cortisol after LDDST (µg/dL)	16.7	—	—	—	—	—	—	—

A 25-year-old woman experienced a 35-kg weight gain, facial rounding, striae, acne, hirsutism, amenorrhea, new-onset hypertension, anxiety, and depression over the course of 9 months. Biochemical testing was compelling for Cushing's disease, and MRI showed a microadenoma. The patient became hypocortisolemic after TSS#1 done in July 2011 (pathology positive for ACTH-adenoma, nadir cortisol reached on postoperative day 5). She required hydrocortisone replacement for 9 months, while Cushing's manifestations resolved. In February 2013, she again developed anxiety and hypertension and laboratory tests indicated recurrence. MRI did not localize a tumor. She underwent TSS#2 in May 2013 (pathology positive for ACTH-adenoma, MIB1 index 7%, no mitoses). Nadir s-cortisol reached on postoperative day 5 was 1.2 mcg/dL. She required hydrocortisone replacement for 3 months. Hypercortisolism recurred in July 2014 along with weight gain, skin manifestations, and hypertension. MRI showed a 3-mm tumor. She underwent stereotactic radiation in August 2014, which rendered her eucortisolemic after 1.3 years. Ketoconazole was used until radiation effect.

Abbreviations: LDDST, low-dose dexamethasone suppression test; s/p TSS, status post transsphenoidal surgery; UFC, urinary free cortisol; UNL, upper normal limit.
[a] Nadir s-cortisol measured in the first few days postoperatively.

indicated that early postoperative s-cortisol thresholds of 2 mcg/dL and 5 mcg/dL, respectively, yielded similar recurrence rates, whereas no single threshold eliminated the risk of recurrence. A study by Costenaro and colleagues,[26] in 103 patients, found an s-cortisol threshold of 5.7 mcg/dL measured within 10 to 12 days postoperatively had a stronger correlation with biochemical remission than a threshold of 3.5 mcg/dL measured within the first 48 hours. Similarly, Asuzu and colleagues'[55] study indicated an s-cortisol threshold of 5 mcg/dL at 10 days postoperatively was predictive of remission. A meta-analysis by Sughrue and colleagues[57] evaluated the implications of immediate postoperative s-cortisol levels for long-term remission in 18 studies through June 2008 involving 786 patients. Recurrence rates in patients who achieved low cortisol levels were significantly lower compared with patients who achieved normals-cortisol levels (9% and 24% respectively). There was significant heterogeneity regarding the length of follow-up and biochemical criteria used to define recurrence.

Mean s-cortisol levels drawn every 6 hours for the first 72 hours postoperatively inversely correlate with the long-term remission in some[5] but not all studies.[52]

With routine measurement of s-cortisol postoperatively, some studies indicated that delayed postoperative remission can also occur. **Table 2** illustrates one of the author's patients who achieved eucortisolism at 3 months postoperatively (see **Table 2**). Valassi and colleagues'[20] study in 620 patients operated at 2 tertiary care centers identified 3 categories of postoperative cortisol response: immediate remission

Table 2
Case illustrating delayed resolution of hypercortisolism after 3 months postoperatively

Date Measurement	August 2012	November 2012	December 2012 (s/p TSS#1)	January 2013 (s/p TSS#2)	April 2013	June 2013	July 2013	November 2014	April 2015	January 2016
AM s-cortisol (6.7–22.6 µg/dL)	28.8	—	31.1[a]	23.0[a]	5.9	7.0	7.9	5.8	5.3	26.0
Plasma ACTH (6–58 pg/mL)	27	—	64	56	—	—	27	39	49	161
UFC (≤45 µg/d)	602	—	415	—	—	—	—	—	—	640
Bedtime salivary cortisol (nmol/L)	—	5 × UNL	—	—	—	Normal	Normal	Normal	—	—
AM cortisol after LDDST (µg/dL)	18.1	—	—	—	—	0.6	—	—	—	22.6

A 35-year-old woman experienced 30-kg weight gain, facial rounding, new striae, acne, hirsutism, amenorrhea and new-onset diabetes mellitus, and hypertension over the course of 9 months. Biochemical testing was compelling for Cushing's disease; MRI showed a pituitary microadenoma, and inferior petrosal sinus sampling yielded a central to periphery ratio.

The patient remained hypercortisolemic and symptomatic after TSS#1 done in December 2012, whereas pathology was negative for adenoma. She underwent hypophysectomy (TSS#2) in January 2013 and no adenoma was identified on pathology. Symptomatic hypercortisolism persisted until April 2013 when cortisol normalized. Over the next 6 months, she lost 30 kg and diabetes and hypertension resolved. Hypercortisolism recurred in 1/2016 along with straie and weight gain. MRI showed a small right cavernous sinus lesion. She underwent fractionated radiation in March 2016, which rendered her eucortisolemic after 1.5 years. Mifepristone was used until radiation effect.

Abbreviations: LDDST, low-dose dexamethasone suppression test; s/p TSS, status post transsphenoidal surgery; UFC, urinary free cortisol; UNL, upper normal limit.

[a] Nadir s-cortisol measured in the first few days postoperatively.

(hypocortisolism or eucortisolism throughout the postoperative follow-up; 70.5% cases), no remission (persistent hypercortisolism, 23.9% cases), and delayed remission (initially high u-cortisol followed by a delayed and persistent decrease, 5.6% cases). The delayed remission group included a higher proportion of older women and macroadenomas and a lower proportion of patients with ACTH-staining adenoma. In addition, the mean postoperative ACTH levels were higher in the delayed-remission versus immediate-remission group.

Interpretation of the immediate postoperative cortisol level has practical consequences, as most centers recommend an early reoperation for patients who do not achieve hypocortisolism. For example, Locatelli and colleagues[60] delineated a protocol for repeating the surgery for patients in whom s-cortisol was greater than 2 mcg/dL in the first 3 days after surgery. Hameed and colleagues[56] recommended early reoperation for postoperative s-cortisol greater than 10 mcg/dL. A review of 14 studies in 786 patients found a low specificity for s-cortisol to predict durable remission (88%–94%). The same review indicated that normal s-cortisol level's positive predictive value to predict recurrence was only 17% to 31%.[57] The Endocrine Society's consensus statement from 2008 points out measurement of u-cortisol can provide useful information when s-cortisol is equivocal, with a u-cortisol less than 20 mcg/24 h suggesting remission.[2] In the author's opinion, the approach of early reoperation is reasonable for patients with persistently elevated cortisol levels. For patients achieving eucortisolism, close clinical and biochemical evaluation is appropriate; a decision regarding reoperation can be made 6 to 12 weeks postoperatively (**Box 2**).

OTHER POSTOPERATIVE PARAMETERS THAT MAY INFLUENCE SURGICAL OUTCOMES

Plasma ACTH levels generally decrease significantly and abruptly from baseline in the first 2 weeks postoperatively. Some studies indicated low serum ACTH levels correlate with sustained remission,[30,56,61] whereas other studies did not confirm this observation.[31,62] One recent study indicated that ACTH and dehydroepiandrosterone sulfate levels measured at the time of nadir hypocortisolism may carry additional prognostic value. An ACTH threshold of 20 ng/L effectively separated the recurrence from sustained remission groups despite similar mean s-cortisol levels.[63]

The normalized early postoperative value (NEPV) cortisol can be calculated based on early postoperative cortisol levels and stimulated post–corticotropin-releasing hormone (CRH) cortisol levels obtained during preoperative testing. NEPV can also be calculated for ACTH levels by the same formula. Asuzu and colleagues'[55] study found that NEPV cortisol and ACTH values correlated with short-term remission (**Box 3**).

Several studies performed dynamic testing with CRH, desmopressin, or metyrapone in the first few weeks following TSS. Invitti and colleagues[59] demonstrated that an increase by more than 50% of s-cortisol or plasma ACTH after CRH

Box 2
Implications of postoperative cortisol levels measured within 14 days from surgery

1. Low: surgical remission likely, glucocorticoid replacement needed, recurrence still possible (even for undetectable levels)

2. Normal: both remission and persistent disease possible, further testing necessary, high risk of recurrence

3. High: remission unlikely, further testing necessary, early reoperation probably needed

---

Box 3
Biochemical parameters associated with biochemical surgical outcomes in different studies

- Preoperative ACTH levels
- Morning s-cortisol level in the first 14 days postoperatively
- Postoperative ACTH levels in the first 14 days postoperatively
- Postoperative mean of s-cortisol sampled every 6 hours in the first 3 days postoperatively
- Postoperative stimulated cortisol and ACTH levels during CRH test done at 10 days postoperatively

---

administration indicated an increased risk of recurrence. Lindsay and colleagues[28] found that patients with higher cortisol and ACTH levels after CRH administration 10 days after surgery had more recurrence. Alwani and colleagues[64] found that CRH-stimulated peak cortisol greater or equal to 21.7 mcg/dL predicted a lack of biochemical remission with a negative predictive value of 100%. Also in this study, a 11-deoxycortisol level greater or equal to 12 mcg/dL predicted a lack of biochemical remission with a negative predictive value of 94%. There are also reports indicating an overlap in recurrence between patients with a positive response and no response to CRH or desmopressin.[65] Van Aken and colleagues[66] demonstrated high specificity of the metyrapone test regarding recurrence. Subsequent studies did not support metyrapone test utility because of the wide range of 11-deoxycortisol values.[64] Dynamic testing is rarely performed in clinical practice in patients recovering from TSS for multiple reasons: they are cumbersome and no clear thresholds exist to predict recurrence.

The studies on predictors of durable remission in patients undergoing surgery for Cushing's disease are retrospective, heterogeneous, and take into consideration a variable number of parameters. Some studies performed multivariable analysis, and others did not. The contribution of each factor was evaluated in a meta-analysis by Abu Dabrh and colleagues[9] published in 2016 that included 87 surgical studies on 8113 treatment-naïve patients with Cushing's disease. The meta-analysis identified the following 2 predictors of short-term remission: smaller adenoma size and positive ACTH tumor histology. When adult-only studies are considered, only a smaller adenoma size remained significant. Other parameters were not significant, including age groups (children vs adults), sex, dural invasion, first versus repeat surgery, biochemical criteria, cutoff points to define outcomes, and preoperative visualization of the tumor on imaging. Unlike remission, recurrence of hypercortisolism was not predicted by any of the aforementioned parameters. The authors pointed out the issue of statistical heterogeneity.

SUMMARY

Cushing's disease is a rare condition that poses many challenges for endocrinologists and neurosurgeons. Most patients achieve biochemical remission after TSS performed by an experienced neurosurgeon, but the risk of recurrence is significant. The individual risk can be evaluated after carefully reviewing preoperative and immediate postoperative clinical, biochemical, radiological, and histologic parameters. Despite extensive study over the past 25 years, further research is needed to unveil additional measurable determinants of recurrence. Long-term endocrinologic surveillance is essential in all patients with Cushing's disease.

REFERENCES

1. Clayton RN, Raskauskiene D, Reulen RC, et al. Mortality and morbidity in Cushing's disease over 50 years in Stoke-on-Trent, UK: audit and meta-analysis of literature. J Clin Endocrinol Metab 2011;96(3):632–42.
2. Biller BM, Grossman AB, Stewart PM, et al. Treatment of adrenocorticotropin-dependent Cushing's syndrome: a consensus statement. J Clin Endocrinol Metab 2008;93(7):2454–62.
3. Clayton RN, Jones PW, Reulen RC, et al. Mortality in patients with Cushing's disease more than 10 years after remission: a multicentre, multinational, retrospective cohort study. Lancet Diabetes Endocrinol 2016;4(7):569–76.
4. Oldfield EH. Surgical management of Cushing's disease: a personal perspective. Clin Neurosurg 2011;58:13–26.
5. Mayberg M, Reintjes S, Patel A, et al. Dynamics of postoperative serum cortisol after transsphenoidal surgery for Cushing's disease: implications for immediate reoperation and remission. J Neurosurg 2017. [Epub ahead of print].
6. Ciric I, Zhao JC, Du H, et al. Transsphenoidal surgery for Cushing disease: experience with 136 patients. Neurosurgery 2012;70(1):70–80 [discussion: 80–1].
7. Dallapiazza RF, Oldfield EH, Jane JA Jr. Surgical management of Cushing's disease. Pituitary 2015;18(2):211–6.
8. Hammer GD, Tyrrell JB, Lamborn KR, et al. Transsphenoidal microsurgery for Cushing's disease: initial outcome and long-term results. J Clin Endocrinol Metab 2004;89(12):6348–57.
9. Abu Dabrh AM, Singh Ospina NM, Al Nofal A, et al. Predictors of biochemical remission and recurrence after surgical and radiation treatments of Cushing disease: a systematic review and meta-analysis. Endocr Pract 2016;22(4):466–75.
10. Ram Z, Nieman LK, Cutler GB Jr, et al. Early repeat surgery for persistent Cushing's disease. J Neurosurg 1994;80(1):37–45.
11. Starke RM, Reames DL, Chen CJ, et al. Endoscopic transsphenoidal surgery for Cushing disease: techniques, outcomes, and predictors of remission. Neurosurgery 2013;72(2):240–7 [discussion: 247].
12. Trainer PJ, Lawrie HS, Verhelst J, et al. Transsphenoidal resection in Cushing's disease: undetectable serum cortisol as the definition of successful treatment. Clin Endocrinol (Oxf) 1993;38(1):73–8.
13. Kari E, Oyesiku NM, Dadashev V, et al. Comparison of traditional 2-dimensional endoscopic pituitary surgery with new 3-dimensional endoscopic technology: intraoperative and early postoperative factors. Int Forum Allergy Rhinol 2012;2(1):2–8.
14. Alahmadi H, Cusimano MD, Woo K, et al. Impact of technique on Cushing disease outcome using strict remission criteria. Can J Neurol Sci 2013;40(3):334–41.
15. Sheth SA, Bourne SK, Tritos NA, et al. Neurosurgical treatment of Cushing disease. Neurosurg Clin N Am 2012;23(4):639–51.
16. Sarkar S, Rajaratnam S, Chacko G, et al. Pure endoscopic transsphenoidal surgery for functional pituitary adenomas: outcomes with Cushing's disease. Acta Neurochir (Wien) 2016;158(1):77–86 [discussion: 86].
17. Jagannathan J, Smith R, DeVroom HL, et al. Outcome of using the histological pseudocapsule as a surgical capsule in Cushing disease. J Neurosurg 2009;111(3):531–9.
18. Alexandraki KI, Kaltsas GA, Isidori AM, et al. Long-term remission and recurrence rates in Cushing's disease: predictive factors in a single-centre study. Eur J Endocrinol 2013;168(4):639–48.

19. Dimopoulou C, Schopohl J, Rachinger W, et al. Long-term remission and recurrence rates after first and second transsphenoidal surgery for Cushing's disease: care reality in the Munich Metropolitan Region. Eur J Endocrinol 2014;170(2): 283–92.

20. Valassi E, Biller BM, Swearingen B, et al. Delayed remission after transsphenoidal surgery in patients with Cushing's disease. J Clin Endocrinol Metab 2010;95(2): 601–10.

21. Oldfield EH. Cushing's disease: lessons learned from 1500 cases. Neurosurgery 2017;64(CN_suppl_1):27–36.

22. Yap LB, Turner HE, Adams CB, et al. Undetectable postoperative cortisol does not always predict long-term remission in Cushing's disease: a single centre audit. Clin Endocrinol (Oxf) 2002;56(1):25–31.

23. Hofmann BM, Fahlbusch R. Treatment of Cushing's disease: a retrospective clinical study of the latest 100 cases. Front Horm Res 2006;34:158–84.

24. Estrada J, Garcia-Uria J, Lamas C, et al. The complete normalization of the adrenocortical function as the criterion of cure after transsphenoidal surgery for Cushing's disease. J Clin Endocrinol Metab 2001;86(12):5695–9.

25. McCance DR, Gordon DS, Fannin TF, et al. Assessment of endocrine function after transsphenoidal surgery for Cushing's disease. Clin Endocrinol (Oxf) 1993;38(1):79–86.

26. Costenaro F, Rodrigues TC, Rollin GA, et al. Evaluation of Cushing's disease remission after transsphenoidal surgery based on early serum cortisol dynamics. Clin Endocrinol (Oxf) 2014;80(3):411–8.

27. Bochicchio D, Losa M, Buchfelder M. Factors influencing the immediate and late outcome of Cushing's disease treated by transsphenoidal surgery: a retrospective study by the European Cushing's Disease Survey Group. J Clin Endocrinol Metab 1995;80(11):3114–20.

28. Lindsay JR, Oldfield EH, Stratakis CA, et al. The postoperative basal cortisol and CRH tests for prediction of long-term remission from Cushing's disease after transsphenoidal surgery. J Clin Endocrinol Metab 2011;96(7):2057–64.

29. Rollin GA, Ferreira NP, Junges M, et al. Dynamics of serum cortisol levels after transsphenoidal surgery in a cohort of patients with Cushing's disease. J Clin Endocrinol Metab 2004;89(3):1131–9.

30. Acebes JJ, Martino J, Masuet C, et al. Early post-operative ACTH and cortisol as predictors of remission in Cushing's disease. Acta Neurochir (Wien) 2007;149(5): 471–7 [discussion 477–9].

31. Esposito F, Dusick JR, Cohan P, et al. Clinical review: early morning cortisol levels as a predictor of remission after transsphenoidal surgery for Cushing's disease. J Clin Endocrinol Metab 2006;91(1):7–13.

32. Simmons NE, Alden TD, Thorner MO, et al. Serum cortisol response to transsphenoidal surgery for Cushing disease. J Neurosurg 2001;95(1):1–8.

33. Blevins LS Jr, Christy JH, Khajavi M, et al. Outcomes of therapy for Cushing's disease due to adrenocorticotropin-secreting pituitary macroadenomas. J Clin Endocrinol Metab 1998;83(1):63–7.

34. Atkinson AB, Kennedy A, Wiggam MI, et al. Long-term remission rates after pituitary surgery for Cushing's disease: the need for long-term surveillance. Clin Endocrinol (Oxf) 2005;63(5):549–59.

35. Aranda G, Ensenat J, Mora M, et al. Long-term remission and recurrence rate in a cohort of Cushing's disease: the need for long-term follow-up. Pituitary 2015; 18(1):142–9.

36. Oki Y. Medical management of functioning pituitary adenoma: an update. Neurol Med Chir (Tokyo) 2014;54(12):958–65.
37. Roelfsema F, Biermasz NR, Pereira AM. Clinical factors involved in the recurrence of pituitary adenomas after surgical remission: a structured review and meta-analysis. Pituitary 2012;15(1):71–83.
38. Rutkowski MJ, Flanigan PM, Aghi MK. Update on the management of recurrent Cushing's disease. Neurosurg Focus 2015;38(2):E16.
39. Carroll TB, Javorsky BR, Findling JW. Postsurgical recurrent Cushing disease: clinical benefit of early intervention in patients with normal urinary free cortisol. Endocr Pract 2016;22(10):1216–23.
40. Fleseriu M, Hamrahian AH, Hoffman AR, et al. American Association of Clinical Endocrinologists and American College of Endocrinology disease state clinical review: diagnosis of recurrence in Cushing disease. Endocr Pract 2016;22(12): 1436–48.
41. Patil CG, Veeravagu A, Prevedello DM, et al. Outcomes after repeat transsphenoidal surgery for recurrent Cushing's disease. Neurosurgery 2008;63(2): 266–70 [discussion: 270–1].
42. Kuo CH, Shih SR, Li HY, et al. Adrenocorticotropic hormone levels before treatment predict recurrence of Cushing's disease. J Formos Med Assoc 2017; 116(6):441–7.
43. Cannavo S, Almoto B, Dall'Asta C, et al. Long-term results of treatment in patients with ACTH-secreting pituitary macroadenomas. Eur J Endocrinol 2003;149(3): 195–200.
44. Anthony JR, Alwahab UA, Kanakiya NK, et al. Significant elevation of growth hormone level impacts surgical outcomes in acromegaly. Endocr Pract 2015;21(9): 1001–9.
45. Chang EF, Zada G, Kim S, et al. Long-term recurrence and mortality after surgery and adjuvant radiotherapy for nonfunctional pituitary adenomas. J Neurosurg 2008;108(4):736–45.
46. Nieman LK, Biller BM, Findling JW, et al. Treatment of Cushing's syndrome: an Endocrine Society clinical practice guideline. J Clin Endocrinol Metab 2015; 100(8):2807–31.
47. Arnaldi G, Angeli A, Atkinson AB, et al. Diagnosis and complications of Cushing's syndrome: a consensus statement. J Clin Endocrinol Metab 2003;88(12): 5593–602.
48. Hofmann BM, Hlavac M, Martinez R, et al. Long-term results after microsurgery for Cushing disease: experience with 426 primary operations over 35 years. J Neurosurg 2008;108(1):9–18.
49. Jagannathan J, Sheehan JP, Jane JA Jr. Evaluation and management of Cushing syndrome in cases of negative sellar magnetic resonance imaging. Neurosurg Focus 2007;23(3):E3.
50. Pouratian N, Prevedello DM, Jagannathan J, et al. Outcomes and management of patients with Cushing's disease without pathological confirmation of tumor resection after transsphenoidal surgery. J Clin Endocrinol Metab 2007;92(9):3383–8.
51. Chee GH, Mathias DB, James RA, et al. Transsphenoidal pituitary surgery in Cushing's disease: can we predict outcome? Clin Endocrinol (Oxf) 2001;54(5): 617–26.
52. Ramm-Pettersen J, Halvorsen H, Evang JA, et al. Low immediate postoperative serum-cortisol nadir predicts the short-term, but not long-term, remission after pituitary surgery for Cushing's disease. BMC Endocr Disord 2015;15:62.

53. Lonser RR, Ksendzovsky A, Wind JJ, et al. Prospective evaluation of the characteristics and incidence of adenoma-associated dural invasion in Cushing disease. J Neurosurg 2012;116(2):272–9.

54. Erfe JM, Perry A, McClaskey J, et al. Long-term outcomes of tissue-based ACTH-antibody assay-guided transsphenoidal resection of pituitary adenomas in Cushing disease. J Neurosurg 2017. [Epub ahead of print].

55. Asuzu D, Chatain GP, Hayes C, et al. Normalized early postoperative cortisol and ACTH values predict nonremission after surgery for Cushing disease. J Clin Endocrinol Metab 2017;102(7):2179–87.

56. Hameed N, Yedinak CG, Brzana J, et al. Remission rate after transsphenoidal surgery in patients with pathologically confirmed Cushing's disease, the role of cortisol, ACTH assessment and immediate reoperation: a large single center experience. Pituitary 2013;16(4):452–8.

57. Sughrue ME, Shah JK, Devin JK, et al. Utility of the immediate postoperative cortisol concentrations in patients with Cushing's disease. Neurosurgery 2010; 67(3):688–95 [discussion: 695].

58. Patil CG, Prevedello DM, Lad SP, et al. Late recurrences of Cushing's disease after initial successful transsphenoidal surgery. J Clin Endocrinol Metab 2008; 93(2):358–62.

59. Invitti C, Pecori Giraldi F, de Martin M, et al. Diagnosis and management of Cushing's syndrome: results of an Italian multicentre study. Study Group of the Italian Society of Endocrinology on the Pathophysiology of the Hypothalamic-Pituitary-Adrenal Axis. J Clin Endocrinol Metab 1999;84(2):440–8.

60. Locatelli M, Vance ML, Laws ER. Clinical review: the strategy of immediate reoperation for transsphenoidal surgery for Cushing's disease. J Clin Endocrinol Metab 2005;90(9):5478–82.

61. Flitsch J, Knappe UJ, Ludecke DK. The use of postoperative ACTH levels as a marker for successful transsphenoidal microsurgery in Cushing's disease. Zentralbl Neurochir 2003;64(1):6–11.

62. Pereira AM, van Aken MO, van Dulken H, et al. Long-term predictive value of postsurgical cortisol concentrations for cure and risk of recurrence in Cushing's disease. J Clin Endocrinol Metab 2003;88(12):5858–64.

63. El Asmar N, Rajpal A, Selman WR, et al. The value of peri-operative levels of ACTH, DHEA and DHEA-S and tumor size in predicting recurrence of Cushing's disease. J Clin Endocrinol Metab 2018;103(2):477–85.

64. Alwani RA, de Herder WW, van Aken MO, et al. Biochemical predictors of outcome of pituitary surgery for Cushing's disease. Neuroendocrinology 2010; 91(2):169–78.

65. Colombo P, Dall'Asta C, Barbetta L, et al. Usefulness of the desmopressin test in the postoperative evaluation of patients with Cushing's disease. Eur J Endocrinol 2000;143(2):227–34.

66. van Aken MO, de Herder WW, van der Lely AJ, et al. Postoperative metyrapone test in the early assessment of outcome of pituitary surgery for Cushing's disease. Clin Endocrinol (Oxf) 1997;47(2):145–9.

Outcomes of Pituitary Radiation for Cushing's Disease

Natasha Ironside, MBChB[a], Ching-Jen Chen, MD[b],
Cheng-Chia Lee, MD[c], Daniel M. Trifiletti, MD[d],
Mary Lee Vance, MD[e], Jason P. Sheehan, MD, PhD[b,*]

KEYWORDS

- Cushing's disease • Stereotactic radiosurgery • Radiation therapy • Endocrine
- Remission

KEY POINTS

- For patients with persistent or recurrent Cushing's disease after transsphenoidal resection, ionizing radiation delivery to the pituitary is the primary adjuvant treatment.
- More recently, single-session stereotactic radiosurgery has been popularized over conventional fractionated external beam radiotherapy as the treatment of choice.
- Endocrine remission rates, times to remission, and tumor control rates between stereotactic radiosurgery and external beam radiotherapy are comparable among major series.
- Heterogeneity in endocrine remission and recurrence rates highlights a need for investigation. Potential contributing factors include differences in patient selection, treatment parameters, and use of adjuvant medication.
- New pituitary hormone deficiency is the most frequent adverse effect after stereotactic radiosurgery and external beam radiotherapy. Other complications, including cranial neuropathy and visual deficit, are uncommon.

INTRODUCTION

Biochemical remission with the preservation of normal pituitary function is the primary goal in the treatment of Cushing's disease.[1] Transsphenoidal resection remains the

---

Disclosure Statement: The authors have nothing to disclose.
[a] Department of Neurosurgery, Auckland City Hospital, Private Bag 92 024, Auckland Mail Center, Auckland 1142, New Zealand; [b] Department of Neurological Surgery, University of Virginia Health System, PO Box 800-212, Charlottesville, VA 22908, USA; [c] Department of Neurosurgery, Taipei Veterans General Hospital, 17 Floor, No. 201, Sec. 2, Shipai Road, Beitou District, Taipei 11217, Taiwan; [d] Department of Radiation Oncology, Mayo Clinic, 4500 San Pablo Road South, Jacksonville, FL 32224, USA; [e] Division of Endocrinology and Metabolism, University of Virginia Health System, 2 Floor, Suite 2100, 415 Ray C Hunt Drive, Charlottesville, VA 22908, USA
* Corresponding author. Department of Neurological Surgery, Health Sciences Center, Box 800-212, Charlottesville, VA 22908.
E-mail address: jps2f@virginia.edu

Endocrinol Metab Clin N Am 47 (2018) 349–365
https://doi.org/10.1016/j.ecl.2018.01.002
0889-8529/18/© 2018 Elsevier Inc. All rights reserved.

gold standard of treatment, offering remission rates that range from 59% to 97%.[2–5] Despite the high rates of initial remission that can be achieved with transsphenoidal resection, delayed recurrences have been reported in up to 50% of patients, as late as 30 years after surgical resection.[6–8] This finding presents a significant challenge to the long-term management of Cushing's disease. Radiation targeting residual tumor cells represents an important adjuvant treatment for patients with persistent or recurrent Cushing's disease.[8] In select patients who are poor surgical candidates or unwilling to undergo surgery, upfront radiation therapy may also be considered.[9,10] The administration of ionizing radiation includes conventional external-beam fractionated radiation therapy (XRT) and stereotactic radiosurgery (SRS), the latter of which can be delivered via linear accelerator-based systems, gamma knife, proton beam, and various other commercially available units.[11] In recent years, for tumors located in the sellar and parasellar regions, SRS has become a modality of choice for radiation delivery. SRS permits the administration of focused, high-dose treatment in a single session, while limiting the exposure of nearby critical neurovascular structures to unwanted radiation.[10,12] This review outlines the indications, outcomes, and adverse effects associated with radiation treatment of Cushing's disease.

Techniques Used for Radiation Delivery to the Pituitary Gland

SRS is characterized by the delivery of a high-dose of hypofractionated radiation to a precise target using a multiheaded cobalt-based unit (Gamma Knife, Elekta AB, Stockholm, Sweden), linear particle accelerator, or proton beam unit.[10,12,13] In gamma knife radiosurgery (GKRS), numerous radiation beams are focused on the target using a crossfire technique.[14] Gamma rays, produced by radioactive decay of cobalt-60 sources, are converged on an isocenter within the tumor using a collimator. A high central radiation dose with submillimeter accuracy can be achieved through various combinations of the beam number, aperture size, and position.[11,15] Typically prescribed at a 50% isodose line, the cobalt system can achieve steep radiation dose fall-off just beyond target margins.[11,14,15] In linear accelerator-based SRS systems (CyberKnife, Edge, Novalis TX, Trilogy, and Axesse), x-rays are derived from the collision of an accelerated electron with a high z target. An isodose line of 80% to 90% is frequently prescribed to encompass the target volume, resulting in a greater penumbra effect and a lower maximum dose when compared with GKRS.[13,14,16,17] Proton beam therapy takes advantage of the Bragg phenomenon, in which the peak energy transferred by an accelerated proton occurs immediately before it comes to rest, sparing the deeper tissues of unwanted radiation.[18] Although proton beam use has increased, most centers do not currently offer this treatment, owing to the size, technical challenges, and cost of construction of these proton beam units for radiosurgical delivery.[10,11,18,19]

XRT delivers ionizing radiation in multiple fractionated doses (25–30 daily treatments) and can be used in patients who are not candidates for SRS owing to safety concerns associated with large tumor size, irregular geometry, extrasellar extension, or proximity to the optic apparatus.[12] However, the use of multisession SRS in treating those with large tumors or tumors in close proximity to critical neurovascular structures has recently demonstrated promising results.[14,20–22]

Illustrative Case

A 43-year-old woman who presented with clinical stigmata of Cushing's disease underwent microscopic transsphenoidal resection of an adrenocorticotropic hormone-secreting pituitary adenoma in April 2006 (**Fig. 1**). She experienced postoperative persistence of hypercortisolism and received GKRS in November 2006. This

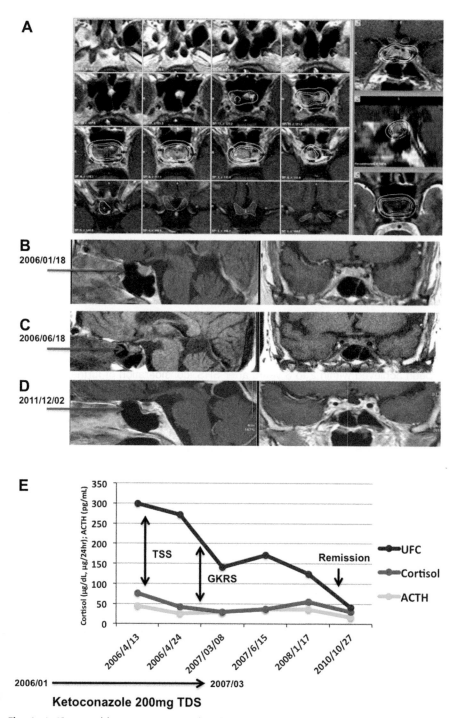

Fig. 1. A 43 year-old woman presented with clinical stigmata of Cushing's disease (moon face, buffalo hump, and ecchymosis) and underwent microscopic transsphenoidal resection (TSR) in April 2006. Postoperatively, endocrine remission was not achieved, and she

persistence resulted in a progressive decrease in urinary free cortisol, serum cortisol, and serum adrenocorticotropic hormone levels. Biochemical remission was achieved after 18 months. The patient developed hypogonadotropic hypogonadism at 24 months after GKRS.

Biochemical Control Outcomes After Stereotactic Radiosurgery

The growing body of literature reporting the outcomes for SRS in the treatment of Cushing's disease is summarized in **Table 1**.[15,20–47] The mean follow-up duration among the major series was 61 months (range, 7.5–204 months). The initial endocrine remission rate was 65.8% (range, 26.7%–100.0%). The durable remission rate at last follow-up (mean, 4.5 years) was achieved in 64.7% (range, 16.7%–100%). For GKRS (n = 18) the mean endocrine remission rate was 65.8%.[15,23,24,26,28,30,31,34,36–38,40–44,46,47] For linear accelerator-based systems and proton beam units, fewer studies were available, and the mean endocrine remission rates were 45.8% and 65.8%, respectively.[25,27,29,32,33,35,39,45] The mean remission rate in a cohort of patients (n = 28) with MRI-negative Cushing's disease treated with whole sellar radiation was 71.4%.[46] A further retrospective comparison of MRI-negative adenomas treated with whole sellar radiation (n = 78) and MRI-visible adenomas treated with targeted SRS (n = 200) reported no significant difference in initial or durable endocrine remission rates ($P = .16$ and $P = .18$, respectively).[23]

The mean time to remission after SRS was 19.9 months (n = 21; range, 7.5–39.6 months),[15,20,22–33,35,37–40,46,47] with no apparent differences among the different SRS modalities. Adjuvant medication is usually necessary to control hypercortisolemia during the latency period. However, in cases where remission has not been achieved within 2 to 3 years after SRS, consideration of further treatment with curative intent is paramount to effectively mitigate the morbidity associated with persistent hypercortisolism.[10] After SRS, observed rates of recurrence ranged between 0% and 36% among studies, up to 8 years after treatment.[15,20,21,23–29,31–33,35,37–42,44] Delayed recurrences are inherent to patients with Cushing's disease treated with either surgery or radiation, and predictors of long-term treatment success are poorly understood. A recent multicenter study by Mehta and colleagues[23] (n = 273) found a lower marginal dose (20.5 Gy vs 45.3 Gy; $P = .003$) and maximal dose (22.7 Gy vs 67.3 Gy; $P = .009$) to be associated with higher long-term recurrence rates. These findings, supported by Losa and colleagues[34] (n = 271; hazard ratio, 0.85; $P<.01$), warrant further investigation, because the use of a higher dose to achieve durable endocrine remission must outweigh the risk of radiation toxicity.[1,8,48,49] Therefore, even in cases of successful endocrine remission, long-term follow-up remains critical.

---

subsequently underwent gamma knife radiosurgery (GKRS) in November 2006. Ketoconazole 200 mg three times daily (TDS) was initiated before surgery in January 2006, and discontinued in March 2007 after experiencing an allergic reaction and associated hepatitis. (A) In the treatment plan shown, the contoured tumor border (pink), optic chiasm (blue), margin dose of 20 Gy and isodose line of 56% (yellow), 16 Gy and 10 Gy isodose lines (green) are outlined. Thin-slice coronal postcontrast T1-weighted MRI sections through the sella demonstrated progressive decrease of residual tumor volume (red arrows) in the right cavernous sinus at the time of GKRS (B), pre-TSR (C), 2 months after TSR (D), and 3 years after GKRS. (E) A progressive decrease in urinary free cortisol, mirrored by serum cortisol and adrenocorticotropic hormone, after GKRS was observed. The patient developed hypogonadotropic hypogonadism at 2 years after GKRS. Remission was achieved at 18 months after GKRS. ACTH, adrenocorticotropic hormone; TSS, transsphenoidal surgery; UFC, urinary free cortisol.

Table 1
Major series (n ≥10 patients) reporting outcomes after stereotactic radiosurgery for Cushing's disease

Study	Type of SRS	Patients (n)	Mean or Median Follow-up (mo)	Margin Dose (Gy)	Maximal Dose (Gy)	Treatment Volume (cm³)	Mean Tumor Size (cm³)	Endocrine Remission Rate (%)	Durable Control (%)	Mean Time to Remission (mo)	Radiologic Response (%)	Recurrence Rate (%)	Mean Time to Recurrence (mo)	Endocrine Criteria for Remission
Mehta et al,[23] 2017	GKRS	278	67	23.7	46.3	2.1	1.7	80	57	14.5	NR	18	38.3	Normalization UFC
Marek et al,[24] 2015	GKRS	26	98.5	NR	65	1.47	0.56	80.7	NR	25	92.3	0	NR	UFC 38–208 nmol/24 h, morning cortisol 118–618 nmol/L serum ACTH 10–60 ng/L
Budyal et al,[20] 2014	Fractionated LINAC	20	37.5	NR	45	NR	NR	75	65	20	95	0	NR	Serum cortisol after dex suppression test <50 nmol/L
Wilson et al,[25] 2014	LINAC	36	66	20	NR	1.4	0.7	36.1	22.2	16.8	83	3	NR	UFC <276 nmol
Grant et al,[26] 2014	GKRS	15	40.2	35	54.9	0.56	NR	73	48	11.7	100	36	21	Normalization UFC
Lee et al,[46] 2014	GKRS	20	41	25	NR	3	NR	81	71.4	10	NR	10	91.5	UFC <45 μg/24 h
Wattson et al,[27] 2014	Proton	79	47	20	NR	1.7	NR	67	67	31	99	1	NR	Normalization UFC
Kim et al,[22] 2013	Fractionated LINAC	15	93.6	NR	50.4	NR	NR	73	68	39.6	NR	NR	NR	Normalization plasma ACTH or UFC
Sheehan et al,[28] 2013	GKRS	96	48	22	47.2	1.8	1.8	78	70	16.6	98	15.6	38	Normalization plasma cortisol or UFC
Wein et al,[29] 2012	LINAC	17	23	18	31	NR	NR	59	NR	23	100	6	24	Normalization UFC

(continued on next page)

Table 1
(continued)

Study	Type of SRS	Patients (n)	Mean or Median Follow-up (mo)	Margin Dose (Gy)	Maximal Dose (Gy)	Treatment Volume (cm³)	Mean Tumor Size (cm³)	Endocrine Remission Rate (%)	Durable Control (%)	Mean Time to Remission (mo)	Radiologic Response (%)	Recurrence Rate (%)	Mean Time to Recurrence (mo)	Endocrine Criteria for Remission
Sheehan et al,[47] 2011	GKRS	82	31	24	NR	NR	NR	54	54	13	NR	NR	NR	Normalization UFC or need for cortisol replacement
Losa et al,[34] 2010	GKRS	49	48	25	NR	NR	NR	53	NR	NR	NR	NR	NR	Normalization UFC
Castinetti et al,[31] 2009	GKRS	18	96	29	NR	0.40	NR	50	50	42.6	100	11	84	Normalization UFC or dex suppression test <5 nmol/L
Tinnel et al,[37] 2008	GKRS	12	37	25	NR	NR	NR	67	50	10	83.3	17	38	Normalization UFC
Aghi et al,[32] 2008	Proton	31	43	20	NR	NR	NR	58	55	21	NR	3	12	UFC <20 µg/24 h, early morning serum cortisol <5 µg/dL
Wan et al,[36] 2009	GKRS	68	67.3	21.9	NR	NR	3.4	27.9	27.9	NR	89.7	NR	NR	UFC <200 µg/dL or serum cortisol <2.4 µg/dL
Petit et al,[33] 2008	Proton	33	62	20	NR	NR	NR	55	52	14	NR	0	NR	Normalization UFC
Voges et al,[35] 2006	LINAC	17	81.9	16.4	NR	NR	2.9	64.7	52.9	36.2	NR	17.6	NR	Normalization UFC or serum cortisol <25 µg/dL
Castinetti et al,[30] 2007	GKRS	40	94	29.5	NR	0.52	NR	42.5	42.5	22	NR	NR	NR	Normalization UFC or dex suppression test <50 nmol/L

Jagannathan et al,[38] 2007	GKRS	90	41.3	23	NR	NR	NR	54	45.6	13	95	20	27	Normalization UFC
Devin et al,[39] 2004	LINAC	35	7.5	14.7	33.7	NR	NR	49	37	7.5	91	11	35.5	Normalization UFC
Colin et al,[21] 2005	Fractionated LINAC	10	82	NR	50.4	NR	NR	100	100	NR	NR	0	NR	Normalization plasma ACTH/cortisol
Jane et al,[40] 2003	GKRS	45	NR	15	NR	NR	NR	73	NR	16	NR	4	NR	Normalization UFC
Kobayashi et al,[41] 2002	GKRS	20	64.1	28.7	49.4	NR	NR	85	35	NR	100	0	NR	Plasma cortisol <10 μg/dL or ACTH <50 pg/mL
Hoybye et al,[42] 2001	GKRS	18	204	NR	NR	NR	NR	83	NR	NR	NR	0	NR	Normalization UFC plasma cortisol or plasma ACTH
Sheehan et al,[15] 2000	GKRS	43	39.1	20	47	NR	NR	63	56	12.1	100	6.9	31.3	Normalization UFC
Izawa et al,[43] 2000	GKRS	12	27.8	22.5	NR	NR	NR	58.3	16.7	NR	83.3	NR	NR	Normalization elevated hormone level
Levy et al,[45] 1991	Proton	64	120	NR	30–150	NR	NR	86	NR	NR	NR	14	NR	Normalization plasma cortisol or dex suppression test <50 nmol/L
Degerblad et al,[44] 1986	GKRS	29	NR	NR	70–100	NR	NR	82.7	76	NR	NR	0	NR	Normalization UFC

Between 1984 and 2017, baseline radiosurgical parameters, rates of endocrine remission, radiologic response, long-term recurrence, and complications, are outlined.

Abbreviations: ACTH, adrenocorticotropic hormone; Dex, dexamethasone; GKRS, gamma knife radiosurgery; LINAC, linear accelerator; NR, not reported; SRS, stereotactic radiosurgery; UFC, urinary free cortisol.

Variability in remission outcomes can be attributed to differences in patient numbers, endocrine remission criteria, quality of available data, and duration of follow-up. There seems to be a trend toward higher rates of endocrine remission in papers published after 2010, which may reflect improvements in radiosurgical techniques, the establishment of higher volume treatment centers, and greater standardization of endocrine follow-up.[50] Baseline tumor characteristics may additionally play a role in overall endocrine outcomes. In a study by Castinetti and colleagues[31] (n = 18), a lower target volume (0.396 mm^3 vs 0.609 mm^3; $P<.05$) and lower urinary free cortisol level (155 μg/24 h vs 470 μg/24 h; $P<.05$) were univariate predictors of remission. In the vast majority of cases, SRS has been used as an adjuvant therapy after failed surgical resection and its effectiveness as an upfront treatment has not been investigated previously in a large patient cohort.

Two studies have reported a favorable relationship between the discontinuation of steroidogenesis inhibitors immediately before SRS and the achievement of remission. Sheehan and colleagues[28] (n = 96) observed a shorter time to remission in patients not receiving ketoconazole at the time of GKRS (12.6 months vs 21.8 months in patients receiving ketoconazole; $P<.012$). Castinetti and colleagues[31] (n = 40) noted an improvement in overall remission rates in patients not receiving ketoconazole at the time of GKRS (n = 25 [48%]), upon comparison with those who were (n = 15 [20%]; $P = .02$). However, Mehta and colleagues[23] (n = 273) did not observe such an association between ketoconazole administration (n = 85), initial remission ($P = .10$), durable remission ($P = .46$), and recurrence ($P = .20$) on univariate analyses. Preradiation use of medications may alter the metabolism and cycling of hyperfunctioning corticotrophs, influencing the discrimination of tumor target and its response to ionizing radiation.[51] Several categories of medications are used in the treatment of Cushing's disease (steroidogenesis inhibitors, somatostatin receptor ligands, and cortisol receptor blockers). Further studies are necessary to understand this issue.

Biochemical Control Outcomes After Conventional External Beam Radiation Therapy

Table 2 summarizes the major series using XRT for Cushing's disease, published between 1984 and 2017. The mean follow-up was 77 months (range, 24–114 months).[52–59] Endocrine remission rates after XRT (mean, 67.5%; range, 46%–89%) were similar to those achieved by SRS.[52–59] The mean time to remission ranged from 15 to 24 months.[53,55,58,59] Upfront XRT for Cushing's disease, reported in 2 studies, achieved endocrine remission rates of 46% (mean, 16 months) and 57%, respectively.[54,55]

Tumor Control Outcomes After Stereotactic Radiosurgery

Tumor control, defined as a decrease in or stability of tumor volume on diagnostic imaging after SRS, was achieved in approximately 94% of patients (range, 77%–100%) among major series.[15,20,24–29,31,36–39,41,43] The disparity between tumor control and endocrine remission rates highlights an opportunity for improvement in outcomes in addition to a better understanding of the relationship between radiation parameters and biochemical response.[60] Among major series, the mean margin dose was 22.6 Gy (range, 14.7–35 Gy) and the mean maximal dose was 47 Gy (range, 31–100 Gy). The mean tumor volume was 1.84 cm^3 (range, 0.56–3.4 cm^3) and the mean dose volume was 1.34 cm^3 (range, 0.4–2.1 cm^3). In a cohort of 418 patients with secretory pituitary adenomas treated with GKRS at the University of Virginia between 1989 and 2006, a trend toward improved endocrine remission rates with each 1 cm^3 decrease in tumor volume was observed (median, 1.9 cm^3; range, 0.1–27 cm^3; odds ratio, 1.30 [95% confidence interval 1.05–1.61]; $P = .072$). The series additionally

Table 2
Summary table of major series (n ≥10 patients) reporting outcomes after fractionated external beam radiotherapy for Cushing's disease

Study	Patients (n)	Mean or Median Follow-up (mo)	Dose (Gy)	Endocrine Remission Rate (%)	Mean Time to Remission (mo)	Tumor Control (%)	Recurrence Rate (%)	Time to Recurrence (mo)	Endocrine Criteria for Remission
Minniti et al,[13] 2007	40	108	45	84	24	93	0	NR	Dex suppression test <50 ng/mL, normalization UFC
Estrada et al,[53] 1997	30	30	50	83	18	NR	0	NR	Dex suppression test <5 μg/dL, normalization UFC
Tsang et al,[56] 1996	29	87.6	45	56	NR	96	NR	NR	UFC < 220 nmol/24 h
Murayama et al,[58] 1992	20	90.5	54	55	10.1	NR	20	60–84	Normalization dex suppression test (μg/dL)
Vicente et al,[57] 1991	14	24	50	70	NR	NR	0	NR	Plasma cortisol <303.5 nmol/L, dex suppression test 138 nmol/L
Littley et al,[55] 1990	24	94.8	20	25	15.9	NR	21	NR	Serum cortisol <400 nmol/L, normalization UFC
Howlett et al,[54] 1989	21	114	45	57	NR	100	NR	NR	Serum cortisol 300–400 nmol/L
Ahmed et al,[52] 1984	19	42	20	42	6–12	NR	NR	NR	UFC (nmol/24 h)

Between 1984 and 2017, baseline radiation treatment parameters, rates of endocrine remission, radiologic response, long-term recurrence, and complications are outlined.

Abbreviations: dex, dexamethasone; NR, not reported; UFC, urinary free cortisol.

found a margin dose of 25 Gy or greater to be associated with an earlier time to remission (P = .019).[47]

Tumor Control Outcomes After Conventional External Beam Radiotherapy

Among XRT series, tumor control rates ranged from 93% to 100%, at a mean follow-up of 8.3 years, which is comparable with those achieved with SRS.[54,56,59] The mean total dose was 41.25 Gy (range, 20–45 Gy), delivered in approximately 20 fractions (range, 8–25 fractions) over 29 days (range, 12–35 days).[52–59] For XRT, the relationship between radiation dose, tumor control, and endocrine remission is not well-defined, because remission rates vary widely among series delivering a similar mean total radiation dose.[53,56,57,59] Despite an early response, delayed recurrence is commonly encountered after radiotherapy for Cushing's disease.[8] Littley and colleagues[55] and Murayama and colleagues,[58] reporting recurrence rates of 20% and 21%, respectively, found no significant differences in tumor or treatment characteristics between patients with and without recurrence. This further underscores the necessity of long-term follow-up in all patients.

Adverse Effects of Pituitary Radiation

The development of new pituitary hormone deficiency or deficiencies is the most commonly encountered adverse effect after SRS, occurring in 29.7% of cases (range, 0%–69%) at a mean of 31 months (range, 4–132 months). Among XRT series, new pituitary hormone deficiency occurred in 38.4% of cases (range, 0%–58%)[52–55,57–59] (**Table 3**). Higher rates of hormone deficiency after XRT in comparison with SRS have been previously acknowledged in the literature.[61,62]

There may be a relationship between margin dose greater than 16 Gy and risk of pituitary hormone deficiency (odds ratio, 1.08; P = .01).[23] Other variables, including whole sella irradiation and cavernous sinus invasion, have not been shown to be significant predictors of deficiency (P = .67 and P = .87, respectively).[63] Additional potential contributing factors include variation in patient characteristics, prior treatment history, and completeness of the endocrine follow-up.[12] Although a balance between dose optimization and the mediation of the risk of pituitary dysfunction should be sought, hormone deficiency is a treatable complication arising from radiosurgery.[46,63] Furthermore, in the treatment of residual or recurrent Cushing's disease, the likelihood of adverse effects associated with SRS must be carefully weighed against the risk of Nelson's syndrome after bilateral adrenalectomy, which ranges from 8% to 66%.[64]

Multiple cranial nerves (II, III, IV, and V) by virtue of their proximity to the sellar region are at risk of inadvertent injury after radiation treatment.[12] Overall, cranial neuropathy occurred in 1.5% of cases among the SRS series (range, 0%–6%) and in no cases among the XRT series.[15,20,21,23–30,32,33,36,38–40,42–44,52–59] The maximum dose to the optic nerve, which is highly sensitive to the effects of radiation, is generally kept at less than 8 to 12 Gy.[26] Additional safety parameters include dose planning with contouring and shielding of critical neurovascular structures.[12] Visual disturbance, defined as either optic nerve injury or symptomatic visual complication, occurred in less than 1% of cases among the SRS series (range, 0%–3%) and no cases among the XRT series.[15,20,21,23–30,32,33,36,38–40,42–44,52–59] Symptomatic optic nerve pallor was observed in 1 patient at a maximum dose of 7.4 Gy.[26]

As a result of hormonal effects on vasculature, the risk of ischemic stroke increases in patients with hypercortisolemia. Radiation itself creates a proinflammatory environment, which can lead to vascular injury.[65] Among major series using SRS, there were no reported ischemic events.[15,20,21,23–30,32,33,36,38–40,42–44] Cerebrovascular events

Table 3
Summary table of major series (n ≥10 patients) reporting adverse events after radiation therapy for Cushing's disease

Study	Patients (n)	New Anterior Pituitary Deficiency, n (%)	TSH (n)	FSH/LH (n)	GH (n)	Panhypopituitarism (n)	Mean Time to New Pituitary Deficiency (mo)	Optic Neuropathy, n (%)	Other Cranial Neuropathy, n (%)	Mean Time to Neuropathy (mo)	Resolution/ Mean Time to Resolution (mo)	Other Adverse Events
SRS												
Mehta et al,[23] 2017	278	70 (25)	46	28	29	0	NR	4 (1.4)	7 (2.5)	NR	NR	Nil
Marek et al,[24] 2015	26	3 (12)	1	1	1	0	70 (12–132)	NR	NR	—	—	Hemorrhage (asymptomatic) n = 1
Budyal et al,[20] 2014	20	8 (40)	5	6	0	0	42 (0–60)	0 (0)	0 (0)	—	—	Nil
Wilson et al,[25] 2014	36	2 (5.6)	0	2	0	0	NR	0 (0)	0 (0)	—	—	Asymptomatic radiation necrosis n = 1
Grant et al,[26] 2014	15	6 (40)	NR	NR	NR	NR	11.7 (6.3–17.1)	NR	NR	—	—	Nil
Wattson et al,[27] 2014	79	NR	—	—	—	—	—	0 (0)	1 (1.3)	NR	Y/9	Temporal lobe seizures n = 3
Sheehan et al,[28] 2013	96	35 (36)	NR	NR	NR	NR	NR	0 (0)	3 (3.1)	6	NR	Nil
Wein et al,[29] 2012	17	1 (5.9)	1	0	0	0	NR	0 (0)	0 (0)	—	—	Nil
Tinnel et al,[37] 2008	12	6 (50)	6	6	0	0	NR	0 (0)	0 (0)	—	—	Nil
Aghi et al,[32] 2008	31	13 (42)	10	2	7	0	NR	0 (0)	0 (0)	—	—	Nil
Wan et al,[36] 2009	68	NR	NR	NR	NR	NR	NR	NR	NR	NR	NR	Persistent vomiting n = 1 Asymptomatic radiation necrosis n = 2

(continued on next page)

Table 3
(continued)

Study	Patients (n)	New Anterior Pituitary Deficiency, n (%)	TSH (n)	FSH/LH (n)	GH (n)	Panhypopituitarism (n)	Mean Time to New Pituitary Deficiency (mo)	Optic Neuropathy, n (%)	Other Cranial Neuropathy, n (%)	Mean Time to Neuropathy (mo)	Resolution/ Mean Time to Resolution (mo)	Other Adverse Events
Petit et al,[33] 2008	38	17 (45)	8	3	7	2	27 (9–60)	0 (0)	0 (0)	—	—	Asymptomatic radiation necrosis n = 2
Castinetti et al,[30] 2007	40	6 (15)	2	0	2	2	60 (12–96)	0 (0)	2 (5)	NR	NR	Nil
Jagannathan et al,[38] 2007	90	20 (22.2)	9	NR	7	NR	16 (4–36)	5 (5.6)	5 (5.6)	6 (2–15)	NR	Nil
Devin et al,[39] 2004	35	14 (40)	7	7	4	0	NR	NR	NR	—	—	Nil
Colin et al,[21] 2005	10	NR	NR	NR	NR	NR	—	1 (2.8)	0 (0)	NR	NR	Nil
Jane et al,[40] 2003	45	14 (31)	NR	NR	NR	NR	—	1 (2.2)	0 (0)	NR	NR	Nil
Hoybe et al,[42] 2001	18	13 (69)	11	1	13	NR	—	0 (0)	0 (0)	—	—	Nil
Sheehan et al,[15] 2000	43	6 (14)	5	1	0	0	21 (8–35)	1 (2.3)	0 (0)	18	—	Nil
Izawa et al,[43] 2000	12	0 (0)	0	0	0	0	—	0 (0)	0 (0)	—	—	Nil
Degerblad et al,[44] 1986	29	12 (41)	8	5	—	—	4–84	0 (0)	0 (0)	—	—	Nil
XRT												
Minniti et al,[13] 2007	40	23 (58)	NR	NR	NR	19	0–120	1 (2.5)	0 (0)	NR	Y	Ischemic stroke n = 2
Estrada et al,[53] 1997	30	17 (57)	3	6	17	1	NR	0 (0)	0 (0)	—	—	Nil

Tsang et al,[56] 1996	20	NR	NR	NR	NR	0	—	0 (0)	0 (0)	—	Nil
Murayama et al,[58] 1992	20	7 (35)	1	2	4	0	NR	NR	NR	—	Nil
Vicente et al,[57] 1991	14	3 (21)	2	1	0	0	33 (24–42)	NR	NR	—	Nil
Littley et al,[55] 1990	24	12 (50)	0	0	12	0	13–171	0 (0)	0 (0)	—	Nil
Howlett et al,[54] 1989	21	10 (48)	2	3	5	NR	96 (34.8–141.6)	NR	NR	—	Nil
Ahmed et al,[52] 1984	19	0 (0)	0	0	0	0	—	NR	NR	—	Nil

Between 1984 and 2017, rates and mean time to onset of new anterior pituitary deficiency and cranial neuropathy are outlined. Other adverse events, including rates of stroke and radiation necrosis, are summarized.

Abbreviations: FSH, follicle-stimulating hormone; GH, growth hormone; LH, luteinizing hormone; NR, not reported; SRS, stereotactic radiosurgery; TSH, thyroid-stimulating hormone; XRT, conventional external beam radiation therapy.

were encountered in 2 patients after XRT, which suggests that targeted single-dose radiation may be associated with a more favorable safety effect profile.[59] Other infrequently reported radiosurgery-related complications, including radiation-induced parenchymal necrosis, internal carotid artery stenosis or occlusion, seizures, and asymptomatic hemorrhage are outlined in **Table 3**. No radiation-induced tumors were observed among SRS or XRT series on long-term follow-up.[15,20,21,23–27,29,30,32,33,36–40,42–44,47] The cumulative tumor risk associated with XRT in general is 2% at 12 years.[66]

SUMMARY

SRS and radiation therapy are reasonable treatment options for persistent or recurrent Cushing's disease and for those patients deemed unsuitable for resection. The growing popularity of SRS over XRT for Cushing's disease treatment can be attributed to the convenience of single-session treatments, and its favorable remission rate and adverse effect profile. Endocrine remission and tumor control rates are similar between SRS and XRT. To date, comparisons have been limited by heterogeneous, retrospectively collected data, and small cohort sizes. The strength of association between the effects of radiation treatment parameters and the coadministration of adjuvant medications on endocrine remission rates warrant further investigation.

REFERENCES

1. Lonser RR, Nieman L, Oldfield EH. Cushing's disease: pathobiology, diagnosis, and management. J Neurosurg 2017;126(2):404–17.
2. Rees DA, Hanna FW, Davies JS, et al. Long-term follow-up results of transsphenoidal surgery for Cushing's disease in a single centre using strict criteria for remission. Clin Endocrinol (Oxf) 2002;56(4):541–51.
3. Dallapiazza RF, Oldfield EH, Jane JA Jr. Surgical management of Cushing's disease. Pituitary 2015;18(2):211–6.
4. Lonser RR, Wind JJ, Nieman LK, et al. Outcome of surgical treatment of 200 children with Cushing's disease. J Clin Endocrinol Metab 2013;98(3):892–901.
5. Nieman LK, Biller BM, Findling JW, et al. Treatment of Cushing's syndrome: an endocrine society clinical practice guideline. J Clin Endocrinol Metab 2015; 100(8):2807–31.
6. Aranda G, Ensenat J, Mora M, et al. Long-term remission and recurrence rate in a cohort of Cushing's disease: the need for long-term follow-up. Pituitary 2015; 18(1):142–9.
7. Alexandraki KI, Kaltsas GA, Isidori AM, et al. Long-term remission and recurrence rates in Cushing's disease: predictive factors in a single-centre study. Eur J Endocrinol 2013;168(4):639–48.
8. Abu Dabrh AM, Singh Ospina NM, Al Nofal A, et al. Predictors of biochemical remission and recurrence after surgical and radiation treatments of Cushing disease: a systematic review and meta-analysis. Endocr Pract 2016;22(4):466–75.
9. Mehta GU, Lonser RR. Management of hormone-secreting pituitary adenomas. Neuro Oncol 2017;19(6):762–73.
10. Starke RM, Williams BJ, Vance ML, et al. Radiation therapy and stereotactic radiosurgery for the treatment of Cushing's disease: an evidence-based review. Curr Opin Endocrinol Diabetes Obes 2010;17(4):356–64.
11. Tritos NA, Biller BM. Update on radiation therapy in patients with Cushing's disease. Pituitary 2015;18(2):263–8.

12. Ding D, Starke RM, Sheehan JP. Treatment paradigms for pituitary adenomas: defining the roles of radiosurgery and radiation therapy. J Neurooncol 2014; 117(3):445–57.

13. Minniti G, Brada M. Radiotherapy and radiosurgery for Cushing's disease. Arq Bras Endocrinol Metabol 2007;51(8):1373–80.

14. McTyre E, Helis CA, Farris M, et al. Emerging indications for fractionated gamma knife radiosurgery. Neurosurgery 2017;80(2):210–6.

15. Sheehan JM, Vance ML, Sheehan JP, et al. Radiosurgery for Cushing's disease after failed transsphenoidal surgery. J Neurosurg 2000;93(5):738–42.

16. Deinsberger R, Tidstrand J. LINAC radiosurgery as a tool in neurosurgery. Neurosurg Rev 2005;28(2):79–88 [discussion: 89–91].

17. Friedman WA, Foote KD. Linear accelerator radiosurgery in the management of brain tumours. Ann Med 2000;32(1):64–80.

18. Chen CC, Chapman P, Petit J, et al. Proton radiosurgery in neurosurgery. Neurosurg Focus 2007;23(6):E5.

19. Paganetti H, Kooy H. Proton radiation in the management of localized cancer. Expert Rev Med Devices 2010;7(2):275–85.

20. Budyal S, Lila AR, Jalali R, et al. Encouraging efficacy of modern conformal fractionated radiotherapy in patients with uncured Cushing's disease. Pituitary 2014; 17(1):60–7.

21. Colin P, Jovenin N, Delemer B, et al. Treatment of pituitary adenomas by fractionated stereotactic radiotherapy: a prospective study of 110 patients. Int J Radiat Oncol Biol Phys 2005;62(2):333–41.

22. Kim JO, Ma R, Akagami R, et al. Long-term outcomes of fractionated stereotactic radiation therapy for pituitary adenomas at the BC Cancer Agency. Int J Radiat Oncol Biol Phys 2013;87(3):528–33.

23. Mehta GU, Ding D, Patibandla MR, et al. Stereotactic radiosurgery for Cushing's disease: results of an international, multicenter study. J Clin Endocrinol Metab 2017;102(11):4284–91.

24. Marek J, Jezkova J, Hana V, et al. Gamma knife radiosurgery for Cushing's disease and Nelson's syndrome. Pituitary 2015;18(3):376–84.

25. Wilson PJ, Williams JR, Smee RI. Cushing's disease: a single centre's experience using the linear accelerator (LINAC) for stereotactic radiosurgery and fractionated stereotactic radiotherapy. J Clin Neurosci 2014;21(1):100–6.

26. Grant RA, Whicker M, Lleva R, et al. Efficacy and safety of higher dose stereotactic radiosurgery for functional pituitary adenomas: a preliminary report. World Neurosurg 2014;82(1–2):195–201.

27. Wattson DA, Tanguturi SK, Spiegel DY, et al. Outcomes of proton therapy for patients with functional pituitary adenomas. Int J Radiat Oncol Biol Phys 2014;90(3): 532–9.

28. Sheehan JP, Xu Z, Salvetti DJ, et al. Results of gamma knife surgery for Cushing's disease. J Neurosurg 2013;119(6):1486–92.

29. Wein L, Dally M, Bach LA. Stereotactic radiosurgery for treatment of Cushing disease: an Australian experience. Intern Med J 2012;42(10):1153–6.

30. Castinetti F, Nagai M, Dufour H, et al. Gamma knife radiosurgery is a successful adjunctive treatment in Cushing's disease. Eur J Endocrinol 2007;156(1):91–8.

31. Castinetti F, Nagai M, Morange I, et al. Long-term results of stereotactic radiosurgery in secretory pituitary adenomas. J Clin Endocrinol Metab 2009;94(9): 3400–7.

32. Aghi MK, Petit J, Chapman P, et al. Management of recurrent and refractory Cushing's disease with reoperation and/or proton beam radiosurgery. Clin Neurosurg 2008;55:141–4.

33. Petit JH, Biller BM, Yock TI, et al. Proton stereotactic radiotherapy for persistent adrenocorticotropin-producing adenomas. J Clin Endocrinol Metab 2008;93(2): 393–9.

34. Losa M, Picozzi P, Redaelli MG, et al. Pituitary radiotherapy for Cushing's disease. Neuroendocrinology 2010;92(Suppl 1):107–10.

35. Voges J, Kocher M, Runge M, et al. Linear accelerator radiosurgery for pituitary macroadenomas: a 7-year follow-up study. Cancer 2006;107(6):1355–64.

36. Wan H, Chihiro O, Yuan S. MASEP gamma knife radiosurgery for secretory pituitary adenomas: experience in 347 consecutive cases. J Exp Clin Cancer Res 2009;28:36.

37. Tinnel BA, Henderson MA, Witt TC, et al. Endocrine response after gamma knife-based stereotactic radiosurgery for secretory pituitary adenoma. Stereotact Funct Neurosurg 2008;86(5):292–6.

38. Jagannathan J, Sheehan JP, Pouratian N, et al. Gamma knife surgery for Cushing's disease. J Neurosurg 2007;106(6):980–7.

39. Devin JK, Allen GS, Cmelak AJ, et al. The efficacy of linear accelerator radiosurgery in the management of patients with Cushing's disease. Stereotact Funct Neurosurg 2004;82(5–6):254–62.

40. Jane JA Jr, Vance ML, Woodburn CJ, et al. Stereotactic radiosurgery for hypersecreting pituitary tumors: part of a multimodality approach. Neurosurg Focus 2003;14(5):e12.

41. Kobayashi T, Kida Y, Mori Y. Gamma knife radiosurgery in the treatment of Cushing disease: long-term results. J Neurosurg 2002;97(5 Suppl):422–8.

42. Hoybye C, Grenback E, Rahn T, et al. Adrenocorticotropic hormone-producing pituitary tumors: 12- to 22-year follow-up after treatment with stereotactic radiosurgery. Neurosurgery 2001;49(2):284–91.

43. Izawa M, Hayashi M, Nakaya K, et al. Gamma knife radiosurgery for pituitary adenomas. J Neurosurg 2000;93(Suppl 3):19–22.

44. Degerblad M, Rahn T, Bergstrand G, et al. Long-term results of stereotactic radiosurgery to the pituitary gland in Cushing's disease. Acta Endocrinol (Copenh) 1986;112(3):310–4.

45. Levy RP, Fabrikant JI, Frankel KA, et al. Heavy-charged-particle radiosurgery of the pituitary gland: clinical results of 840 patients. Stereotact Funct Neurosurg 1991;57(1–2):22–35.

46. Lee CC, Chen CJ, Yen CP, et al. Whole-sellar stereotactic radiosurgery for functioning pituitary adenomas. Neurosurgery 2014;75(3):227–37 [discussion: 237].

47. Sheehan JP, Pouratian N, Steiner L, et al. Gamma Knife surgery for pituitary adenomas: factors related to radiological and endocrine outcomes. J Neurosurg 2011;114(2):303–9.

48. Lindsay JR, Oldfield EH, Stratakis CA, et al. The postoperative basal cortisol and CRH tests for prediction of long-term remission from Cushing's disease after transsphenoidal surgery. J Clin Endocrinol Metab 2011;96(7):2057–64.

49. Asuzu D, Chatain GP, Hayes C, et al. Normalized early postoperative cortisol and ACTH values predict nonremission after surgery for Cushing disease. J Clin Endocrinol Metab 2017;102(7):2179–87.

50. Rutkowski MJ, Flanigan PM, Aghi MK. Update on the management of recurrent Cushing's disease. Neurosurg Focus 2015;38(2):E16.

51. Kondziolka D. Cushing's disease and stereotactic radiosurgery. J Neurosurg 2013;119(6):1484–5 [discussion: 1485].
52. Ahmed SR, Shalet SM, Beardwell CG, et al. Treatment of Cushing's disease with low dose radiation therapy. Br Med J (Clin Res Ed) 1984;289(6446):643–6.
53. Estrada J, Boronat M, Mielgo M, et al. The long-term outcome of pituitary irradiation after unsuccessful transsphenoidal surgery in Cushing's disease. N Engl J Med 1997;336(3):172–7.
54. Howlett TA, Plowman PN, Wass JA, et al. Megavoltage pituitary irradiation in the management of Cushing's disease and Nelson's syndrome: long-term follow-up. Clin Endocrinol (Oxf) 1989;31(3):309–23.
55. Littley MD, Shalet SM, Beardwell CG, et al. Long-term follow-up of low-dose external pituitary irradiation for Cushing's disease. Clin Endocrinol (Oxf) 1990; 33(4):445–55.
56. Tsang RW, Brierley JD, Panzarella T, et al. Role of radiation therapy in clinical hormonally-active pituitary adenomas. Radiother Oncol 1996;41(1):45–53.
57. Vicente A, Estrada J, de la Cuerda C, et al. Results of external pituitary irradiation after unsuccessful transsphenoidal surgery in Cushing's disease. Acta Endocrinol (Copenh) 1991;125(5):470–4.
58. Murayama M, Yasuda K, Minamori Y, et al. Long term follow-up of Cushing's disease treated with reserpine and pituitary irradiation. J Clin Endocrinol Metab 1992;75(3):935–42.
59. Minniti G, Osti M, Jaffrain-Rea ML, et al. Long-term follow-up results of postoperative radiation therapy for Cushing's disease. J Neurooncol 2007;84(1):79–84.
60. Sheehan J. Stereotactic radiosurgery for functioning pituitary adenomas–a higher dose is better but only up to a point. World Neurosurg 2014;82(1–2):e75–6.
61. Landolt AM, Haller D, Lomax N, et al. Stereotactic radiosurgery for recurrent surgically treated acromegaly: comparison with fractionated radiotherapy. J Neurosurg 1998;88(6):1002–8.
62. Becker G, Kocher M, Kortmann RD, et al. Radiation therapy in the multimodal treatment approach of pituitary adenoma. Strahlenther Onkol 2002;178(4): 173–86.
63. Xu Z, Lee Vance M, Schlesinger D, et al. Hypopituitarism after stereotactic radiosurgery for pituitary adenomas. Neurosurgery 2013;72(4):630–7, 636–7.
64. Barber TM, Adams E, Ansorge O, et al. Nelson's syndrome. Eur J Endocrinol 2010;163(4):495–507.
65. van Westrhenen A, Muskens IS, Verhoeff JJC, et al. Ischemic stroke after radiation therapy for pituitary adenomas: a systematic review. J Neurooncol 2017; 135(1):1–11.
66. Minniti G, Traish D, Ashley S, et al. Risk of second brain tumor after conservative surgery and radiotherapy for pituitary adenoma: update after an additional 10 years. J Clin Endocrinol Metab 2005;90(2):800–4.

New Molecular Targets for Treatment of Cushing's Disease

Elizabeth Foulkes, BMedSci, John Newell-Price, MA, PhD, FRCP*

KEYWORDS

- Cushing's disease • Therapy • ACTH • Cortisol • Pituitary

KEY POINTS

- Cushing's disease is the result of pituitary corticotroph adenomas autonomously secreting ACTH, with a disruption of the normal hypothalamic-pituitary-adrenal axis and uncontrolled hypercortisolism.
- Until recently, the mechanisms causing the development of Cushing's disease remained largely unknown.
- Emerging discoveries have made major progress into the understanding of the molecular pathogenesis of Cushing's disease in a significant proportion of corticotroph adenomas.
- Developments in the understanding of glucocorticoid resistance in Cushing's disease, through the identification of interactions between TR4 and HSP90 with the glucocorticoid receptor, could provide promising new therapeutic approaches in treatment.

NORMAL PHYSIOLOGY OF THE HYPOTHALAMIC-PITUITARY-ADRENAL AXIS

In considering potential new molecular targets for the treatment of Cushing's disease, it is useful to consider first the normal physiologic regulation of ACTH synthesis and release. The normal hypothalamic-pituitary-adrenal axis relies on regulatory negative feedback from circulating cortisol levels.[1] Corticotropin-releasing hormone (CRH) and arginine vasopressin (AVP) are released from the paraventricular nucleus of the hypothalamus and act on pituitary corticotroph cells, in the anterior pituitary, to ultimately stimulate the release of adrenocorticotropic hormone (ACTH) into the circulation.[2] CRH acts by binding to the CRH-R1 receptor on the surface of the corticotroph cells, activating a stimulatory G-protein alpha subunit, and causing a downstream signaling cascade.[3,4] The outcome of this signaling cascade is the promotion of proopiomelanocortin (POMC) gene transcription, resulting in the synthesis of POMC and ACTH

Disclosure Statement: The authors have nothing to disclose.
Department of Oncology and Metabolism, The Medical School, University of Sheffield, Beech Hill Road, Sheffield S10 2RX, UK
* Corresponding author.
E-mail address: j.newellprice@sheffield.ac.uk

Endocrinol Metab Clin N Am 47 (2018) 367–373
https://doi.org/10.1016/j.ecl.2018.02.006
0889-8529/18/© 2018 Elsevier Inc. All rights reserved.

release. POMC is the polypeptide precursor of ACTH; cleaved by prohormone convertases (PC1) in the corticotroph cells of the anterior pituitary to produce peptide fragments, including ACTH.[5,6] ACTH is then packaged into vesicles and released from the cells by exocytosis.

Once in the circulation, ACTH binds to melanocortin 2 receptor on the surface of the adrenocortical cells, particularly in the zona fasciculata, to stimulate the steroidogenesis pathway and the release of cortisol into the circulation. Normally, cortisol then exhibits negative feedback to inhibit its own synthesis by transrepression of hypothalamic CRH and synthesis and release of anterior pituitary ACTH.[7] Cortisol acts at the level of the hypothalamus and anterior pituitary by binding to the glucocorticoid receptor type 2 (NR3C1) to form a NR3C1/cortisol complex. Subsequently, this complex translocates from the cytoplasm to the nucleus to bind to regulatory areas on the DNA and inhibit the synthesis of *POMC, CRH*, and *AVP* mRNA, thereby reducing the secretion of ACTH and regulating the hypothalamic-pituitary-adrenal axis.[8] In Cushing's disease, there is excess *POMC* expression and ACTH secretion that is resistant to the normal glucocorticoid negative feedback mechanisms, resulting in excess serum and urinary cortisol, which clinically manifests as Cushing's syndrome.

CURRENT MEDICAL THERAPIES

Current medical therapies for Cushing's disease can be divided into 3 main categories based on their site of action: at the level of the pituitary, by inhibiting ACTH secretion; at the adrenal gland to inhibit steroidogenesis; and at the target tissue by blocking the glucocorticoid receptor.[9–11] All therapies have drawbacks and there is a real clinical need for new medical therapies directed at the pituitary. Such therapies may, in the future, be based on recently identified novel molecular targets.

TESTICULAR ORPHAN NUCLEAR RECEPTOR 4

Glucocorticoid binding to the NR3C1 glucocorticoid receptor (GR) in the hypothalamus and anterior pituitary results in the translocation of the ligand-bound GR to negatively repress *POMC* transcription, and reduce ACTH secretion. In Cushing's disease, corticotroph tumor cells exhibit relative resistance to the inhibitory action of glucocorticoids on ACTH secretion.[7,12] Recently, it has been identified that testicular orphan nuclear receptor 4 (TR4) is strongly expressed in corticotroph tumor cell nuclei, and acts to reduce the effects of glucocorticoids and GR inhibition of *POMC* expression.[7,13] TR4, is also known as nuclear receptor subfamily 2, group C, member 2 (NR2C2) and is a member of the nuclear receptor superfamily and is a transcriptional regulator in a variety of processes including *POMC* transcription.[13] TR4 is expressed in the *cytosol* of normal pituitary corticotroph cells, and expression is markedly increased in ACTH-secreting corticotroph tumors in both humans and mice. Furthermore, immunocytochemistry studies revealed no expression of TR4 in the nuclei of normal corticotroph cells, in contrast to corticotroph tumors, which showed abundant expression and redistribution of TR4 from the cytosol to the nucleus,[13] suggesting a pathologic alteration of function of TR4 in corticotroph adenomas compared with normal corticotroph cells.

Studies in vitro using *POMC*-expressing AtT20 cells revealed that overexpression of TR4 correlated with an increase in *POMC* transcription and ACTH secretion. In contrast to these findings, knockdown of TR4 using a small interfering RNA showed reduced *POMC*-luciferase reporter activity, reduced *POMC* mRNA and protein expression, and a reduction in the amount of ACTH secreted by the corticotroph tumor cells. To examine if TR4 has an effect on the in vivo growth of corticotroph tumors, nude mice were inoculated with AtT20 cells that had TR4-knocked down. Compared with control mice that had been inoculated with unaltered AtT20 cells, there were significantly reduced levels of circulating ACTH and reduced expression of *POMC* and *TR4* in the tumors formed from the TR4-knockdown cells.[13] Overexpression of TR4 also caused resistance to GR-induced inhibition of *POMC* expression[7]: following transfection of AtT20 cells with a *POMC*-promoter luciferase reporter with and without TR4-expressing plasmids, dexamethasone treatment caused prompt inhibition of *POMC* expression when TR4 was not overexpressed, but *POMC* expression was not suppressed in the presence of TR4 overexpression. Further data using specific short hairpin RNA (shRNA) toward TR4 revealed a reduction in *POMC* reporter activity, suggesting TR4 directly contributes to *POMC* expression.

Together, these studies indicate that TR4 interacts with the GR (NR3C1) to override the negative regulation of *POMC* transcription by glucocorticoids, and also contributes to *POMC* expression. These data indicate that TR4 may be a potential target for therapy in Cushing's disease, but more data are needed to dissect the relative importance of TR4 in comparison with other factors and pathways in *POMC* transcription.

HEAT SHOCK PROTEIN 90

A further target for the treatment of Cushing's disease also relates to the action of the GR, and its interaction with the chaperone protein heat shock protein 90 (HSP90). Interaction between HSP90 and the NR3C1 GR facilitates the binding of glucocorticoids and aids the translocation of the NR3C1-ligand complex to the nucleus, where it binds to DNA and alters gene transcription.[14]

HSP90 action and binding to GR can be influenced at either its N-terminal or C-terminal; 17-AAG is an N-terminal HSP90 inhibitor and novobiocin inhibits HSP90 at the C-terminal. In addition, the recently identified HSP90 inhibitor silibinin also acts via the C-terminal of HSP90 and allows separation of GR from HSP90.[15] HSP90 is overexpressed in corticotroph adenomas compared with the normal pituitary corticotroph cells, leading to impaired ability of glucocorticoids to suppress *POMC* transcription, so enhancing glucocorticoid resistance at the level of the pituitary.[15] Cultures of human corticotroph adenomas treated with silibinin showed restored sensitivity to the inhibitory effect of glucocorticoids; following addition of exogenous dexamethasone, the resistance to glucocorticoid regulation was decreased and suppression of endogenous ACTH secretion was enhanced.[15] These results suggest that HSP90 may be a new molecular target for medical therapy in Cushing's disease; however, the sample size was small and this study only analyzed the effects of HSP90 inhibition on glucocorticoid resistance in 6 primary cultures of human corticotroph adenomas. Potentially, HSP90-inhibition using silibinin might be used to restore glucocorticoid sensitivity in patients with Cushing's disease. Because silibinin is used in the treatment of drug-induced hepatotoxicity and prostate cancer, and has a proven safety profile in humans,[16] it may be an easier compound to investigate for the treatment of Cushing's disease, but formal trials are needed.

Similarly, 2 HSP90 inhibitors, 17-AAG and CCT018159, reduced cell proliferation, *POMC* mRNA levels and ACTH secretion in AtT20 cells.[17] Data in vivo are awaited.

EPITHELIAL GROWTH FACTOR RECEPTOR

Pituitary corticotroph cell adenomas express highly the epidermal growth factor receptor (EGFR).[18] Therefore, this receptor has been investigated as a new molecular target in the treatment of Cushing's disease.

Gefitinib is a tyrosine kinase inhibitor that targets the EGFR and is effective in treating other cancers that overexpress EGFR.[19] Gefitinib treatment of primary cell cultures from surgically resected human corticotroph tumors suppressed *POMC* mRNA expression, suggesting that EGFR-inhibition could be a novel strategy for suppressing ACTH secretion from corticotroph adenomas in Cushing's disease. Mechanistically, although EGFR activation induces *POMC*-promoter activity, this was inhibited following treatment with U0126, a MAP kinase (MAPK) pathway inhibitor, but not by S31 to 201 (a STAT3 inhibitor). These results suggest that epidermal growth factor (EGF) induces *POMC* transcriptional activity via the MAPK pathway, and that EGFR signaling induces *POMC* mRNA expression and ACTH secretion in corticotroph tumors. Therefore, the EGFR could be a new molecular target for treating patients with Cushing's disease. Unfortunately, gefitinib has considerable toxicity when treating patients with other cancers and these may limit usefulness in Cushing's disease, but clinical trials are in progress.[19,20] Moreover, recent data implicate further the role of EGFR signaling in the pathogenesis of Cushing's disease and reinforce the possible application of therapies targeting this pathway as a potential treatment.

UBIQUITIN-SPECIFIC PROTEASE 8

Until recently, the genetic basis driving tumor growth of corticotroph adenoma cells in Cushing's disease was unknown. As Cushing's disease rarely occurs in the context of familial genetic syndromes, and patients do not usually have a family history of Cushing's disease, it seems likely that it is most likely due to a sporadic somatic mutation rather than germline mutations.

Whole-exome sequencing of tumor and germline DNA sample pairs from patients with CD revealed that 40% had somatic missense mutations in the gene encoding ubiquitin-specific protease 8 (USP8).[21] Further studies using larger cohorts of patients with CD also analyzed the prevalence of USP8 mutations in corticotroph adenomas and found a prevalence of 36%.[22,23] Furthermore, all of the mutations of USP8 were found to cluster in a hotspot region of exon 14.[22,23] These mutations have not been found in any other form of pituitary tumor.[22]

The USP8 gene is located on chromosome 15q21.2 and codes for USP8 protein, a deubiquitinating enzyme. Ubiquitination is the reversible, posttranslational process of binding ubiquitin to target proteins, such as cell surface proteins, thereby marking them for degradation by the endosome-lysosome system.[21] The USP8 enzyme catalyzes the cleavage of the ubiquitin tags, thus protecting growth factor receptors, including EGFR, from degradation, leading to receptor recycling to the cell surface.[8,23] Ubiquitination of the EGFR occurs following EGF binding to the cell surface. EGF binds to and activates EGFR, leading to rapid transportation of the receptor from the membrane into the cell, where it is degraded during the process of receptor downregulation.[18] This process is essential in ensuring that the cell does not respond excessively to EGF stimulation, which could have potentially damaging consequences. In Cushing's disease, mutations in USP8 were shown to target the 14-3-3 protein-binding domain, which leads to impaired binding of 14-3-3 proteins. This results in enhanced deubiquitinating enzyme activation, impaired EGFR downregulation, and increased EGFR stability and signaling.[18,21,24] EGF has been shown to act directly on pituitary cells to increase POMC mRNA transcription, cell proliferation, and ACTH secretion.[19,25] ACTH-secreting pituitary adenomas exhibiting the USP8 mutant express a higher level of EGFR and produce an increased amount of *POMC* mRNA and ACTH compared with tumors with wild-type USP8.[21,23] It is possible

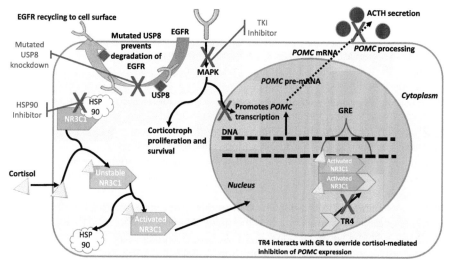

Fig. 1. Novel targets for potential therapy in Cushing's disease. Schematic representation of potential novel targets discussed in text. Sites where inhibitors may act are shown by red "X." GRE, glucocorticoid response element; TKI, tyrosine kinase inhibitor.

that specific targeting of the mutated USP8 might be a therapeutic strategy: shRNA knockdown of mutated *USP8* gene expression caused a significant reduction in the ACTH secreted from cells with the mutant USP8, but had no effect on cells with wild-type USP8.[23]

SUMMARY

Cushing's disease is the result of pituitary corticotroph adenomas autonomously secreting ACTH, with a disruption of the normal hypothalamic-pituitary-adrenal axis and uncontrolled hypercortisolism. Until recently, the mechanisms causing the development of Cushing's disease remained largely unknown. Emerging discoveries have made major progress into the understanding of the molecular pathogenesis of Cushing's disease in a significant proportion of corticotroph adenomas. Developments in the understanding of glucocorticoid resistance in Cushing's disease, through the identification of interactions between TR4 and HSP90 with the GR, could provide promising new therapeutic approaches in the treatment of CD. The identification of a somatic mutational hotspot in *USP8* also provides insight into the role of EGFR on causing excess synthesis of ACTH, and may serve as a new molecular focal point for future development of effective tumor-target therapies **(Fig. 1)**.

REFERENCES

1. Wondisford FE. A new medical therapy for Cushing disease? J Clin Invest 2011; 121(12):4621–3.
2. Vale W, Spiess J, Rivier C, et al. Characterization of a 41-residue ovine hypothalamic peptide that stimulates secretion of corticotropin and beta-endorphin. Science 1981;213(4514):1394–7.
3. Aguilera G, Nikodemova M, Wynn PC, et al. Corticotropin releasing hormone receptors: two decades later. Peptides 2004;25(3):319–29.

4. Grammatopoulos DK, Chrousos GP. Functional characteristics of CRH receptors and potential clinical applications of CRH-receptor antagonists. Trends Endocrinol Metab 2002;13(10):436–44.

5. Raffin-Sanson ML, de Keyzer Y, Bertagna X. Proopiomelanocortin, a polypeptide precursor with multiple functions: from physiology to pathological conditions. Eur J Endocrinol 2003;149(2):79–90.

6. Moisiadis VG, Matthews SG. Glucocorticoids and fetal programming part 1: outcomes. Nat Rev Endocrinol 2014;10(7):391–402.

7. Zhang DY, Du L, Heaney AP. Testicular receptor-4: novel regulator of glucocorticoid resistance. J Clin Endocrinol Metab 2016;101(8):3123–33.

8. Daniel E, Newell-Price J. Recent advances in understanding Cushing disease: resistance to glucocorticoid negative feedback and somatic USP8 mutations. F1000Res 2017;6:613.

9. Lau D, Rutledge C, Aghi MK. Cushing's disease: current medical therapies and molecular insights guiding future therapies. Neurosurg Focus 2015;38(2):10.

10. Langlois F, McCartney S, Fleseriu M. Recent progress in the medical therapy of pituitary tumors. Endocrinol Metab (Seoul) 2017;32(2):162–70.

11. Nieman LK, Biller BMK, Findling JW, et al. Treatment of Cushing's syndrome: an endocrine society clinical practice guideline. J Clin Endocrinol Metab 2015; 100(8):2807–31.

12. Newell-Price J, Bertagna X, Grossman AB, et al. Cushing's syndrome. Lancet 2006;367(9522):1605–17.

13. Du L, Bergsneider M, Mirsadraei L, et al. Evidence for orphan nuclear receptor TR4 in the etiology of Cushing disease. Proc Natl Acad Sci U S A 2013; 110(21):8555–60.

14. Echeverria PC, Picard D. Molecular chaperones, essential partners of steroid hormone receptors for activity and mobility. Biochim Biophys Acta 2010;1803(6): 641–9.

15. Riebold M, Kozany C, Freiburger L, et al. A C-terminal HSP90 inhibitor restores glucocorticoid sensitivity and relieves a mouse allograft model of Cushing disease. Nat Med 2015;21(3):276–80.

16. Ramasamy K, Agarwal R. Multitargeted therapy of cancer by silymarin. Cancer Lett 2008;269(2):352–62.

17. Sugiyama A, Kageyama K, Murasawa S, et al. Inhibition of heat shock protein 90 decreases ACTH production and cell proliferation in AtT-20 cells. Pituitary 2015; 18(4):542–53.

18. Theodoropoulou M, Reincke M, Fassnacht M, et al. Decoding the genetic basis of Cushing's disease: USP8 in the spotlight. Eur J Endocrinol 2015;173(4):M73–83.

19. Fukuoka H, Cooper O, Ben-Shlomo A, et al. EGFR as a therapeutic target for human, canine, and mouse ACTH-secreting pituitary adenomas. J Clin Invest 2011; 121(12):4712–21.

20. Jian FF, Cao YA, Bian LG, et al. USP8: a novel therapeutic target for Cushing's disease. Endocrine 2015;50(2):292–6.

21. Reincke M, Sbiera S, Hayakawa A, et al. Mutations in the deubiquitinase gene USP8 cause Cushing's disease. Nat Genet 2015;47(1):31–8.

22. Perez-Rivas LG, Reincke M. Genetics of Cushing's disease: update. J Endocrinol Invest 2016;39(1):29–35.

23. Ma ZY, Song ZJ, Chen JH, et al. Recurrent gain-of-function USP8 mutations in Cushing's disease. Cell Res 2015;25(3):306–17.

24. Jian FF, Li YF, Chen YF, et al. Inhibition of ubiquitin-specific peptidase 8 suppresses adrenocorticotropic hormone production and tumorous corticotroph cell growth in AtT20 cells. Chin Med J 2016;129(17):2102–8.
25. Childs GV, Patterson J, Unabia G, et al. Epidermal growth factor enhances ACTH secretion and expression of POMC mRNA by corticotropes in mixed and enriched cultures. Mol Cell Neurosci 1991;2(3):235–43.

Recent Advances on Subclinical Hypercortisolism

Guido Zavatta, MD, Guido Di Dalmazi, MD*

KEYWORDS

• Subclinical • Mild • Cushing's • Hypercortisolism • Adrenal

KEY POINTS

- The most recent guidelines suggest the use of 1-mg dexamethasone suppression test in all patients with adrenal incidentalomas.
- Mass spectrometry–based steroid profiling is useful in evaluation of subclinical hypercortisolism.
- Adrenal protocol computed tomography scan provides morphologic information that may be predictive of cortisol hypersecretion.
- Subclinical hypercortisolism is associated with increased incidence of cardiovascular diseases and increased mortality from cardiovascular events and infections.
- Adrenalectomy in patients with subclinical hypercortisolism and unilateral adenomas has some beneficial effects on associated comorbidities, as shown by retrospective studies.

INTRODUCTION

The term "adrenal incidentaloma" refers to an adrenal mass discovered during imaging performed for reasons unrelated to adrenal disorders. Even though most adrenal incidentalomas do not show biochemical evidence of hormonal excess, up to 30% of those tumors are associated with subclinical hypercortisolism (SH).[1] SH is a pathologic condition defined as biochemical evidence of hypercortisolism in patients without typical signs or symptoms of Cushing's syndrome.[1] In recent years, this condition has been evaluated in several studies that increased the understanding regarding its natural history and the outcomes of available therapeutic options. The refined radiological techniques and the introduction of metabolomic profiling by mass spectrometry have improved the performance of current diagnostic criteria and provided new insights regarding the pathogenesis of subtle cortisol excess. The purpose of this review is to present the most recent advances in SH.

Disclosure Statement: The authors have nothing to disclose.
Division of Endocrinology, Department of Medical and Surgical Sciences, Alma Mater Studiorum University of Bologna, S. Orsola-Malpighi Hospital, Via Massarenti 9, Bologna 40138, Italy
* Corresponding author.
E-mail address: guido.didalmazi@unibo.it

BIOCHEMICAL DIAGNOSIS OF SUBCLINICAL HYPERCORTISOLISM

Considering that SH occurs in patients without overt signs of cortisol excess, laboratory tests plays a pivotal role in the diagnosis of this condition (**Box 1**). Cortisol suppression to 1-mg dexamethasone suppression test (DST) has been traditionally considered the most reliable parameter to screen for endogenous Cushing's syndrome. The cortisol value that defines SH has been a topic of controversy.[2] The sensitivity and the specificity of the different cutoffs for cortisol vary across different studies.[3] The European Society of Endocrinology (ESE) clinical guidelines on the management of adrenocortical tumors published in 2016 introduced some important points.[1] First, the 1-mg DST is recommended in all patients with adrenal incidentalomas, with a cutoff for serum cortisol of greater than 5 μg/dL defining SH, whereas suppression to 1.8 to 5 μg/dL indicates possible SH. The usefulness of the 1-mg DST has been proven in several studies investigating the natural history of SH. Patients with cortisol levels greater than 1.8 μg/dL are at increased risk for cardiovascular diseases.[4,5] Moreover, patients with SH had a lower survival rate than those with nonsecreting adrenal tumors, because of cardiovascular events and infectious complications.[4,6] Second, the ESE experts' panel recommended that cortisol levels after DST should be considered a continuous rather than a categorical variable, supporting the concept of a continuum of progression of hypercortisolism over time. Finally, even though several additional tests can help with the diagnosis of SH in patients with cortisol suppression between 1.8 and 5 μg/dL, the presence of comorbidities related to hypercortisolism should be carefully considered when making therapeutic recommendations. These recommendations include diabetes mellitus, hypertension, and cardiovascular disease.[7]

Additional tests for patients with abnormal DST include basal adrenocorticotropic hormone (ACTH) levels (helpful in diagnosing ACTH-independent hypercortisolism when suppressed <10 pg/mL). However, ACTH is inhibited in a variable proportion of patients with adrenal incidentalomas and is sometimes detectable in patients with ACTH-independent Cushing's syndrome.[8] Moreover, ACTH immunoassays are vulnerable to interference of endogenous antibodies.[9] Unlike overt Cushing's syndrome, SH patients do not benefit much from urinary free cortisol (UFC) measurement,[8] mainly because of the low sensitivity in detecting mild cortisol excess. However, a recent study showed that high UFC levels measured by mass spectrometry might be a biomarker of cardiovascular risk in patients with SH.[10] Dehydroepiandrosterone-sulfate (DHEAS) levels are frequently reduced in patients with hypercortisolism for 2 reasons: reduced activity of the 17,20-lyase in hyperfunctioning tumors[11] and reduced stimulation of adrenal cortex adjacent/contralateral to the tumor by the low levels of pituitary ACTH. A large retrospective study showed that DHEAS levels less than 40 μg/dL had a specificity of 75% and a sensitivity of 68% in identifying SH.[12] Moreover, DHEAS offered comparable sensitivity and greater specificity to the 1-mg DST for the detection of SH.[13]

Box 1
Diagnostic testing for subclinical hypercortisolism

- All patients with adrenal incidentalomas should undergo a 1-mg DST.
- Cortisol suppression less than 1.8 μg/dL indicates a normal response, whereas values greater than 5 μg/dL define subclinical hypercortisolism.
- For cortisol suppression between 1.8 and 5 μg/dL, additional tests include late-night salivary cortisol and DHEAS, whereas ACTH and UFC levels seem less helpful.
- Reduced levels of adrenal androgens measured by mass spectrometry may be used as markers of SH.

The main limitation of studies investigating DHEAS as a diagnostic tool is related to the low accuracy of traditional immunometric assays in measuring reduced androgen levels. Indeed, mass spectrometry has proven to be superior to immunometric assays in the range close to the lower limit of detection.[14] Late-night salivary cortisol (LNSC) as a single hormonal parameter is not sufficient to make the diagnosis of SH.[15,16] However, LNSC combined with cortisol after 1-mg DST greater than 1.8 μg/dL has 89% sensitivity and 85% specificity for detection of SH.[17] In addition, the analysis of daily salivary cortisol rhythm measured by mass spectrometry showed that patients with 1-mg DST cortisol levels greater than 1.8 μg/dL had higher cortisol levels in the morning, and no significant impairment of cortisol circadian rhythm.[18]

RADIOLOGICAL DIAGNOSIS

The size of a normal adrenal gland has been systematically defined in a cohort of 55 patients more than 20 years ago.[19] By using an old-generation 10-mm-thick-sections computed tomographic (CT) scanner, Vincent and colleagues[19] showed that the thickness of normal adrenal limbs was ≤5 mm. Schneller and colleagues,[20] by using a modern 5-mm-thick slice CT scanner, highlighted that the median width of right and left adrenal lateral limb in 105 patients was 4.0 mm and 4.6 mm, respectively. Linear measurement of the width of the adrenal limbs was positively associated with adrenal gland total volume. Even with the limitations concerning the small number of patients, those studies raise the hypothesis that adrenal limb thickness greater than 5 mm, with or without distinct micronodules, might be considered a pathologic finding and should be further investigated by hormonal tests. Nonetheless, the ESE guidelines suggest performing additional diagnostic workup only for lesions ≥1 cm, unless there is clinical evidence of hormone excess.[1] The guidelines do not provide recommendations on management of smaller adrenal lesions.

Incidentally discovered bilateral adrenal lesions can be classified as bilateral adenomas, macronodular hyperplasia, and distinct bilateral nodules with normal or atrophic adjacent adrenal tissue.[1] In some instances, it may be challenging to distinguish those conditions by performing standard radiological imaging techniques. A retrospective study by Park and colleagues[21] analyzed CT densitometry and percentage washout in 424 histologically confirmed adrenal tumors. Even though standard CT parameters were not useful in differentiating adenoma from hyperplasia, a larger tumor size was suggestive of adenoma and the presence of ≥3 nodules increased the likelihood of hyperplasia. Notably, by using the adrenal protocol, all cases of nodular hyperplasia were diagnosed as multiple adenomas preoperatively.

The increasing precision in the radiological techniques has led to investigate the possibility that CT scan may be used to characterize the functional status of an adrenal tumor. The authors' group first presented a score calculated by using several radiological parameters to differentiate nonsecreting adrenal adenomas from those associated with SH.[22] The diagnostic accuracy in classifying patients with abnormal cortisol suppression to DST (>1.8 μg/dL) was 85%, with sensitivity and specificity of 81% and 87%, respectively. Contrast-enhanced venous phase and tumor diameter were identified as significant parameters. In a multicentric study, Olsen and colleagues[23] found that SH was positively associated with the size of adenoma and inversely correlated to unenhanced CT attenuation. In contrast, a recent study showed that unenhanced CT attenuation was positively associated with cortisol hypersecretion.[24] However, no subgroup analysis was performed for SH.

The ESE guidelines recommend that all patients should undergo a noncontrast CT scan (**Box 2**). In those cases of lipid-rich adenomas (ie, homogeneous lesions with

---

Box 2
Radiological diagnosis of adrenal incidentalomas

- Adrenal incidentaloma definition refers to lesions that are larger than 1 cm in diameter.
- CT should be used as a first-line imaging technique.
- The region of interest for measurement of CT attenuation should include at least 75% of the lesion and precontrast Hounsfield Units (HU) $\leq$10 in a homogeneous mass define a lipid-rich adenoma.
- Tumors with precontrast HU >10 should undergo CT scan with delayed contrast washout at 10 or 15 minutes to calculate absolute washout (AWO) and relative washout (RWO).
- AWO greater than 60% and/or RWO greater than 40% suggest a benign adrenal mass.

---

unenhanced CT attenuation $\leq$10 HU) that are smaller than 4 cm, no further imaging is required.[1] However, this recommendation has a very low quality of evidence and further studies should address this issue.

MASS SPECTROMETRY–BASED METABOLOMIC PROFILING IN SUBCLINICAL HYPERCORTISOLISM

Adrenal tumors associated with SH have been found to cosecrete other steroids, defined as "minor" in the past. The clinical relevance of a broad spectrum of steroid excess has not yet been clarified. A recent study by the authors' group analyzed a panel of 10 steroids in adrenal incidentalomas and controls, by means of liquid chromatography-tandem mass spectrometry (LC-MS/MS).[25] Androgen reduction (DHEA, androstenedione, and testosterone) resulted as a marker of SH. Notably, higher levels of corticosterone, 11-deoxycorticosterone, and 21-deoxycortisol were also found in SH than in nonsecreting adenomas after Synacthen test, which may implicate these steroids with glucocorticoid and mineralocorticoid activity in the pathogenesis of cardiovascular diseases encountered in patients with SH. In a recent paper, Kotłowska and colleagues[26] analyzed a total of 19 urinary steroids in patients with Cushing's syndrome, nonfunctioning adrenal incidentalomas, and controls, by using gas chromatography-mass spectrometry (GC/MS). A panel of 6 steroids was identified as a potential biomarker of hypercortisolism. Interestingly, adrenal incidentalomas had a defined steroid profiling, well-separated form of Cushing's syndrome, and minimally overlapped that of controls.

The urinary steroid profiling has also provided novel insights into the pathogenesis of cortisol hypersecretion. The 24-hour urinary steroid profiling by GC/MS in a large cohort of subjects with primary aldosteronism, adrenal incidentalomas, Cushing's syndrome, and healthy controls revealed that glucocorticoid output of patients with primary aldosteronism was at least as high as in those with SH.[27] The excessive glucocorticoid production was correlated with several metabolic parameters, such as waist circumference, high-density lipoprotein, and diastolic blood pressure. Therefore, the previously unrecognized glucocorticoid excess in primary aldosteronism may be a major determinant of the well-known increased metabolic risk associated with this condition. If those findings will be confirmed in independent cohorts, treatment options for tumors cosecreting aldosterone and cortisol should be reviewed, given that mineralocorticoid receptor blockers may not be sufficient to contrast the glucocorticoid-mediated adverse metabolic effects. Recently, plasma steroid profiling by LC-MS/MS also proved to be useful in differentiating the subtypes of Cushing's syndrome. The 10-steroid panel showed a discriminatory power close to that of LNSC, UFC, cortisol after 1-mg DST, and ACTH.[28]

Mass spectrometry has also been applied to the study of the metabolic consequences of hypercortisolism. Recently, the targeted metabolomic profiling of a large cohort of patients showed that several alterations in amino acid metabolism, urea cycle, and beta-oxidation were tightly related to the excessive cortisol production, independently of potential confounding factors, mainly diabetes.[29] Interestingly, some features specific to Cushing's syndrome, like alterations of acetyl-carnitine, hydroxy-tetradecadienylcarnitine, branched-chain amino acids, histidine, tyrosine, and kynurenine, were confirmed in patients with SH, leading to the speculation that protein catabolism and alterations of beta-oxidation may be relevant pathogenetic pathways even in patients without overt signs of Cushing's syndrome.[29]

MOLECULAR PATHOGENESIS OF SUBCLINICAL HYPERCORTISOLISM

In most patients with bilateral macronodular adrenal hyperplasia (BMAH), steroidogenesis is driven by activation of overexpressed aberrant G protein–coupled receptors, which induce the intracellular events that are normally triggered by ACTH.[30] Different receptors have been implicated in the pathogenesis of cortisol overproduction, including those for gastric inhibitory polypeptide (GIP), vasopressin, angiotensin type 1, luteinizing hormone/human chorionic gonadotropin, serotonin, and glucagon. Aberrant receptors have been identified in up to 50% of patients with unilateral adenomas associated with hypercortisolism, with higher prevalence in those patients with mild Cushing's syndrome and SH. A recent study showed that GIP receptor expression in adenomas is driven by monoallelic overexpression of *GIPR*, because of alterations of *GIPR* regulatory regions and chromosome rearrangements.[31]

Recent advances on the pathogenesis of BMAH have been made after identification of germline mutation of *ARMC5* in about 30% of apparently sporadic cases, suggesting that hypercortisolism was related to increased tumor proliferation rather than altered steroidogenesis.[32–35] Interestingly, despite that the prevalence of SH is higher in patients with bilateral lesions versus unilateral adenomas, the prevalence of associated comorbidities is not different between these 2 conditions.[36] Therefore, hypercortisolism in bilateral tumors might be less severe or have a slower progression.

Recent advances have also been made in understanding the genetic background of unilateral adrenal adenomas. Unlike clinically manifest Cushing's syndrome, the role of somatic *PRKACA* mutations seems to be irrelevant in SH (4% of cases).[37] Whole-exome sequencing revealed a high prevalence of mutations of *CTNNB1* in patients with SH, which was not different from that of nonsecreting tumors.[38] The differential expression of genes involved in Ca^{++}-signaling pathway could discriminate tumors associated with overt Cushing's syndrome from those associated with mild hypercortisolism, including SH, providing novel pathogenetic insights that should be investigated in targeted molecular studies.[38]

TREATMENT OF SUBCLINICAL HYPERCORTISOLISM

The ESE guidelines suggest that adrenalectomy may be performed in patients with unilateral adenomas with lack of suppression to DST (cortisol >5 μg/dL) and at least 2 comorbidities potentially related to hypercortisolism. However, no agreement has been reached for surgical indication in the remaining cases, and a personalized approach has been suggested.[1] Overall, the quality of evidence supporting adrenalectomy in SH was very low. Indeed, studies investigating the surgical outcomes are limited by the nonrandomized and retrospective design, patients' selection, and different criteria to define SH. Nonetheless, a recent meta-analysis has shown an over-all improvement of cardiovascular risk factors, such as hypertension and diabetes mellitus, in surgically treated patients versus those undergoing conservative manage-ment.[39] To date, only one randomized controlled trial (RCT) has been performed, high-lighting normalization or improvement of diabetes and hypertension in 63% and 67% of the patients, respectively, in patients undergoing surgery.[40] However, the improve-ment was significant only for hypertension.

The long-term retrospective data on the natural history of SH provide insights regarding what patients are at risk of developing cardiovascular diseases. Sub-jects with previous cardiovascular events, hypertension, and increasing cortisol levels after 1-mg DST over time showed a higher incidence of cardiovascular diseases.[4] Moreover, the higher the cortisol after 1-mg DST, the higher the mortality of patients with SH.[4,6] Altogether, those studies highlighted that SH should be considered a cardiovascular risk factor.[4–6] Further targeted RCTs are needed to investigate the benefits of surgery in SH patients with a high cardiovascular risk.

Unilateral adrenalectomy has been proposed for patients with BMAH associated with SH to avoid life-long adrenal insufficiency induced by bilateral adrenalectomy. However, when unilateral approach is preferred, difficulties come from the lateraliza-tion of the source of cortisol hypersecretion. To this scope, adrenal scintigraphy with radiolabeled norcholesterol has been proposed as a promising technique.[41] However, the scarce availability of radiotracers has limited its applications. Adrenal vein sam-pling has also been considered a useful alternative,[42] even though this technique has not gained popularity so far because of the well-known technical difficulties of the catheterization of the right adrenal vein. The removal of the adrenal gland harboring larger nodules is considered the preferred option.[43]

Adrenal steroidogenesis inhibitors, such as ketoconazole, metyrapone, and less frequently etomidate, have been used for the treatment of overt hypercortisolism.[44] To date, evidence supporting the use of medical treatment of improvement of cardio-vascular and metabolic outcomes in patients with SH is missing. Nevertheless, Debono and colleagues[45] recently published the results of a pilot study showing data on the efficacy of metyrapone in patients with SH. Treatment with metyrapone 500 mg at 18:00 hours and 250 mg at 22:00 hours induced a restoration of circadian rhythm of cortisol and a decrease of the cardiovascular risk marker interleukin-6. The study included a small number of patients, requiring confirmation by larger studies.

Novel steroidogenesis inhibitors are currently being tested.[44] Osilodrostat (LCI699) is a potent and selective inhibitor of CYP11B2 and CYP11B1. Considering the double ac-tion of this compound, it may be a promising treatment in patients with aldosterone and cortisol cosecretion. The glucocorticoid receptor antagonism mifepristone has been used in patients with overt Cushing's syndrome and hyperglycemia and is currently un-der evaluation in patients with SH (ClinicalTrials.gov identifier: NCT01990560).

SUMMARY

A unique definition for the diagnosis of SH, as proposed by the current guidelines, is a step forward in the management of patients with adrenal incidentalomas. Metabolo-mic profiling by mass spectrometry is a promising tool for a more precise diagnosis as well as classification and management of SH. Finally, the advances regarding the pathogenesis of SH is opening new avenues for drug development in SH. Future studies are needed to understand the effects of novel pharmacologic compounds approved for overt Cushing's syndrome in patients with SH.

REFERENCES

1. Fassnacht M, Arlt W, Bancos I, et al. Management of adrenal incidentalomas: European Society of Endocrinology Clinical Practice Guideline in collaboration with the European Network for the Study of Adrenal Tumors. Eur J Endocrinol 2016; 175(2):G1–34.
2. Chiodini I, Albani A, Ambrogio AG, et al. Six controversial issues on subclinical Cushing's syndrome. Endocrine 2017;56(2):262–6.
3. Chiodini I. Diagnosis and treatment of subclinical hypercortisolism. J Clin Endocrinol Metab 2011;96(5):1223–36.
4. Di Dalmazi G, Vicennati V, Garelli S, et al. Cardiovascular events and mortality in patients with adrenal incidentalomas that are either non-secreting or associated with intermediate phenotype or subclinical Cushing's syndrome: a 15-year retrospective study. Lancet Diabetes Endocrinol 2014;2:396–405.
5. Morelli V, Reimondo G, Giordano R, et al. Long-term follow-up in adrenal incidentalomas: an Italian multicenter study. J Clin Endocrinol Metab 2014;99:827–34.
6. Debono M, Bradburn M, Bull M, et al. Cortisol as a marker for increased mortality in patients with incidental adrenocortical adenomas. J Clin Endocrinol Metab 2014;99:4462–70.
7. Di Dalmazi G. Update on the risks of benign adrenocortical incidentalomas. Curr Opin Endocrinol Diabetes Obes 2017;24(3):193–9.
8. Chiodini I, Morelli V. Subclinical hypercortisolism: how to deal with it? Front Horm Res 2016;46:28–38.
9. Yener S, Demir L, Demirpence M, et al. Interference in ACTH immunoassay negatively impacts the management of subclinical hypercortisolism. Endocrine 2017; 56(2):308–16.
10. Ceccato F, Antonelli G, Frigo AC, et al. First-line screening tests for Cushing's syndrome in patients with adrenal incidentaloma: the role of urinary free cortisol measured by LC-MS/MS. J Endocrinol Invest 2017;40(7):753–60.
11. Sakai Y, Yanase T, Hara T, et al. Mechanism of abnormal production of adrenal androgens in patients with adrenocortical adenomas and carcinomas. J Clin Endocrinol Metab 1994;78(1):36–40.
12. Yener S, Yilmaz H, Demir T, et al. DHEAS for the prediction of subclinical Cushing's syndrome: perplexing or advantageous? Endocrine 2015;48(2):669–76.
13. Dennedy MC, Annamalai AK, Prankerd Smith O, et al. Low DHEAS: a sensitive and specific test for detection of subclinical hypercortisolism in adrenal incidentalomas. J Clin Endocrinol Metab 2017;102(3):786–92.
14. Fanelli F, Belluomo I, Di Lallo VD, et al. Serum steroid profiling by isotopic dilution-liquid chromatography-mass spectrometry: comparison with current immunoassays and reference intervals in healthy adults. Steroids 2011; 76(3):244–53.
15. Masserini B, Morelli V, Bergamaschi S, et al. The limited role of midnight salivary cortisol levels in the diagnosis of subclinical hypercortisolism in patients with adrenal incidentaloma. Eur J Endocrinol 2009;160(1):87–92.
16. Nunes M-L, Vattaut S, Corcuff J-B, et al. Late-night salivary cortisol for diagnosis of overt and subclinical Cushing's syndrome in hospitalized and ambulatory patients. J Clin Endocrinol Metab 2009;94(2):456–62.
17. Palmieri S, Morelli V, Polledri E, et al. The role of salivary cortisol measured by liquid chromatography-tandem mass spectrometry in the diagnosis of subclinical hypercortisolism. Eur J Endocrinol 2013;168(3):289–96.

18. Ceccato F, Barbot M, Albiger N, et al. Daily salivary cortisol and cortisone rhythm in patients with adrenal incidentaloma. Endocrine 2017;1–10. https://doi.org/10.1007/s12020-017-1421-3.

19. Vincent JM, Morrison ID, Armstrong P, et al. The size of normal adrenal glands on computed tomography. Clin Radiol 1994;49(7):453–5.

20. Schneller J, Reiser M, Beuschlein F, et al. Linear and volumetric evaluation of the adrenal gland–MDCT-based measurements of the adrenals. Acad Radiol 2014;21(11):1465–74.

21. Park SY, Park BK, Park JJ, et al. Differentiation of adrenal hyperplasia from adenoma by use of CT densitometry and percentage washout. Am J Roentgenol 2016;206(1):106–12.

22. Mosconi C, Vicennati V, Papadopoulos D, et al. Can imaging predict subclinical cortisol secretion in patients with adrenal adenomas? A CT predictive score. Am J Roentgenol 2017;209(1):122–9.

23. Olsen H, Nordenström E, Bergenfelz A, et al. Subclinical hypercortisolism and CT appearance in adrenal incidentalomas: a multicenter study from Southern Sweden. Endocrine 2012;42(1):164–73.

24. Chambre C, McMurray E, Baudry C, et al. The 10 Hounsfield units unenhanced computed tomography attenuation threshold does not apply to cortisol secreting adrenocortical adenomas. Eur J Endocrinol 2015;173:325–32.

25. Di Dalmazi G, Fanelli F, Mezzullo M, et al. Steroid profiling by LC-MS/MS in nonsecreting and subclinical cortisol-secreting adrenocortical adenomas. J Clin Endocrinol Metab 2015;100(9):3529–38.

26. Kotłowska A, Puzyn T, Sworczak K, et al. Metabolomic biomarkers in urine of Cushing's syndrome patients. Int J Mol Sci 2017;18(2):294.

27. Arlt W, Lang K, Sitch AJ, et al. Steroid metabolome analysis reveals prevalent glucocorticoid excess in primary aldosteronism. JCI Insight 2017;2(8) [pii:93136].

28. Eisenhofer G, Masjkur J, Peitzsch M, et al. Plasma steroid metabolome for diagnosis and subtyping patients with Cushing syndrome. Clin Chem 2017. https://doi.org/10.1373/clinchem.2017.282582.

29. Di Dalmazi G, Quinkler M, Deutschbein T, et al. Cortisol-related metabolic alterations assessed by mass spectrometry assay in patients with Cushing's syndrome. Eur J Endocrinol 2017;177(2):227–37.

30. El Ghorayeb N, Bourdeau I, Lacroix A. Multiple aberrant hormone receptors in Cushing's syndrome. Eur J Endocrinol 2015;173(4):M45–60.

31. Lecoq A-L, Stratakis CA, Viengchareun S, et al. Adrenal GIPR expression and chromosome 19q13 microduplications in GIP-dependent Cushing's syndrome. JCI Insight 2017;2(18) [pii:92184].

32. Assié G, Libé R, Espiard S, et al. ARMC5 mutations in macronodular adrenal hyperplasia with Cushing's syndrome. N Engl J Med 2013;369(22):2105–14.

33. Faucz FR, Zilbermint M, Lodish MB, et al. Macronodular adrenal hyperplasia due to mutations in an armadillo repeat containing 5 (ARMC5) gene: a clinical and genetic investigation. J Clin Endocrinol Metab 2014;99(6):E1113–9.

34. Espiard S, Drougat L, Libé R, et al. ARMC5 mutations in a large cohort of primary macronodular adrenal hyperplasia: clinical and functional consequences. J Clin Endocrinol Metab 2015;100(6):E926–35.

35. Albiger NM, Regazzo D, Rubin B, et al. A multicenter experience on the prevalence of ARMC5 mutations in patients with primary bilateral macronodular adrenal hyperplasia: from genetic characterization to clinical phenotype. Endocrine 2017;55(3):959–68.

36. Paschou SA, Kandaraki E, Dimitropoulou F, et al. Subclinical Cushing's syndrome in patients with bilateral compared to unilateral adrenal incidentalomas: a systematic review and meta-analysis. Endocrine 2016;51(2):225–35.
37. Di Dalmazi G, Beuschlein F. PRKACA mutations in adrenal adenomas: genotype/phenotype correlations. Horm Metab Res 2017;49(4):301–6.
38. Ronchi CL, Di Dalmazi G, Faillot S, et al. Genetic landscape of sporadic unilateral adrenocortical adenomas without PRKACA p.Leu206Arg mutation. J Clin Endocrinol Metab 2016;101(9):3526–38.
39. Bancos I, Alahdab F, Crowley RK, et al. Improvement of cardiovascular risk factors after adrenalectomy in patients with adrenal tumors and subclinical Cushing's syndrome: a systematic review and meta-analysis. Eur J Endocrinol 2016; 175(6):R283–95.
40. Toniato A, Merante-Boschin I, Opocher G, et al. Surgical versus conservative management for subclinical Cushing syndrome in adrenal incidentalomas: a prospective randomized study. Ann Surg 2009;249(3):388–91.
41. Papierska L, Ćwikła J, Rabijewski M, et al. Adrenal 131I-6β-iodomethylnorcholesterol scintigraphy in choosing the side for adrenalectomy in bilateral adrenal tumors with subclinical hypercortisolemia. Abdom Imaging 2015;40(7):2453–60.
42. Lee S, Ha MS, Eom YS, et al. Role of unilateral aderenalectomy in ACTH-independent macronodular adrenal hyperplasia. World J Surg 2009;33(1): 157–8 [author reply: 159].
43. Albiger NM, Ceccato F, Zilio M, et al. An analysis of different therapeutic options in patients with Cushing's syndrome due to bilateral macronodular adrenal hyperplasia: a single-centre experience. Clin Endocrinol (Oxf) 2015;82(6):808–15.
44. Fleseriu M, Castinetti F. Updates on the role of adrenal steroidogenesis inhibitors in Cushing's syndrome: a focus on novel therapies. Pituitary 2016;19(6):643–53.
45. Debono M, Harrison RF, Chadarevian R, et al. Resetting the abnormal circadian cortisol rhythm in adrenal incidentaloma patients with mild autonomous cortisol secretion. J Clin Endocrinol Metab 2017;102(9):3461–9.

Adrenal Surgery for Cushing's Syndrome
An Update

Guido Di Dalmazi, MD[a], Martin Reincke, MD[b],*

KEYWORDS

- Cushing's • Surgery • Adrenalectomy • Hypercortisolism • Bilateral adrenalectomy
- Adrenal

KEY POINTS

- The laparoscopic approach is superior to all other available techniques for surgical removal of adrenal glands except for tumors with radiologic evidence of malignancy or signs of local invasion.
- Unilateral adrenalectomy is the gold standard for treatment of Cushing's syndrome because of unilateral adenomas.
- Bilateral adrenalectomy should be restricted to well-selected patients who are poorly responsive to standard treatments, in the emergency setting, or in standard clinical care.
- Unilateral adrenalectomy may be considered a potential treatment option in patients with bilateral macronodular adrenal hyperplasia.

INTRODUCTION

The recent discoveries on the genetic and molecular background of hypercortisolism have radically improved the knowledge of the pathophysiology of Cushing's syndrome and promoted the research for promising pharmacologic compounds that might change treatment strategies in the coming years. Moreover, the increasing popularity of disease-specific registries across and within Europe led to the creation of large retrospective databases with reliable data even on a rare condition like Cushing's syndrome. Therefore, the long-term data on the natural history of Cushing's syndrome allowed a critical revision of the clinical practice on the management of this condition.

Disclosure Statement: The authors have nothing to disclose.
[a] Division of Endocrinology, Department of Medical and Surgical Sciences, Alma Mater Studiorum University of Bologna, S. Orsola-Malpighi Hospital, Via Massarenti 9, Bologna 40138, Italy; [b] Department of Medicine IV, Klinikum der Universität, Ludwig-Maximilians-Universität München, Ziemssenstraße 1, München 80336, Germany
* Corresponding author.
E-mail address: martin.reincke@med.uni-muenchen.de

Endocrinol Metab Clin N Am 47 (2018) 385–394
https://doi.org/10.1016/j.ecl.2018.01.004
0889-8529/18/© 2018 Elsevier Inc. All rights reserved.

This review summarizes the current role of adrenalectomy as a treatment option for different subtypes of Cushing's syndrome.

HISTORY AND EVOLUTION OF ADRENALECTOMY TECHNIQUES

Since the first report published in 1890 by Thornton,[1] the number of surgical interventions for removal of adrenal glands has increased at the same pace with the knowledge of the importance of adrenal hormones and their alterations. Open adrenalectomy (O-Adx) has been the treatment of choice for adrenal tumors until the early 1990s, when Gagner and colleagues[2] published a pioneering study introducing the laparoscopic adrenalectomy (L-Adx). The increasing skill of surgeons and the improvement of surgical devices over time allowed this technique to become the gold standard for the treatment of adrenal tumors, replacing O-Adx in most cases. L-Adx has shown several advantages over O-Adx in length of hospital stay, postoperative morbidity, and time of recovery to normal daily life.[3] A very recent study showed that L-Adx may be a safe option also in well-selected elderly patients.[4] During the last few years, L-Adx has evolved to more technically challenging approaches, such as single-incision minimally invasive and robot-assisted procedures, which have been claimed to reduce postoperative pain and shorten hospital stay, with respect to traditional multiport L-Adx (**Box 1**).[5–7] However, in a recent comprehensive review, Nomine-Criqui and colleagues[8] failed to prove the superiority of robot-assisted L-Adx over L-Adx in morbidities and mortalities. In addition, one of the most recent evolutions of this technique, single-port robot-assisted L-Adx, did not show difference in postoperative morbidity, when compared with L-Adx.[9] The higher cost of robot-assisted L-Adx, which doubles that of L-Adx, still represents the main limitation to a widespread use of this technique.[7]

The improvement of L-Adx over the last 25 years has recently led to the proposal that some patients may undergo adrenalectomy as outpatients.[10] Data on fast-track L-Adx have been reported in several case series, showing favorable outcomes in terms of postoperative morbidity and patient's recovery to normal life.[11–13] Fast-track L-Adx should however be restricted to well-selected cases, such as young patients without pheochromocytoma, with tumors less than 6 cm, and predicted favorable surgical outcome.[14]

LAPAROSCOPIC VERSUS OPEN ADRENALECTOMY

In the absence of randomized controlled trials, the main data on the comparison of postoperative outcomes of L-Adx and O-Adx come from retrospective evidence in large-scale studies, which highlighted a higher rate of postoperative complications in open versus laparoscopic procedures. In their analysis of a large cohort of patients

---

Box 1
Laparoscopic adrenalectomy modalities

- Anterior laparoscopic adrenalectomy
- Posterior (retroperitoneal) adrenalectomy
- Single-port minimally invasive adrenalectomy
- Robot-assisted laparoscopic adrenalectomy
- Fast-track (outpatient) laparoscopic adrenalectomy

undergoing either L-Adx or O-Adx, Elfenbein and colleagues[15] showed a lower rate of 30-day postoperative morbidity after the former (6.4% vs 18.8%, P<.001). Eichhorn-Wharry and colleagues[16] highlighted that patients undergoing O-Adx had higher mortality and increased risk of developing severe complications requiring recovery in the intensive care unit than those treated with L-Adx, independently of other risk factors. Barreca and colleagues[17] showed that patients undergoing L-Adx had a faster recovery to normal daily-life activity than those treated by O-Adx. Finally, L-Adx has been considered more cost-effective than O-Adx,[18] even though the calculation of tangible and intangible costs of adrenalectomy may vary widely, according to the National Health System and insurance policies of different countries.

Therefore, all the evidence claims the superiority of L-Adx versus O-Adx, even with the limitations related to the retrospective design of the studies. Despite the substantial number of patients included in those reports, no subgroup analysis has been performed to investigate the potential impact of the diverse types of hormonal excess on postoperative morbidity and mortality. Considering the clinical picture of patients with Cushing's syndrome (ie, hypercoagulable state, infections, and delayed wound healing, among others), it is expected that a more extensive surgical procedure might lead to a higher rate of postoperative morbidity. Unfortunately, only a few small-scale studies have addressed this issue, and none of them highlighted differences in postoperative complications between L-Adx and O-Adx in patients with Cushing's syndrome.[19–21] A recent study compared 3 different surgical approaches in patients undergoing bilateral adrenalectomy (Bil-Adx) for Cushing's syndrome (transabdominal L-Adx, simultaneous posterior retroperitoneoscopic L-Adx, and robot-assisted L-Adx), failing to show superiority of one of those techniques in reducing postoperative morbidity.[22] Similarly, a recent study focused on long-term outcomes of Bil-Adx showed comparable morbidities and mortalities in ectopic Cushing's syndrome, Cushing's disease, and bilateral macronodular hyperplasia (BMAH).[23]

O-Adx is considered the preferred choice in specific conditions, such as contraindication to laparoscopy (eg, severe coagulopathies, cardiac disease, or glaucoma), and in the presence of large adrenal tumors, with a cutoff of 5 to 6 cm considered reasonable by several investigators.[24] Indeed, a tumor size greater than 5 cm has been identified as a predictive factor for conversion from laparoscopic to open surgery (up to 14% of the cases).[24] A recent nationwide retrospective analysis of 659 adrenalectomies performed in Sweden showed that the conversion rate to O-Adx was 5.6%, with tumor size and presence of malignant tumors as the most important predictive factors.[25] Surprisingly, patients with hypercortisolism were not affected by a higher rate of postoperative infections, wound healing, and bleeding, even though the study was not focused on addressing this specific issue.[25] Independently of the size of the mass, O-Adx has been suggested to be a better choice over L-Adx for the treatment of adrenocortical carcinoma, because of the possibility of obtaining a more complete resection and a lower risk of local recurrence and peritoneal spread.[26]

UNILATERAL ADRENALECTOMY FOR CORTISOL-PRODUCING ADENOMA

Unilateral adrenalectomy (Uni-Adx) is the gold standard for the definitive treatment of Cushing's syndrome because of adrenocortical adenoma. Very recent studies have supported the hypothesis of the monoclonal origin of those tumors, by showing that somatic mutations of *PRKACA*, *GNAS*, and *CTNNB1* are the most common alterations in greater than 50% of the cases.[27] Therefore, Uni-Adx may be curative in virtually all patients.

> **Box 2**
> **Key features of unilateral adrenalectomy for cortisol-producing adenoma with Cushing's syndrome**
>
> • Rate of postoperative adrenal insufficiency: 100%
>
> • Mean time to recovery of the hypothalamus-pituitary-adrenal axis: 18 to 30 months
>
> • Recommended initial dose of hydrocortisone for treatment of postsurgical adrenal insufficiency: 12 to 15 mg/m^2/d
>
> • Most frequent adverse events after surgery: steroid withdrawal syndrome (arthralgia, whole body pain, fatigue, nausea, appetite loss, disturbed night-day rhythm and depression)

Following Uni-Adx, the obvious consequence is the onset of adrenal insufficiency due to contralateral adrenal atrophy, because of prolonged adrenocorticotropic hormone (ACTH) suppression (**Box 2**). The prevalence of recovery and the timing of restoring a normal adrenal function have been recently reviewed.[28] Among studies published during the last 30 years, the prevalence of postoperative adrenal insufficiency was 100% in all but one study, whereas recovery of the hypothalamus-pituitary-adrenal (HPA) axis was reported in 92% of patients, with a mean time of 18 months. Recovery of eucortisolism was documented by normal stimulated cortisol values after short Synacthen testing in 20% of the cases, whereas it was not defined in 73% of cases, strongly limiting the interpretation of the results about time of recovery. In a recent report, patients with unilateral adenomas showed a recovery to a normal HPA axis function in a mean time of 2.5 years (interquartile range [IQR] 1.6–5.4 years), which was slower than that of patients with Cushing's disease (1.4 years, IQR 0.9–3.4) and ectopic Cushing's syndrome (0.6 years, IQR 0.03–1.1) ($P = .002$).[29]

Unfortunately, all the studies failed to identify the potential preoperative factors that may predict the time of recovery the HPA axis function. The heterogeneity of the study designs, the lack of a standardized definition of HPA axis recovery, and the different schemes of glucocorticoid replacement therapy are among the main reasons for this unanswered question. Indeed, perioperative and postoperative management of patients undergoing Uni-Adx has not been standardized yet, and the management of adrenal insufficiency may be highly heterogenous among different centers.[30] The recommended dose of hydrocortisone to treat postsurgical adrenal insufficiency is 12 to 15 mg/m^2/d, because it has been validated on a clinical basis.[31] Patients undergoing Uni-Adx may suffer from a steroid withdrawal syndrome characterized by arthralgia, whole body pain, fatigue, nausea, appetite loss, disturbed night-day rhythm, and depression, among other symptoms. It is commonly treated with larger doses of hydrocortisone, even though no studies have proven the efficacy of this strategy. The cause of steroid withdrawal syndrome is still poorly understood.[32]

BILATERAL ADRENALECTOMY IN ADRENOCORTICOTROPIC HORMONE–DEPENDENT CUSHING'S SYNDROME

Bil-Adx has been traditionally considered a safe option to achieve a radical and fast treatment of hypercortisolism in well-selected patients with ACTH-dependent Cushing's syndrome (ADCS). Data on the outcomes of Bil-Adx are available from retrospective studies, involving small cohorts of highly heterogeneous patients, with a variable length of follow-up. Moreover, Bil-Adx is usually performed as the last treatment option, when all other therapeutic options have failed to control hypercortisolism. In a meta-analysis of 23 studies, 30-day morbidity and mortality were acceptable (18%

Box 3
Key facts of bilateral adrenalectomy

- Surgical morbidity: 18%
- Surgical mortality: 3%
- Clinical remission of Cushing's syndrome: greater than 95%
- Clinically significant adrenal remnants after Bil-Adx less than 5%
- Improved health-related quality of life in 82% to 89%
- Need for lifelong glucocorticoid and mineralocorticoid replacement therapy
- Risk of adrenal crisis: 4.1 to 9.1 per 100 patient-years
- Risk of corticotroph tumor progression (Nelson syndrome): median incidence 21%

---

and 3%, respectively).[33] Several studies proved that Bil-Adx for ADCS led to complete biochemical remission in most of the patients (reviewed in Ref.[33]; **Box 3**). The presence of adrenal remnants after Bil-Adx has been reported in up to 27% of the patients, with a rate of clinically significant recurrence of disease in a negligible number of patients (<5%).[34] Clinical disease remission of typical phenotypic stigmata was reported in most of the patients after Bil-Adx.[33] Moreover, long-term studies showed improvement of health-related quality of life (QOL) after Bil-Adx,[33] although QOL remains impaired compared with a healthy population.[23] Finally, several studies showed that mortality after Bil-Adx in ADCS was recorded in a median of 17% of the patients.[33] As expected, patients suffering from ectopic Cushing's syndrome had the lowest survival rate.[23]

The downside of Bil-Adx includes the obvious necessity for life-long steroid replacement therapy (glucocorticoid and mineralocorticoid) and the risk of developing Nelson syndrome (NS). A reliable analysis of the prevalence of NS after Bil-Adx is impaired by the heterogeneity of the studies, the small number of patients in most of the studies, the different follow-up protocols, and the variable definition of NS. Therefore, NS has been reported in a wide range of patients after surgery (0%–50% of the cases, median 21%). Among all potential predictive factors for development of NS, young age and baseline ACTH levels have been identified as the most reliable.[33]

Considering all the mentioned data, the usefulness of Bil-Adx has been recently reconsidered and restricted to nonresponders to conventional treatments for hypercortisolism. Bil-Adx may also be considered an additional strategy in an emergency setting, in patients with ectopic Cushing's syndrome and severe clinical picture, after failure of medical therapy.[34]

BILATERAL MACRONODULAR HYPERPLASIA: UNILATERAL OR BILATERAL ADRENALECTOMY?

Bil-Adx has been considered the treatment of choice to achieve cure of hypercortisolism in patients with BMAH.[35] However, in patients with mild hypercortisolism, Uni-Adx has been proposed as a feasible and safe alternative to Bil-Adx.[36] A total of 12 studies (7 case reports and 5 case series with ≥4 patients) reported data on the outcome of 58 patients undergoing Uni-Adx (**Table 1**). Remission of hypercortisolism was documented in most of the patients, during a follow-up range of 7 to 137 months since adrenalectomy. Studies reporting data on a reliable number of patients[37–40] showed a variable prevalence of remission ranging from 25%[38] up to 92%.[40]

Table 1
Studies showing the outcomes of patients with bilateral macronodular adrenal hyperplasia treated with unilateral adrenalectomy

Author, Year (Ref.)	No. of Patients	Outcome	Follow-up (mo)	Adrenal Insufficiency	HPA Axis Recovery
Lacroix et al,[50] 1997	1	Remission	36	Yes	Yes
N'Diaye et al,[51] 1999	1	Remission	12	Yes	Yes
Lamas et al,[52] 2002	4	Remission	74 (30–137)	2/4	Yes
Ogura et al,[53] 2003	1	Remission	10	No	—
Sato et al,[54] 2006	1	Remission	8	Yes	Yes
Vezzosi et al,[55] 2007	1	Remission	7	Yes	Yes
Iacobone et al,[39] 2008	7	Remission[6] Persistence[1]	50 (27–42) —	2/6 —	Yes —
Mazzuco et al,[56] 2009	1	Remission	84	No	—
Kobayashi et al,[57] 2012	1	Recurrence	60	No	—
Xu et al,[40] 2013	13 BMAH	Remission[12] Persistence[1]	69 (23–120) —	2/12 —	Yes —
	12 PPNAD	Remission[12] Recurrence[1]	47 (16–113)	1/12	Yes
Debillon et al,[37] 2015	15	Remission[13] Recurrence[2]	60 (39–105)	5/13 1/2	3/5 yes (+2/5 "latent" adrenal insufficiency)
Albiger et al,[38] 2015	12	Remission[3] Recurrence[8] Persistence[1]	106 (80–135) 54 (12–180) —	2/3 Not reported —	Yes Not reported —

Abbreviation: PPNAD, primary pigmented nodular adrenocortical disease.

Recurrence was documented in 2 case series in 2 of 15[37] and in 1 of 12[38] patients, respectively. Persistence of hypercortisolism, requiring contralateral adrenalectomy, has been described in 3 studies, in 1 of 7,[41] in 1 of 13,[42] and 1 of 12 patients,[38] respectively. A few additional studies reported the results of Uni-Adx in patients with BMAH. However, no data on remission or recurrence of Cushing's syndrome were clearly reported.[41,42] Although the most recent guidelines on the treatment of Cushing's syndrome recommend Bil-Adx in BMAH, with low quality of evidence, no clear direction is given on Uni-Adx.[43] Indeed, the available data on the outcomes of Uni-Adx rely on small case series with a high heterogeneity in the selection of the patients.

An additional source of uncertainty is the selection of the adrenal gland that should be removed. Adrenal scintigraphy has been evaluated as a potential tool to identify the hypersecreting tumor in BMAH,[44] even though the low imaging resolution and the scarce availability of radiotracers have strongly limited the use of this technique. Adrenal vein sampling has been proposed as an alternative strategy,[45] however, with the well-known limitations related to the presence of anatomic variants that make catheterization of the right adrenal vein challenging. In the absence of straightforward evidence, the removal of the larger tumor has been advocated as a reliable procedure to achieve normalization of hypercortisolism. Recent data have shown that mutations of *ARMC5*, which are found in 30% of the patients,[46–49] may lead to hypercortisolism due to an increased adrenal mass rather than enhanced steroidogenic ability.[46]

Therefore, the choice of removing the bigger adrenal tumor in BMAH seems to be supported by pathogenetic and clinical evidence. Indeed, a recent study proved that patients with the longest recurrence-free time were those with marked asymmetry of the tumors who underwent removal of the bigger adrenal.[38]

Two case series with more than 10 patients showed a prevalence of postoperative adrenal insufficiency after Uni-Adx in BMAH of 16%[40] and 40%,[37] followed by complete recovery of a normal HPA axis function. Whether the absence of adrenal insufficiency after Uni-Adx may be a predictor of early recurrence has not been investigated.

SUMMARY

Laparoscopic adrenal surgery for Cushing's syndrome is a safe and effective option for treatment of several pathologic conditions associated with Cushing's syndrome, in primis unilateral adrenocortical adenomas. Despite the continuous evolution of the surgical technique, L-Adx has been shown to perform better than any other procedure available up to now, when efficacy and cost-effectiveness are taken into account. The increased expertise of surgeons and the very low rate of complications have paved the way to the application for fast-track surgery, whose potential should be investigated also in patients with hypercortisolism.

The progress on the pathogenetic molecular mechanisms underlying Cushing's syndrome in BMAH is boosting the research on targeted pharmacologic compounds, progressively restricting the indication for Bil-Adx to patients who do not respond to conventional treatments, in the emergency setting, as well as in routine clinical practice. However, prospective studies are needed to understand the efficacy of cortisol-lowering medical treatments in disease control in a long-term setting, and their superiority over Bil-Adx. Finally, targeted studies in larger cohorts of patients are needed to identify the predictive factors of recurrence/persistence of hypercortisolism after Uni-Adx in BMAH, in order to standardize the surgical approach, trying to avoid life-long steroid replacement therapy.

REFERENCES

1. Thorton JK. Abdominal nephrectomy for large sarcoma of the left suprarenal capsule. Clin Soc Trans (London) 1890;23:150–3.
2. Gagner M, Lacroix A, Bolté E. Laparoscopic adrenalectomy in Cushing's syndrome and pheochromocytoma. N Engl J Med 1992;327:1033.
3. Shen WT, Sturgeon C, Duh QY. From incidentaloma to adrenocortical carcinoma: the surgical management of adrenal tumors. J Surg Oncol 2005;89:186–92.
4. Weinandt M, Gaujoux S, Khayat A, et al. Laparoscopic adrenalectomy in elderly patients. Surg Laparosc Endosc Percutan Tech 2017;27(6):e132–5.
5. Wang L, Wu Z, Li M, et al. Laparoendoscopic single-site adrenalectomy versus conventional laparoscopic surgery: a systematic review and meta-analysis of observational studies. J Endourol 2013;27:743–50.
6. Vidal Ó, Astudillo E, Valentini M, et al. Single-incision transperitoneal laparoscopic left adrenalectomy. World J Surg 2012;36:1395–9.
7. Taskin HE, Arslan NC, Aliyev S, et al. Robotic endocrine surgery: state of the art. World J Surg 2013;37:2731–9.
8. Nomine-Criqui C, Germain A, Ayav A, et al. Robot-assisted adrenalectomy: indications and drawbacks. Updates Surg 2017;69:127–33.
9. Arghami A, Dy BM, Bingener J, et al. Single-port robotic-assisted adrenalectomy: feasibility, safety, and cost-effectiveness. JSLS 2015;19. e2014.00218.

10. Nehs MA, Ruan DT. Minimally invasive adrenal surgery: an update. Curr Opin Endocrinol Diabetes Obes 2011;18:193–7.

11. Rayan SS, Hodin RA. Short-stay laparoscopic adrenalectomy. Surg Endosc 2000; 14:568–72.

12. Edwin B, Raeder I, Trondsen E, et al. Outpatient laparoscopic adrenalectomy in patients with Conn's syndrome. Surg Endosc 2001;15:589–91.

13. Gill IS, Hobart MG, Schweizer D, et al. Outpatient adrenalectomy. J Urol 2000; 163:717–20.

14. Mohammad WM, Frost I, Moonje V. Outpatient laparoscopic adrenalectomy: a Canadian experience. Surg Laparosc Endosc Percutan Tech 2009;19:336–7.

15. Elfenbein DM, Scarborough JE, Speicher PJ, et al. Comparison of laparoscopic versus open adrenalectomy: results from American College of Surgeons-National Surgery Quality Improvement Project. J Surg Res 2013;184:216–20.

16. Eichhorn-Wharry LI, Talpos GB, Rubinfeld I. Laparoscopic versus open adrenalectomy: another look at outcome using the Clavien classification system. Surgery 2012;152:1090–5.

17. Barreca M, Presenti L, Renzi C, et al. Expectations and outcomes when moving from open to laparoscopic adrenalectomy: multivariate analysis. World J Surg 2003;27:223–8.

18. Hobart MG, Gill IS, Schweizer D, et al. Financial analysis of needlescopic versus open adrenalectomy. J Urol 1999;162:1264–7.

19. Acosta E, Pantoja JP, Gamino R, et al. Laparoscopic versus open adrenalectomy in Cushing's syndrome and disease. Surgery 1999;126:1111–6.

20. Porpiglia F, Fiori C, Bovio S, et al. Bilateral adrenalectomy for Cushing's syndrome: a comparison between laparoscopy and open surgery. J Endocrinol Invest 2004;27:654–8.

21. Guazzoni G, Montorsi F, Bocciardi A, et al. Transperitoneal laparoscopic versus open adrenalectomy for benign hyperfunctioning adrenal tumors: a comparative study. J Urol 1995;153:1597–600.

22. Raffaelli M, Brunaud L, De Crea C, et al. Synchronous bilateral adrenalectomy for Cushing's syndrome: laparoscopic versus posterior retroperitoneoscopic versus robotic approach. World J Surg 2014;38:709–15.

23. Oßwald A, Plomer E, Dimopoulou C, et al. Favorable long-term outcomes of bilateral adrenalectomy in Cushing's disease. Eur J Endocrinol 2014;171:209–15.

24. Taffurelli G, Ricci C, Casadei R, et al. Open adrenalectomy in the era of laparoscopic surgery: a review. Updates Surg 2017;69:135–43.

25. Thompson LH, Nordenström E, Almquist M, et al. Risk factors for complications after adrenalectomy: results from a comprehensive national database. Langenbecks Arch Surg 2017;402:315–22.

26. Kulke MH, Benson AB 3rd, Bergsland E, et al. Neuroendocrine tumors. J Natl Compr Canc Netw 2012;10:724–64.

27. Di Dalmazi G, Beuschlein F. PRKACA mutations in adrenal adenomas: genotype/phenotype correlations. Horm Metab Res 2017;49:301–6.

28. Di Dalmazi G, Berr CM, Fassnacht M, et al. Adrenal function after adrenalectomy for subclinical hypercortisolism and Cushing's syndrome: a systematic review of the literature. J Clin Endocrinol Metab 2014;99:2637–45.

29. Berr CM, Di Dalmazi G, Osswald A, et al. Time to recovery of adrenal function after curative surgery for Cushing's syndrome depends on etiology. J Clin Endocrinol Metab 2015;100:1300–8.

30. Murray RD, Ekman B, Uddin S, et al. Management of glucocorticoid replacement in adrenal insufficiency shows notable heterogeneity - data from the EU-AIR. Clin Endocrinol (Oxf) 2017;86:340–6.
31. Doherty GM, Nieman LK, Cutler GB Jr, et al. Time to recovery of the hypothalamic-pituitary-adrenal axis after curative resection of adrenal tumors in patients with Cushing's syndrome. Surgery 1990;108:1085–90.
32. Margolin L, Cope DK, Bakst-Sisser R, et al. The steroid withdrawal syndrome: a review of the implications, etiology, and treatments. J Pain Symptom Manage 2007;33:224–8.
33. Ritzel K, Beuschlein F, Mickisch A, et al. Clinical review: outcome of bilateral adrenalectomy in Cushing's syndrome: a systematic review. J Clin Endocrinol Metab 2013;98:3939–48.
34. Guerin C, Taieb D, Treglia G, et al. Bilateral adrenalectomy in the 21st century: when to use it for hypercortisolism? Endocr Relat Cancer 2016;23:R131–42.
35. Lacroix A, Feelders RA, Stratakis CA, et al. Cushing's syndrome. Lancet 2015; 386:913–27.
36. Lacroix A. ACTH-independent macronodular adrenal hyperplasia. Best Pract Res Clin Endocrinol Metab 2009;23:245–59.
37. Debillon E, Velayoudom-Cephise FL, Salenave S, et al. Unilateral adrenalectomy as a first-line treatment of Cushing's syndrome in patients with primary bilateral macronodular adrenal hyperplasia. J Clin Endocrinol Metab 2015;100:4417–24.
38. Albiger NM, Ceccato F, Zilio M, et al. An analysis of different therapeutic options in patients with Cushing's syndrome due to bilateral macronodular adrenal hyperplasia: a single-centre experience. Clin Endocrinol (Oxf) 2015;82:808–15.
39. Iacobone M, Albiger N, Scaroni C, et al. The role of unilateral adrenalectomy in ACTH-independent macronodular adrenal hyperplasia (AIMAH). World J Surg 2008;32:882–9.
40. Xu Y, Rui W, Qi Y, et al. The role of unilateral adrenalectomy in corticotropin-independent bilateral adrenocortical hyperplasias. World J Surg 2013;37:1626–32.
41. Li J, Yang CH. Diagnosis and treatment of adrenocorticotrophic hormone-independent macronodular adrenocortical hyperplasia: a report of 23 cases in a single center. Exp Ther Med 2015;9:507–12.
42. Zhang Y, Li H. Classification and surgical treatment for 180 cases of adrenocortical hyperplastic disease. Int J Clin Exp Med 2015;8:19311–7.
43. Nieman LK, Biller BM, Findling JW, et al. Treatment of Cushing's syndrome: an Endocrine Society clinical practice guideline. J Clin Endocrinol Metab 2015; 100:2807–31.
44. Wong KK, Komissarova M, Avram AM, et al. Adrenal cortical imaging with I-131 NP-59 SPECT-CT. Clin Nucl Med 2010;35:865–9.
45. Lee S, Ha MS, Eom YS, et al. Role of unilateral aderenalectomy in ACTH-independent macronodular adrenal hyperplasia. World J Surg 2009;33:157–8.
46. Assié G, Libé R, Espiard S, et al. ARMC5 mutations in macronodular adrenal hyperplasia with Cushing's syndrome. N Engl J Med 2013;369:2105–14.
47. Faucz FR, Zilbermint M, Lodish MB, et al. Macronodular adrenal hyperplasia due to mutations in an armadillo repeat containing 5 (ARMC5) gene: a clinical and genetic investigation. J Clin Endocrinol Metab 2014;99:E1113–9.
48. Espiard S, Drougat L, Libé R, et al. ARMC5 mutations in a large cohort of primary macronodular adrenal hyperplasia: clinical and functional consequences. J Clin Endocrinol Metab 2015;100:E926–35.
49. Albiger NM, Regazzo D, Rubin B, et al. A multicenter experience on the prevalence of ARMC5 mutations in patients with primary bilateral macronodular

adrenal hyperplasia: from genetic characterization to clinical phenotype. Endocrine 2017;55:959–68.

50. Lacroix A, Tremblay J, Rousseau G, et al. Propranolol therapy for ectopic beta-adrenergic receptors in adrenal Cushing's syndrome. N Engl J Med 1997;337: 1429–34.

51. N'Diaye N, Hamet P, Tremblay J, et al. Asynchronous development of bilateral nodular adrenal hyperplasia in gastric inhibitory polypeptide-dependent Cushing's syndrome. J Clin Endocrinol Metab 1999;84:2616–22.

52. Lamas C, Alfaro JJ, Lucas T, et al. Is unilateral adrenalectomy an alternative treatment for ACTH-independent macronodular adrenal hyperplasia?: long-term follow-up of four cases. Eur J Endocrinol 2002;146:237–40.

53. Ogura M, Kusaka I, Nagasaka S, et al. Unilateral adrenalectomy improves insulin resistance and diabetes mellitus in a patient with ACTH-independent macronodular adrenal hyperplasia. Endocr J 2003;50:715–21.

54. Sato M, Soma M, Nakayama T, et al. A case of adrenocorticotropin-independent bilateral adrenal macronodular hyperplasia (AIMAH) with primary hyperparathyroidism (PHPT). Endocr J 2006;53:111–7.

55. Vezzosi D, Cartier D, Régnier C, et al. Familial adrenocorticotropin-independent macronodular adrenal hyperplasia with aberrant serotonin and vasopressin adrenal receptors. Eur J Endocrinol 2007;156:21–31.

56. Mazzuco TL, Chaffanjon P, Martinie M, et al. Adrenal Cushing's syndrome due to bilateral macronodular adrenal hyperplasia: prediction of the efficacy of beta-blockade therapy and interest of unilateral adrenalectomy. Endocr J 2009;56: 867–77.

57. Kobayashi T, Miwa T, Kan K, et al. Usefulness and limitations of unilateral adrenalectomy for ACTH-independent macronodular adrenal hyperplasia in a patient with poor glycemic control. Intern Med 2012;51:1709–13.

Adrenocortical Carcinoma with Hypercortisolism

Soraya Puglisi, MD, Paola Perotti, BS, Anna Pia, MD, Giuseppe Reimondo, MD, PhD, Massimo Terzolo, MD*

KEYWORDS

- Adrenocortical carcinoma • Cortisol • Cushing's syndrome • Mitotane

KEY POINTS

- Adrenocortical carcinoma (ACC) is a rare cause of Cushing's syndrome.
- Prompt diagnosis and treatment are important because of its aggressive behavior. Clinical presentation of Cushing's syndrome may be atypical because of cancer-related signs.
- The biochemical hallmarks of Cushing's syndrome caused by ACC are adrenocorticotropic hormone (ACTH)-independent hypercortisolism and frequent concomitant hypersecretion of other steroids (precursors and/or androgens).
- The radiological phenotype of ACC on the computed tomography (CT) scan features its large size, high-density, intratumoral necrosis.
- Surgery is the treatment of choice and should be attempted whenever a radical resection is feasible.

INTRODUCTION

Adrenocortical carcinoma (ACC) is a rare and aggressive tumor with an annual incidence between 0.7 and 2 cases per million population. ACC is more frequently detected in women (55%–60%) and certain age groups (fourth and fifth decades); however, ACC can occur at any age.[1] ACC can affect children, with an exceedingly high incidence reported in southern Brazil because of the high prevalence of a TP53 germline mutation.[2] ACCs most frequently present as sporadic tumors, but can be encountered in the setting of hereditary tumor syndromes, such as Li Fraumeni (TP53 germline and somatic mutations), familial adenomatous polyposis coli (β-catenin somatic mutations), and Beckwith–Wiedeman (IGF-2 overexpression).[3]

Patients with ACC have an extremely poor prognosis, with an overall 5-year survival rate between 16% and 47%.[4] Prognosis is mainly influenced by completeness of surgical removal and tumor stage at diagnosis, with a 5-year stage-dependent survival of

Internal Medicine, Department of Clinical and Biological Sciences, San Luigi Gonzaga Hospital, Regione Gonzole 10, Orbassano 10043, Italy
* Corresponding author.
E-mail address: terzolo@usa.net

Endocrinol Metab Clin N Am 47 (2018) 395–407
https://doi.org/10.1016/j.ecl.2018.02.003
0889-8529/18/© 2018 Elsevier Inc. All rights reserved.

81%, 61%, 50%, and 13%, respectively, from stage 1 to stage 4.[5] However, ACC is a heterogeneous disease with variable survival at any stage depending on molecular, pathologic, and clinical factors that have only been partially ellucidated.[6] One of the factors influencing the clinical phenotype of ACC patients is the functional activity of the tumor, which may result in different endocrine syndromes.[3,4,6] Manifestations of adrenal steroid hormone excess represent the most common presentation of ACC in up to 60% of cases[4] (**Fig. 1**). Patients with nonfunctioning ACC present with back or abdominal pain, nausea, vomiting, or less frequently fever and weigh loss. Also, in an increasing number of patients, ACC is discovered serendipitously, due to the widespread application of high-resolution cross-sectional scans.[7]

CLINICAL PRESENTATION

ACC has the propensity to produce and secrete steroids; thus, in all patients with a suspected ACC, signs and symptoms of cortisol, aldosterone, and sex steroids should be actively investigated[4] (**Box 1**). Concomitant secretion of different steroids is a hallmark of ACC. Pure estrogen excess is rare and may cause gynecomastia, loss of libido, and testicular atrophy in men.[8]

Patients with cortisol-secreting ACC exhibit facial plethora, easy bruising, weight gain, proximal myopathy, severe hypertension, and uncontrolled diabetes mellitus. Hypokalemia is common with severe hypercortisolism, because mineralocorticoid receptors are triggered by the large amount of cortisol that overwhelms the inactivating capacity of corticosteroid 11β-dehydrogenase isoenzyme 2 (HSD11B2). Women frequently complain of acne, hirsutism, and oligomenorrhea.[4] The differential diagnosis in these situations is polycystic ovary syndrome (PCOS), especially with mild or subclinical hypercortisolism. Clinical clues that are helpful to the diagnosis of ACC are the concomitant existence of Cushingoid phenotype with signs of marked androgen excess, or Cushing's phenotype along with cancer-related symptoms (eg, anorexia, cachexia, or mass effect). With rapidly growing tumors, cancer-related features dominate the clinical presentation. ACC can also cause deep venous thrombosis or pulmonary embolism because of either cortisol excess or malignancy.[4] Cortisol

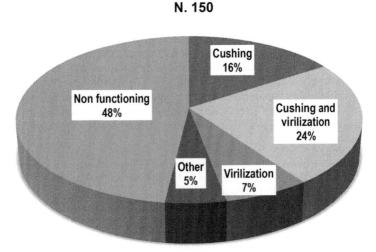

N. 150

Cushing 16%

Non functioning 48%

Cushing and virilization 24%

Other 5%

Virilization 7%

Fig. 1. Hormonal secretion in patients with ACC (S. Luigi series).

Box 1
Clinical manifestations

- Concomitant secretion of multiple steroids is a hallmark of adrenocortical carcinoma

- Hypercortisolism in the most frequent endocrine abnormality in ACC, although can present with catabolic features due to rapidly progressive malignancy

- Manifestations of hypercortisolism in ACC can be mild or subclinical, and erroneously attributed of PCOS

- Flank pain and constitutive symptoms are frequent in incidental ACC

---

excess should be excluded in all patients with suspected ACC, even if they do not harbor typical Cushingoid features.[9] Specific findings at CT scan, such as large mass size, high density (>10 Hounsfield units), intratumoral necrosis, irregular shape, and margins should raise the suspect of an ACC (**Fig. 2**).

ENDOCRINE ASSESSMENT

A detailed hormonal work-up (**Table 1**) should be performed preoperatively in all patients with suspected ACC for several reasons:

Demonstration of hypersecretory steroid profile establishes the adrenocortical origin of the tumor, while other differential diagnoses are being ruled out (ie, lymphoma or sarcoma)

The steroid profile may be helpful with evaluation of the malignant potential (ie, estradiol excess in males, high concentration of dehydroepiandrosterone sulfate [DHEAS] or steroid precursors)

Presence of autonomous cortisol secretion in a patient with ACC indicates a risk of postoperative adrenal insufficiency, which can be potentially life-threatening

Demonstration of steroid excess at baseline establishes tumor markers that can be useful to detect persistence or recurrence of disease postoperatively[4,8]

In patients without overt steroid overproduction, ACC may still secrete excessive amounts of adrenal steroid precursors due to decreased expression of several steroidogenic enzymes.[10] Increased secretion of urinary metabolites of several steroids, and precursors of androgens, glucocorticoids, or mineralcorticoids can be detected

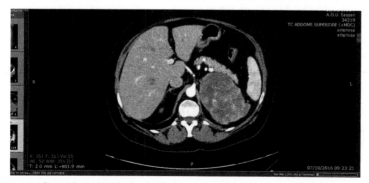

Fig. 2. CT scan of an adrenocortical carcinoma showing a large left adrenal mass of irregular shape and heterogeneous density.

Table 1
Endocrine assessment in patients with suspected or proven adrenocortical carcinoma

Condition	Tests
Cortisol excess	Serum cortisol following 1 mg DST If >1.8 μg/dL: Urinary free cortisol (24 h collection) Morning plasma ACTH Night-time salivary cortisol
Aldosterone excess	Serum potassium If hypokalemia and/or arterial hypertension: Plasma aldosterone and plasma renin activity (PRA) or direct renin
Sex steroid excess	Androstenedione Testosterone (in women) 17β-estradiol (in men and postmenopausal women)
Steroid precursors excess	DHEAS 17OH-progesterone
Catecholamine excess	Urinary fractionated metanephrines (24-hour collection) or free plasma metanephrines

even in the absence of a clinically or biochemically overt steroid excess by the use of sensitive methods such as gas chromatography/mass spectrometry. When applying this methodology, more than 95% of all patients with ACC were found to autonomously secrete steroids or steroid precursors.[11]

A standard 1 mg overnight dexamethasone test (1 mg DST) is recommended to exclude hypercortisolism in ACC, similar with adrenal incidentaloma. This test has higher sensitivity (95% at a cortisol threshold of 1.8 μg/dL), compared with 24-hour urinary-free cortisol (UFC), which is not helpful in cases of mild hypercortisolism.[12] If cortisol levels following the 1 mg DST are not suppressed despite lack of overt Cushing's phenotype, the condition of autonomous cortisol secretion may be present. The recent guidelines of the European Society of Endocrinology and the European Network for the Study of Adrenal Tumors (ENSAT) promoted this definition to the classic subclinical Cushing's syndrome.[9] Autonomous cortisol secretion is certain for cortisol levels above 5 μg/dL after 1 mg DST, while values between 1.8 μg/dL and 5 μg/dL require additional investigation to confirm the diagnosis. These include plasma adrenocorticotropic hormone (ACTH) and UFC levels, as well as a thorough evaluation of clinical conditions potentially associated with cortisol excess (ie, arterial hypertension, diabetes, or obesity). Recognizing asymptomatic cortisol excess preoperatively identifies patients who benefit from glucocorticoid replacement after adrenalectomy.[13]

Aldosterone-producing ACC is rare and generally associated with severe hypertension and marked hypokalemia.[14] Screening for hyperaldosteronism by measuring of plasma aldosterone and plasma renin activity (PRA) (or direct renin concentration) is recommended in all hypertensive and/or hypokalemic patients with adrenal masses.[15] In some cases, pseudoaldosteronism is present, due to increased production of deoxycorticosterone.

Hypersecretion of sexual steroids is frequently observed in ACC patients. Estrogen excess should be ascertained in males (especially in cases of gynecomastia) and postmenopausal women. Baseline 17-OH progesterone levels are frequently increased, as well as androstenedione and DHEAS, leading to increased plasma testosterone in females.[4] Measurement of steroid precursors in blood or urine may be exploited for diagnostic purposes. However, the value of increased DHEAS levels to predict malignancy of an adrenal mass is rather low.[16] More recently, it has been demonstrated that serum steroid paneling by LC-MS/MS is a useful tool to discriminate ACC from other adrenal tumor lesions. In this study, both the number of steroids secreted in high amounts and the marked elevation of several steroid intermediates without biological activity was characteristic of ACC and useful for the differential diagnosis. The cortisol precursor 11-deoxycortisol was found the most discriminating between ACC and non-ACC adrenal lesions.[17]

Assessment of plasma or urine fractionated metanephrines is recommend in patients with suspected ACC to exclude a pheochromocytoma, and avoid misdiagnosis and unexpected intraoperative complications.[4,7,9] Pertinently, a pheochromocytoma may appear as a large, heterogeneous and hypervascularized mass mimicking ACC.

PROGNOSTIC FACTORS

ACC stage and a margin-free resection are important and validated prognostic factors.[3,4] Currently, the ENSAT staging system is the most frequently used and allows a clear stratification of prognosis by stage. In particular, a 5-year stage-dependent survival of 81%, 61%, 50%, and 13%, respectively, from stage 1 to stage 4, has been demonstrated[5] Because surgery still represents the only curative treatment for ACC, an incomplete resection results in shorter survival within the same stage.[3–5] Resection status Rx (unknown), R1 (microscopically positive margins), and R2 (macroscopically positive margins) are associated with progressively reduced survival, irrespective of other risk factors.[3–5] It has been recently established that the proliferation activity of the tumor influences the risk of recurrence following R0 surgery. Assessment of the proliferation index Ki-67 is currently used to assess proliferation, despite some problems harmonizing immunohistochemical readings among different pathologists. In a European multicenter study, a Ki-67 value of 10% was found to separate patients at good or worse prognosis with a hazard ratio of recurrence of 1.042 per each % increase.[18]

The role of overt cortisol excess as a negative prognostic factor was first suggested in an Italian study,[19] including 72 patients with metastatic or locally advanced ACC, submitted to chemotherapy with etoposide, doxorubicin, and cisplatin plus mitotane. Patients with cortisol hypersecretion had shorter overall survival, both in univariate and multivariate analysis (hazard ratio [HR]: 0.64, 0.42–0.97; $P<.04$). This finding was confirmed by a French study,[20] including 202 patients with ACC at different stages. In this large series from a single endocrine center, 135 patients presented with hypercortisolism, and multivariate analysis identified cortisol overproduction as an independent prognostic factor associated with shorter survival (HR 3.90; $P<.0001$). In this subgroup of patients with cortisol-secreting tumors, adjuvant mitotane treatment had a positive effect on the risk of death (HR 0.40; $P<.04$). However, another study in 124 patients with metastatic ACC did not find an association between cortisol secretion and prognosis.[21]

The interaction between cortisol excess and adjuvant mitotane therapy was investigated by Berruti and colleagues[22] in a multicenter, retrospective series of 524 patients with completely resected ACC, of whom 197 patients (37.6%) had overt Cushing's syndrome. After adjustment for sex, age, tumor stage, and adjuvant mitotane therapy, hypercortisolism remained a strong independent predictor for both recurrence (HR: 1.30, 1.04–2.62; $P=.02$) and death (HR: 1.55, 1.15–2.09; $P=.004$). Efficacy of adjuvant mitotane treatment was not affected by the secretory status. The study did not provide information on the impact of subclinical Cushing's on prognosis.

More recently, a study carried out in US surgical institutions[23] demonstrated an association between cortisol secretion and risk of postoperative complications (HR: 2.25, 1.04–4.88; $P=.04$). Moreover, the study confirmed that hypercortisolism was an independent prognostic factor associated with shorter recurrence-free survival (HR: 2.05, 1.16–3.60; $P=.01$).

There are several possible underlying mechanisms by which excess cortisol influences the prognosis in ACC patients. First, hypercortisolism is associated with increased morbidity and mortality,[24] complicating the management of ACC patients (**Box 2**). Second, although an association between cortisol secretion and tumor grading has not been demonstrated so far, tumors with cortisol production may be more aggressive. This was supported by a French study evaluating the role of SKG1 protein expression in ACC.[25] SKG1 is a glucocorticoid-inducible kinase involved in cell cycle progression, acting as an antiapoptotic factor. The study demonstrated an inverse association between SGK1 expression and cortisol overproduction.[25] Low SGK1 protein level was identified as a negative prognostic factor in ACC patients, being associated with reduced OS (HR: 2.0, 1.24–3.24; $P<.005$). Third, the immunosuppressive effects of overt cortisol excess before surgery may favor the development of ACC micrometastases and recurrences.

Of note, studies implicating hypercortisolism as a negative predictive factor were retrospective and used variable methods to confirm cortisol excess. However, they suggest that cortisol excess in ACC may identify a cluster of patients who need more active surveillance and treatment (**Fig. 3**).

TREATMENT

The therapeutic approach in ACC varies according with the stage at diagnosis and performance status. Surgery is the main option in ACC without evidence of metastatic disease (stages I–III) and the only possibility of cure; when a radical resection is feasible, the 5-year survival rate is approximately 55%.[26] Surgery also has a role in the management of stage IV ACC, provided the metastatic spread is confined to a single organ and can be treated with radical intent.[27] The role of tumor debulking is disputed, and this approach is now rarely employed; however, it may have an indication in case of severe hypercortisolemia to reduce the mass of secreting cells.[3,4,28]

Surgery for ACC consists of adrenalectomy, which is performed by open approach in patients with infiltrative tumors or invasion of lymph nodes. On the other hand, stage I-II localized ACC can be removed by either laparoscopic or open adrenalectomy.[3,9] Whatever the surgical approach, surgery must be performed by a skilled surgical team, in centers with a high volume of adrenalectomies per year,[29] with the goal of a R0 resection (microscopically free margins). A radical resection induces temporary cortisol deficiency in patients with cortisol-secreting ACC, who require glucocorticoid replacement postoperatively. This is also the case after removal of a tumor causing autonomous cortisol secretion in patients without overt Cushing's features.[7]

Box 2
Implications of cortisol excess on adrenocortical carcinoma prognosis

- Most studies indicated that overt cortisol excess is associated with a detrimental prognosis
- Risk of recurrence after surgery is higher for cortisol-secreting ACC
- Comorbidities associated to Cushing's decrease life expectancy and complicate management of ACC patients

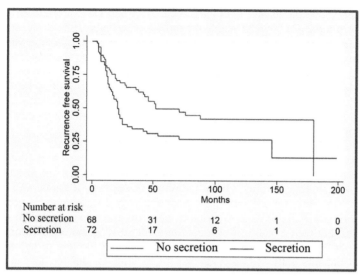

Fig. 3. Recurrence-free survival in patients with cortisol-secreting ACC versus patients with non-functioning ACC (S. Luigi series).

The risk for recurrence is lower for patients who undergo surgery by expert surgeons[30] but cannot be completely prevented. More than 50% of the tumors that have been completely extirpated are doomed to relapse,[31] and most patients with ACC recurrence experience further tumor progression and eventually die of the disease. These outcomes and the significant propensity of ACC to recur provide a rationale for adjuvant therapies.

Mitotane (o,p'-DDD, an isomer of the insecticide dichlorodiphenyltrichloroethane - DDT), is an orally administered adrenolytic drug. The first report of the destruction of the zona fasciculata and zona reticularis in the adrenal gland of dogs receiving mitotane was written in 1960 and demonstrated a marked reduction of glucocorticoids and 17-hydroxycorticosteroids in basal conditions and after ACTH stimulation.[32] Following this observation, it was found that mitotane is able to inhibit gene expression of a variety of cytochrome P450-dependent mitochondrial enzymes of the steroidogenetic pathway, including 20,22 desmolase (CYP11A1), 11β-hydroxylase (CYP11B1), and 18β-hydrolase (CYP11B2).[33] Critical steps of the inhibitory effects on steroidogenesis may occur in mitochondria possibly involving CYP11A1, a mitochondrial enzyme that catalyzes the transformation of cholesterol to pregnenolone.[34] The net effect is an inhibition of adrenal steroid production; thus, mitotane may ameliorate signs and symptoms of cortisol excess, and for this reason this adrenolytic drug has been used as a medical treatment of all causes of Cushing's syndrome.[35]

Although randomized controlled trials on the use of adjuvant mitotane in ACC patients following radical surgery are still unavailable, a large retrospective case-control study reported that patients treated with adjuvant mitotane had a significantly longer recurrence-free survival and overall survival compared with 2 independent groups of patients left untreated following surgery.[36] Recently, the same group updated the follow-up of these cohorts of patients with almost 10 years of additional observation, confirming that adjuvant mitotane treatment is associated with a significant benefit in terms of recurrence-free survival regardless of the hormone secretory status.[37] In this study, median recurrence-free survival was of 42 months in the adjuvant group compared with 17 months in control group 1 (P<.001) and 26 months in the control group 2 (P<.005).[37] Despite its retrospective nature, this study remains the most informative positive study on the topic and represents a reference for decision making on adjuvant therapy. However, literature is conflicting, and there is also evidence of a relative ineffectiveness of adjuvant mitotane. A recent multicenter study concluded that adjuvant mitotane was associated with decreased recurrence-free survival and overall survival. However, patients treated with mitotane had worse prognostic factors than untreated patients (more stage IV and more secreting ACCs in the mitotane group).[38]

During the 1960s and 1970s, mitotane was used for the treatment of patients with nonoperable ACC, with evidence of reduction of the tumor mass and control of the symptoms related to hormonal hypersecretion. However, despite some isolated cases of complete tumor regression,[39] most patients showed only a partial and transient response.[40] In 1982, for the first time, Schteingart and colleagues[41] proposed to extend treatment with mitotane to patients who had undergone complete resection of the mass, but with a high risk of recurrence, introducing the concept of adjuvant treatment. In 2012, the ESMO guidelines recommended the use of mitotane after surgery in patients with ACC at high risk of recurrence, defined as stage III, or Ki-67 greater than 10%, or R1 or Rx resection. For patients at low risk, characterized by stage I or II, Ki-67 less than 10%, and R0 resection, adjuvant therapy with mitotane is not mandatory. An international, multicenter, prospective, randomized trial (ADIUVO trial) is currently enrolling low-risk ACC patients, who are randomized to mitotane or observation, in order to establish the efficacy of adjuvant mitotane in this cohort of patients.[42]

In patients with inoperable or metastatic disease, mitotane is the mainstay of treatment and can be used as a single agent or in combination with classic cytostatic drugs. A key concept of mitotane treatment in patients with advanced/metastatic ACC is that disease responses are mainly confined in patients whose plasma mitotane concentrations are ranging between 14 and 20 mg/L.[43,44] The concept of a therapeutic range has been validated more recently in a retrospective series of 91 patients receiving mitotane for unresectable or metastatic ACC.[45] In this study, mitotane level above 14 mg/L was associated with tumor response and better survival irrespective of whether mitotane was administered as monotherapy or in combination with chemotherapy. Owing to the latency to attain the therapeutic range, mitotane monotherapy is indicated in the management of patients with a low tumor burden and less rapid disease. For ACC showing an aggressive course of disease or with many metastatic sites, cytotoxic chemotherapy is usually recommended. Chemotherapy in association with mitotane is also reserved for patients with advanced ACC at diagnosis or in patients whose disease is progressing on mitotane therapy, when mitotane is usually maintained, if tolerated.[6] Studies have shown a synergism of action between mitotane and chemotherapy due to its ability to reverse multidrug resistance mediated by P-glycoprotein expression. Overcoming multidrug resistance (MDR) gene, mitotane may enhance the cytotoxicity of anthracyclines, etoposide, and taxanes[46,47] whose activity is hampered by enhanced MDR gene expression by ACC.

The management of ACC patients poses unique challenges to the treating physicians who have to deal with both oncological or endocrinological issues.[48] Hypercortisolism requires prompt treatment to ensure rapid correction of the metabolic complications that may be life threatening. A rapid control of the endocrine syndrome may also improve the tolerance for antineoplastic therapy. Pertinently, cortisol-induced immunosuppression increases the risk of severe infections during chemotherapy. Mitotane has a compelling indication in patients with hormone-secreting

ACC, since it has both an inhibitory effect on adrenal steroidogenesis and a cytotoxic effect on the tumor, although its success rate in controlling hormone excess is not well known.[3,10] Mitotane is characterized by a slow onset of action, linked to the building of adequate plasma levels, which means treatment should initially include rapidly effective steroidogenesis inhibitors such as metyrapone, ketoconazole, and etomidate.[28] However, mitotane is a strong inducer of CYP3A4 activity,[49] and this may cause drug interactions when used in a combination therapy. The safety profile of the accompanying drugs should also be carefully considered to avoid cumulative toxicity with mitotane (ie, gastrointestinal and liver toxicity). A series of 14 patients with severe hypercortisolism, including 8 ACC patients, have been treated with a combination of metyrapone and ketoconazole in 2 tertiary-care university hospitals. In patients with ACC, median UFC after 1 week of treatment fell from 16.0 to 1.0 ULN (upper limit of the normal range), and after 1 month, UFC values were normal in 86% of patients. Also, important improvements of clinical status, potassium, glycemia, and blood pressure were reported, with a decrease in drugs used for comorbidities. Adverse effects were minimal, and only 1 patient with ACC had an increase in plasma transaminase, necessitating ketoconazole withdrawal.[50]

Recently, Claps and colleagues[51] reported 3 cases of advanced ACC patients with Cushing's syndrome treated with a combination of metyrapone with the regimen EDP-M, including etoposide, doxorubicin, cisplatin, and mitotane. EDP-M represents the current standard of chemotherapy treatment for advanced ACC.[52] Metyrapone is an adrenolytic molecule targeting the 11-beta-hydroxylase that is currently used to treat Cushing's syndrome of different etiologies.[53] The drug inhibits the conversion of 11-deoxycortisol into cortisol obtaining the reduction of cortisol synthesis within 2 hours after the first drug administration.[54] Metyrapone metabolism and elimination are not altered by concomitant mitotane. Indeed, metyrapone is mainly metabolized by hepatic reduction; then, metyrapone and reduced metyrapone are conjugated to the corresponding glucuronides, and nearly 40% of the administered dose is excreted in the urine within 2 days. Metyrapone per se does not have antineoplastic activity.[28,53] In this study, the addition of metyrapone to EDP-M led to a rapid resolution of symptoms and signs of Cushing's syndrome and a significant improvement of the patient conditions. This finding has to be underlined, because EDP-M usually requires several weeks to attain a control of hypercortisolism. Metyrapone was well tolerated, did not increase the toxicity of the EDP-M regimen, and did not alter EDP-M efficacy in terms of tumor control. Therefore, this combination may represent a rapid, effective, and well-tolerated treatment of overt Cushing's sustained by ACC.

Because of the adrenolytic effect of mitotane, all patients should receive glucocorticoid replacement to prevent adrenal insufficiency. Steroid doses are typically higher than in Addison disease, due to an enhanced metabolic clearance rate of glucocorticoids induced by mitotane.[3,4] It was calculated that mitotane is able to inactivate 50% of administered hydrocortisone through enhanced CYP3A enzyme activity.[55] An inadequate treatment of adrenal insufficiency increases mitotane-related toxicity, particularly gastrointestinal adverse effects, and reduces tolerance.[56] Mineralocorticoid supplementation is not mandatory in all patients, because the zona glomerulosa is partly spared by the toxic effect of mitotane.[56]

SUMMARY

Adrenocortical carcinoma may present frequently with Cushing's syndrome that may have atypical features. Cushing's syndrome is ACTH-independent, and the concomitance of cortisol and androgen excess is a clue to suspect the diagnosis.

Box 3
Therapy for adrenocortical carcinoma with hypercortisolemia

- Surgery is the treatment of choice of ACC when radical resection is feasible and is associated with improved oncological and endocrinological outcomes
- Despite radical surgery, ACC has a high recurrence rate, and mitotane is frequently used as a post-operative adjunctive treatment
- Advanced or inoperable ACC is treated with mitotane alone or in combination with chemotherapy depending on patient and tumor characteristics
- Mitotane is the medical treatment of choice of Cushing's syndrome associated to ACC, but combination with steroidogenesis inhibitors with more rapid onset of action is initially required.

When an adrenocortical carcinoma is associated with cortisol excess, its prognosis is worse compared with nonsecretory tumors, even if complete resection is attained. Tumors causing hypercortisolism have a higher risk of recurrence. Moreover, Cushing's syndrome carries a huge disease burden in case of advanced adrenocortical carcinoma and complicates management. Controlling cortisol excess is an urgent need that may be accomplished before giving chemotherapy to overcome the enhanced risk of infections. Mitotane is the mainstay of medical treatment of hypercortisolism; however, its delayed action calls for associating more rapid agents. The inhibitor of steroidogenesis metyrapone has been used successfully in this context (**Box 3**).

REFERENCES

1. Fassnacht M, Kroiss M, Allolio B. Update in adrenocortical carcinoma. J Clin Endocrinol Metab 2013;98(12):4551–64.
2. Ribeiro RC, Sandrini F, Figueiredo B, et al. An inherited p53 mutation that contributes in a tissue-specific manner to pediatric adrenal cortical carcinoma. Proc Natl Acad Sci U S A 2001;98(16):9330–5.
3. Fassnacht M, Libé R, Kroiss M, et al. Adrenocortical carcinoma: a clinician's update. Nat Rev Endocrinol 2011;7(6):323–35.
4. Stigliano A, Chiodini I, Giordano R, et al. Management of adrenocortical carcinoma: a consensus statement of the Italian Society of Endocrinology (SIE). J Endocrinol Invest 2016;39(1):103–21.
5. Fassnacht M, Johanssen S, Quinkler M, et al. Limited prognostic value of the 2004 international union against cancer staging classification for adrenocortical carcinoma. Cancer 2009;115(2):243–50.
6. Terzolo M, Daffara F, Ardito A, et al. Management of adrenal cancer: A 2013 update. J Endocrinol Invest 2014;37(3):207–17.
7. Terzolo M, Stigliano A, Chiodini I, et al. AME position statement on adrenal incidentaloma. Eur J Endocrinol 2011;164(6):851–70.
8. Else T, Kim AC, Sabolch A, et al. Adrenocortical carcinoma. Endocr Rev 2014; 35(2):282–326.
9. Fassnacht M, Arlt W, Bancos I, et al. Management of adrenal incidentalomas: European Society of Endocrinology clinical practice guideline in collaboration with the European Network for the Study of Adrenal Tumors. Eur J Endocrinol 2016; 175(2):G1–34.

10. Bourdeau I, MacKenzie-Feder J, Lacroix A. Recent advances in adrenocortical carcinoma in adults. Curr Opin Endocrinol Diabetes Obes 2013;20(3):192–7.

11. Arlt W, Biehl M, Taylor AE, et al. Urine steroid metabolomics as a biomarker tool for detecting malignancy in adrenal tumors. J Clin Endocrinol Metab 2011;96(12): 3775–84.

12. Terzolo M, Bovio S, Pia A, et al. Management of adrenal incidentaloma. Best Pract Res Clin Endocrinol Metab 2009;23(2):233–43.

13. Eller-Vainicher C, Morelli V, Salcuni AS, et al. Accuracy of several parameters of hypothalamic-pituitary-adrenal axis activity in predicting before surgery the metabolic effects of the removal of an adrenal incidentaloma. Eur J Endocrinol 2010; 163(6):925–35.

14. Seccia TM, Fassina A, Nussdorfer GG, et al. Aldosterone-producing adrenocortical carcinoma: An unusual cause of Conn's syndrome with an ominous clinical course. Endocr Relat Cancer 2005;12(1):149–59.

15. Funder JW, Carey RM, Mantero F, et al. The management of primary aldosteronism: case detection, diagnosis, and treatment: an endocrine society clinical practice guideline. J Clin Endocrinol Metab 2016;101(5):1889–916.

16. Terzolo M, Alì A, Osella G, et al. The value of dehydroepiandrosterone sulfate measurement in the differentiation between benign and malignant adrenal masses. Eur J Endocrinol 2000;142(6):611–7.

17. Taylor DR, Ghataore L, Couchman L, et al. A 13-steroid serum panel based on LC-MS/MS: use in detection of adrenocortical carcinoma. Clin Chem 2017; 63(12):1836–46.

18. Beuschlein F, Weigel J, Saeger W, et al. Major prognostic role of Ki67 in localized adrenocortical carcinoma after complete resection. J Clin Endocrinol Metab 2015;100(3):841–9.

19. Berruti A, Terzolo M, Sperone P, et al. Etoposide, doxorubicin and cisplatin plus mitotane in the treatment of advanced adrenocortical carcinoma: a large prospective phase II trial. Endocr Relat Cancer 2005;12(3):657–66.

20. Abiven G, Coste J, Groussin L, et al. Clinical and biological features in the prognosis of adrenocortical cancer: poor outcome of cortisol-secreting tumors in a series of 202 consecutive patients. J Clin Endocrinol Metab 2006;91(7): 2650–5.

21. Assié G, Antoni G, Tissier F, et al. Prognostic parameters of metastatic adrenocortical carcinoma. J Clin Endocrinol Metab 2007;92(1):148–54.

22. Berruti A, Fassnacht M, Haak H, et al. Prognostic role of overt hypercortisolism in completely operated patients with adrenocortical cancer. Eur Urol 2014;65(4): 832–8.

23. Margonis GA, Kim Y, Tran TB, et al. Outcomes after resection of cortisol-secreting adrenocortical carcinoma. Am J Surg 2016;211(6):1106–13.

24. Dekkers OM, Horváth-Puhó EE, Jørgensen JOL, et al. Multisystem morbidity and mortality in cushing's syndrome: a cohort study. J Clin Endocrinol Metab 2013; 98(6):2277–84.

25. Ronchi CL, Sbiera S, Leich E, et al. Low SGK1 expression in human adrenocortical tumors is associated with ACTH-independent glucocorticoid secretion and poor prognosis. J Clin Endocrinol Metab 2012;97(12):E2251–60.

26. Schulick RD, Brennan MF. Long-term survival after complete resection and repeat resection in patients with adrenocortical carcinoma. Ann Surg Oncol 1999;6(8): 719–26.

27. Wängberg B, Khorram-Manesh A, Jansson S, et al. The long-term survival in adrenocortical carcinoma with active surgical management and use of monitored mitotane. Endocr Relat Cancer 2010;17(1):265–72.

28. Veytsman I, Nieman L, Fojo T. Management of endocrine manifestations and the use of mitotane as a chemotherapeutic agent for adrenocortical carcinoma. J Clin Oncol 2009;27(27):4619–29.

29. Ayala-Ramirez M, Jasim S, Feng L, et al. Adrenocortical carcinoma: clinical outcomes and prognosis of 330 patients at a tertiary care center. Eur J Endocrinol 2013;169(6):891–9.

30. Hermsen IGC, Kerkhofs TMA, den Butter G, et al. Surgery in adrenocortical carcinoma: Importance of national cooperation and centralized surgery. Surgery 2012;152(1):50–6.

31. Bellantone R, Ferrante A, Boscherini M, et al. Role of reoperation in recurrence of adrenal cortical carcinoma: results from 188 cases collected in the Italian National Registry for Adrenal Cortical Carcinoma. Surgery 1997;122(6):1212–8.

32. Nelson AA, Woodard G. Severe adrenal cortical atrophy (cytotoxic) and hepatic damage produced in dogs by feeding 2,2-bis(parachlorophenyl)-1,1-dichloroethane (DDD or TDE). Arch Pathol 1949;48(5):387–94.

33. Young RB, Bryson MJ, Sweat ML, et al. Complexing of DDT and o,p'DDD with adrenal cytochrome P-450 hydroxylating systems. J Steroid Biochem 1973;4(6):585–91.

34. Cai W, Counsell RE, Schteingart DE, et al. Adrenal proteins should be a reactive intermediate of mitotane. Cancer Chemother Pharmacol 1997;39(6):537–40.

35. Trainer PJ, Besser M. Cushing's syndrome. Therapy directed at the adrenal glands. Endocrinol Metab Clin North Am 1994;23(3):571–84.

36. Terzolo M, Angeli A, Fassnacht M, et al. Adjuvant mitotane treatment for adrenocortical carcinoma. N Engl J Med 2007;356(23):2372–80.

37. Berruti A, Grisanti S, Pulzer A, et al. Long-term outcomes of adjuvant mitotane therapy in patients with radically resected adrenocortical carcinoma. J Clin Endocrinol Metab 2017;102(4):1358–65.

38. Postlewait LM, Ethun CG, Tran TB, et al. Outcomes of adjuvant mitotane after resection of adrenocortical carcinoma: a 13-Institution Study by the US Adrenocortical Carcinoma Group. J Am Coll Surg 2016;222:480–90.

39. Boven E, Vermorken JB, van Slooten H, et al. Complete response of metastasized adrenal cortical carcinoma with o,p'-DDD. Case report and literature review. Cancer 1984;53(1):26–9.

40. Wooten MD, King DK. Adrenal cortical carcinoma. Epidemiology and treatment with mitotane and a review of the literature. Cancer 1993;72(11):3145–55.

41. Schteingart DE, Motazedi A, Noonan RA, et al. Treatment of Adrenal Carcinomas. Arch Surg 1982;117(9):1142–6.

42. Available at: www.adiuvo-trial.org.

43. Baudin E, Pellegriti G, Bonnay M, et al. Impact of monitoring plasma 1,1-dichlorodiphenildichloroethane (o,p'DDD) levels on the treatment of patients with adrenocortical carcinoma. Cancer 2001;92(6):1385–92.

44. Haak HR, Hermans J, van de Velde CJH, et al. Optimal treatment of adrenocortical carcinoma with mitotane: results in a consecutive series of 96 patients. Br J Cancer 1994;69(5):947–51.

45. Hermsen IG, Fassnacht M, Terzolo M, et al. Plasma concentrations of o,p'DDD, o,p'DDA, and o,p'DDE as predictors of tumor response to mitotane in adrenocortical carcinoma: Results of a retrospective ENS@T multicenter study. J Clin Endocrinol Metab 2011;96(6):1844–51.

46. Bates SE, Shieh CY, Mickley LA, et al. Mitotane enhances cytotoxicity of chemotherapy in cell lines expressing a multidrug resistance gene (mdr -1/P-Glycoprotein) which is also expressed by adrenocortical carcinomas. J Clin Endocrinol Metab 1991;73(1):18–29.
47. Villa R, Orlandi L, Berruti A, et al. Modulation of cytotoxic drug activity by mitotane and lonidamine in human adrenocortical carcinoma cells. Int J Oncol 1999;14(1):133–8.
48. Berruti A, Baudin E, Gelderblom H, et al. Adrenal cancer: ESMO clinical practice guidelines for diagnosis, treatment and follow-up. Ann Oncol 2012;23(Suppl. 7):vii131–8.
49. Kroiss M, Quinkler M, Lutz WK, et al. Drug interactions with mitotane by induction of CYP3A4 metabolism in the clinical management of adrenocortical carcinoma. Clin Endocrinol (Oxf) 2011;75(5):585–91.
50. Corcuff JB, Young J, Masquefa-Giraud P, et al. Rapid control of severe neoplastic hypercortisolism with metyrapone and ketoconazole. Eur J Endocrinol 2015;172(4):473–81.
51. Claps M, Cerri S, Grisanti S, et al. Adding metyrapone to chemotherapy plus mitotane for Cushing's syndrome due to advanced adrenocortical carcinoma. Endocrine 2017. https://doi.org/10.1007/s12020-017-1428-9.
52. Fassnacht M, Terzolo M, Allolio B, et al. Combination chemotherapy in advanced adrenocortical carcinoma. N Engl J Med 2012;366(23):2189–97.
53. Daniel E, Aylwin S, Mustafa O, et al. Effectiveness of metyrapone in treating Cushing's syndrome: a retrospective multicenter study in 195 patients. J Clin Endocrinol Metab 2015;100(11):4146–54.
54. Verhelst JA, Trainer PJ, Howlett TA, et al. Short and long-term responses to metyrapone in the medical management of 91 patients with Cushing's syndrome. Clin Endocrinol (Oxf) 1991;35(2):169–78.
55. Chortis V, Taylor AE, Schneider P, et al. Mitotane therapy in adrenocortical cancer induces CYP3A4 and inhibits 5α-reductase, explaining the need for personalized glucocorticoid and androgen replacement. J Clin Endocrinol Metab 2013;98(1):161–71.
56. Daffara F, de Francia S, Reimondo G, et al. Prospective evaluation of mitotane toxicity in adrenocortical cancer patients treated adjuvantly. Endocr Relat Cancer 2008;15(4):1043–53.

The Ectopic Adrenocorticotropic Hormone Syndrome
Rarely Easy, Always Challenging

Aimee R. Hayes, BSc, MBBS (Hons), MMed (Clin Epi), FRACP,
Ashley B. Grossman, BA, BSc, MD, FRCP, FMedSci*

KEYWORDS

- Ectopic • Cushing's • ACTH • Carcinoid • Neuroendocrine tumor
- Small cell lung cancer

KEY POINTS

- Historically, patients with the ectopic adrenocorticotropic hormone (ACTH) syndrome (EAS) presented with aggressive tumors, such as small cell lung cancer, and the abrupt onset of symptoms and signs of severe hypercortisolism; however, the pulmonary carcinoid tumor is now recognized as the most frequent cause of the EAS.
- ACTH-secreting pulmonary carcinoids, like the corticotroph tumors causing Cushing's disease, are often small and difficult to detect; patients typically present with a gradual onset of the classical signs and symptoms of Cushing's syndrome, usually indistinguishable from the presentation of Cushing's disease.
- Differentiating the EAS from Cushing's disease therefore remains challenging and requires a combination of clinical assessment, dynamic biochemical tests, inferior petrosal sinus sampling, and multimodal imaging, each with their own caveats and pitfalls.
- All testing procedures should be considered to be probabilistic rather than algorithmic.

INTRODUCTION

The ectopic adrenocorticotropic hormone (ACTH) syndrome (EAS) comprises around 10% to 20% of ACTH-dependent Cushing's syndrome and 5% to 10% of all types of Cushing's syndrome.[1,2] In the past, most EAS patients presented with small cell lung cancer (SCLC).[3,4] However, because of improved imaging techniques and changing referral patterns, over the past 50 years, the spectrum of malignancies associated with the EAS has broadened to include other neuroendocrine tumors (NETs), predominantly pulmonary, thymic, and pancreatic carcinoids, and more rarely, medullary

Conflicts of Interest: The authors have nothing to disclose.
Neuroendocrine Tumour Unit, Royal Free Hospital, Pond Street, London NW3 2QG, UK
* Corresponding author.
E-mail address: ashley.grossman@ocdem.ox.ac.uk

Endocrinol Metab Clin N Am 47 (2018) 409–425
https://doi.org/10.1016/j.ecl.2018.01.005
0889-8529/18/© 2018 Elsevier Inc. All rights reserved.

endo.theclinics.com

thyroid carcinoma (MTC) and pheochromocytoma.[1,2,5] However, virtually any tumor may develop neuroendocrine differentiation and cause the EAS.

The EAS causes significant comorbidity in a patient with a background malignancy. Furthermore, untreated hypercortisolism contributes to excess mortality. In patients with nonmalignant causes of Cushing's syndrome, mortality is increased with a standard mortality ratio between 2.0 and 4.0 with cardiovascular deaths most common.[6,7] Hence, the EAS should be managed aggressively with every effort to establish rapid eucortisolemia and identify the tumor source, which may frequently be amenable to curative surgery.

PREVALENCE OF ECTOPIC ADRENOCORTICOTROPIC HORMONE SYNDROME

The EAS is rare. Studies show the prevalence of EAS is approximately 1% to 5% in patients with SCLC,[8,9] 3% in patients with thoracic or gastroenteropancreatic carcinoids (excluding MEN1),[10] and 0.7% in patients with MTC,[11] although the prevalence may be higher in patients with thymic carcinoids.[12]

MOLECULAR PATHOPHYSIOLOGY

The EAS is caused by abnormal expression of the pro-opiomelanocortin (*POMC*) gene product arising from non–pituitary tumors in response to ectopic activation of the pituitary-specific promoter of this gene.[13] This promoter is embedded within a defined CpG island and, in contrast to somatically expressed CpG island promoters, is methylated in nonexpressing tissues but specifically unmethylated in expressing tissues.[14] POMC promoter activity and its methylation status have been studied in ACTH-secreting thymic carcinoids, with an association demonstrated between hypomethylation of the POMC promoter region and POMC overexpression.[13]

Genetic mutations associated with the EAS are largely unknown. ACTH-secreting carcinoid tumors may harbor germline *MENIN* mutations,[6] and ACTH-secreting MTC or pheochromocytoma may be associated with germline *RET* mutations, although they are much more frequently sporadic.[1,2]

CLINICAL AND BIOCHEMICAL PRESENTATION OF THE ECTOPIC ADRENOCORTICOTROPIC HORMONE SYNDROME

There are epidemiological and clinical features that can help discriminate between the EAS and Cushing's disease (**Table 1**). The age of onset is normally higher in EAS compared with Cushing's disease,[1,15,16] and the gender ratio also differs, with EAS occurring only slightly more often in women compared with the marked female predominance in Cushing's disease.[1,2,6]

In terms of the clinical features of EAS, there is significant heterogeneity related to the malignant potential of the underlying tumor and the severity of the hypercortisolism. SCLCs and other aggressive tumors are usually associated with much higher ACTH and cortisol levels compared with Cushing's disease and subsequently present with rapid onset of clinical signs and symptoms, including hyperpigmentation, weight loss, and mineralocorticoid effects, as opposed to the classical Cushing's syndrome phenotype.[1,2] Moreover, the detection of EAS in a patient with rapidly progressing SCLC with significant catabolic features can sometimes go unnoticed, contributing to significant comorbidity.[5] In contrast, patients with ACTH-secreting carcinoid tumors more often have a gradual onset of the broad classical signs and symptoms of Cushing's syndrome, indistinguishable from the presentation of Cushing's disease.[1,2]

Table 1
Causes of adrenocorticotropic hormone–dependent Cushing's syndrome

	Proportion (%)	Age (Peak)	Female: Male	Features
ACTH-dependent	70–80	—	—	—
Cushing's disease	60–70	—	—	—
Corticotroph adenoma	60–70	3rd-4th decades	3–5:1	Roughly 50% nonvisible on MRI
Corticotroph hyperplasia	Very rare	—	—	—
Ectopic ACTH[a]	5–10	—	—	—
Malignant neuroendocrine tumors	About 4	5th-6th decades	0.6–1:1	Might have very high ACTH
Benign neuroendocrine tumors	About 6	3rd-4th decades	—	Might respond to dexamethasone, CRH, desmopressin
Occult neuroendocrine tumors	About 2	—	—	—
Ectopic CRH	Very rare	—	—	Causes pituitary corticotroph hyperplasia
ACTH-independent	20–30	—	—	—
Unilateral adrenal	—	—	—	—
Adenoma	10–22	4th-5th decades	4–8:1	Most pure cortisol secretion
Carcinoma	5–7	1st, 5th-6th decades	1.5–3:1	Mixed cortisol and androgen frequent
Bilateral adrenal	1–2	—	—	—
Bilateral macronodular adrenal hyperplasia[b]	<2	5th-6th decades	2–3:1	Modest cortisol secretion compared with size; raised steroid precursors; might have combined androgen and mineralocorticoid cosecretion
Aberrant G protein–coupled receptors	—	—	—	—
Autocrine ACTH production	—	—	—	—
Sporadic or familial (ARMC5)	—	—	—	—
Bilateral micronodular adrenal hyperplasias	<2	—	—	Adrenal size often normal
Primary pigmented nodular adrenocortical disease	Rare	1st-3rd decades	0.5:1 <12 y 2:1 >12 y	Frequent paradoxic increase of urine free cortisol with Liddle's oral dexamethasone suppression test
Isolated or familial with Carney complex	Rare	1st-3rd decades	—	—
Isolated micronodular adrenocortical disease	Very rare	Infants	—	Nonpigmented adrenal micronodules

(continued on next page)

	Proportion (%)	Age (Peak)	Female: Male	Features
Table 1 *(continued)*				
Primary bimorphic adrenocortical disease	Very rare	Infants	—	—
McCune-Albright syndrome	Rare	Infants (<6 mo)	1:1	Internodular adrenal atrophy
Bilateral adenomas or carcinomas	Rare	4th–5th decades	2–4:1	—

[a] Most frequent sources of EASs are small cell lung carcinoma and neuroendocrine tumors of lung, thymus, and pancreas. Less frequent causes include medullary thyroid carcinoma, gastrinoma, pheochromocytoma, prostate carcinoma, and several others.
[b] In bilateral macronodular adrenal hyperplasia tissues, autocrine and paracrine ACTH might be produced and contribute to cortisol secretion. If confirmed by in-vivo studies, the ACTH-independent classification will need to be modified in the future.
From Lacroix A, Feelders RA, Stratakis CA, et al. Cushing's syndrome. The Lancet 2015;386(9996):914; *Reprinted with permission from* Elsevier (The Lancet).

It should be noted, however, that although patients with the EAS, especially secondary to SCLC, tend to have higher ACTH and cortisol levels, there remains significant overlap between the EAS and Cushing's disease cohorts. In 2 consecutive series of EAS patients,[1,2] basal plasma ACTH levels were between 9 and 52 ng/L in 32% and less than 200 ng/L in 50%, respectively, and both series were composed of a significant number of pulmonary carcinoid patients. Conversely, patients with pituitary macroadenomas have been shown to occasionally have very high ACTH levels.[17] It should also be noted that although disease activity in Cushing's disease can be highly fluctuant, this may also occur in the EAS.[1,18]

SOURCE OF ADRENOCORTICOTROPIC HORMONE SECRETION

The lung is the most likely organ to harbor an ectopic source of ACTH. In a review of some of the largest published series (n = 383),[5] the lung was the site of the ACTH-secreting tumor in more than 45% of cases, with pulmonary carcinoids (also referred to as bronchial carcinoids and lung NETs) being the most common (>25%) followed by SCLC (approximately 20%). When SCLCs were excluded from the analysis, the frequency of pulmonary carcinoids was as high as 32% with approximately equal numbers of *typical* and *atypical* morphology. The next most common tumors were thymic (11%) and pancreatic NETs (8%), followed by MTC (6%), and pheochromocytomas (5%).

Importantly, however, despite repeated evaluation, up to 20% of ACTH-secreting tumors remain occult,[1,2,19] although progressively smaller numbers are reported in recent studies because of more sophisticated imaging techniques and, probably, longer follow-up intervals.[5] The major occult source where tumors are eventually demonstrated remains the lung, and ACTH-secreting pulmonary carcinoids or carcinoid tumorlets have been documented as small as 2 to 3 mm.[2,15] However, other elusive sites, such as the appendix, have also been rarely described.[10,20]

DIAGNOSIS OF ECTOPIC ADRENOCORTICOTROPIC HORMONE SECRETION

Discriminating between the EAS and Cushing's disease is challenging because both pulmonary carcinoids and pituitary corticotroph tumors are often small and difficult to detect, even with sophisticated imaging.[2,17] Furthermore, up to 10% of the population will have incidental nonsecreting tumors of the pituitary demonstrable on magnetic resonance imaging (MRI), and pituitary imaging should be interpreted with caution.[21] Hence, there is a reliance on biochemical testing to direct the imaging to the appropriate site, although even this may be challenging because small ectopic sources may still contain many of the intrinsic regulatory mechanisms of corticotroph tumors.[22]

DYNAMIC NONINVASIVE TESTS

Initial tests must first confirm endogenous hypercortisolism (overnight dexamethasone suppression testing or low-dose dexamethasone suppression testing [LDDST], urinary free cortisol, and midnight serum or salivary cortisol assessments) and the demonstration of detectable plasma ACTH to exclude primary adrenal disease. Once the diagnosis of ACTH-dependent Cushing's syndrome has been confirmed, the next challenge is to determine the source (**Fig. 1**).

The rationale for most biochemical tests is that most pituitary corticotroph tumors retain relative sensitivity to corticotrophin-releasing hormone (CRH) stimulation and negative feedback regulation by glucocorticoids, whereas ectopic ACTH-secreting tumors typically do not,[4,23] although this distinction is far from absolute, especially for small carcinoid tumors, usually pulmonary carcinoids.[1,2,10,24]

The most commonly used dynamic tests to discriminate patients with EAS from Cushing's disease are the high-dose dexamethasone suppression test (HDDST), the CRH stimulation test, or the desmopressin stimulation test either alone or in combination with CRH.

The HDDST (2 mg given every 6 hours for 48 hours, or a single 8 mg overnight dose) is considered indicative of Cushing's disease when serum or urinary cortisol suppresses by greater than 50% of the baseline value, with a variable sensitivity and specificity of 60% to 100% and 65% to 100%, respectively.[25–31] Higher sensitivity for the diagnosis of the EAS is obtained using serum cortisol assessment and a higher cutoff for cortisol suppression.[1,32] However, EAS series have demonstrated between 5% and 25% of ACTH-secreting carcinoid tumors show suppressibility of serum or urinary steroid values during dexamethasone suppression testing.[1,2,33] Conversely, approximately 20% of patients with Cushing's disease will fail to show suppressibility of steroid levels greater than 50% of baseline values during dexamethasone testing.[34,35] Hence, the diagnostic accuracy of the HDDST is less than that of the pretest probability of Cushing's disease in patients with ACTH-dependent Cushing's syndrome (80%–90%) and is therefore of low predictive value when interpreted in isolation.[35]

In the CRH stimulation test, recombinant human or ovine-sequence CRH is given as an intravenous bolus of either 1 μg/kg or, more typically, 100 μg. An ACTH increase of at least 35% (sensitivity 93%, specificity 100%) and cortisol increase of at least 20% (sensitivity 91%, specificity 88%) above baseline values is considered indicative of Cushing's disease when ovine CRH is used,[36] and at least a 105% ACTH increase (sensitivity 70%, specificity 100%) and a 14% cortisol increase (85% sensitivity; 100% specificity) when human CRH is used.[37] However, diagnostic errors (false positives and false negatives) occur in 7% to 15% of patients even if the best discriminating criteria are applied, with most errors being false negative results in Cushing's disease patients who fail to respond.[38–41] Therefore, neither the HDDST nor the CRH stimulation tests alone consistently discriminate between Cushing's disease and the EAS, although responses to either clearly shift the probability in favor of Cushing's disease.

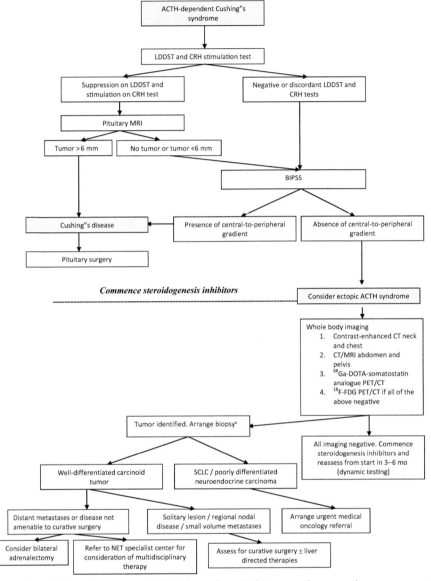

Fig. 1. Establishing the cause of ACTH-dependent Cushing's syndrome and management.
[a] with SSTA cover if there is suspicion of metastatic carcinoid.

Desmopressin can stimulate ACTH secretion from a high proportion of corticotroph adenomas via activation of vasopressin receptors (AVP-R2 and AVP-R1B).[42,43] However, because many ectopic ACTH-secreting tumors also express these receptors, the desmopressin test has even less utility than CRH in the differential diagnosis of ACTH-dependent Cushing's syndrome,[43,44] even when combined with CRH.[45]

Although each test on its own may have limited diagnostic accuracy, the combination of the results of HDDST and CRH testing has more discriminatory power.[26,46] In one study of 245 patients with ACTH-dependent Cushing's syndrome, the combination of cortisol suppression on HDDST and stimulation on CRH had a sensitivity of 95% and a specificity of 93% to detect Cushing's disease.[32] Furthermore, when using optimal criteria, the combination of the LDDST and CRH test had similar diagnostic accuracy (sensitivity 94%, specificity 97%) compared with the combination of the HDDST and CRH test, and it can be argued that the HDDST provides little additional information.[32] Nevertheless, up to 25% of EAS patients may have discordant dynamic test results.[1,2]

INVASIVE TESTING

Most clinicians will diagnose Cushing's disease if a patient with ACTH-dependent Cushing's syndrome has concordant results on the HDDST and CRH test suggestive of Cushing's disease, and the demonstration of a focal lesion of 6 mm or more on pituitary MRI.[22] However, lack of a demonstrable tumor on MRI is not uncommon and has been reported in up to 40% of patients with proven Cushing's disease.[47]

Bilateral inferior petrosal sinus sampling (BIPSS), in experienced hands, is the gold-standard test to identify a pituitary versus ectopic source of ACTH with sensitivity and specificity of approximately 95%.[22,48] A pituitary source is identified by a central-to-peripheral ACTH gradient of more than 2 at baseline and more than 3 following CRH or desmopressin administration.[22] However, false negative[49,50] and rare false positive results have been described.[51,52] False positive responses can occur in EAS patients with mild hypercortisolism,[51,53] and some centers recommend documentation of a 2-fold or greater increase in urinary free cortisol for 6 to 8 weeks prior to BIPSS to ensure suppression of normal corticotrophs. The authors would simply check the serum cortisol within 24 hours of the test to ensure it remained elevated. Treatment with cortisol-lowering agents may also theoretically cause desuppression of normal corticotrophs and subsequent responsivity to CRH or desmopressin.[51] Other rare causes of false positive results in EAS patients include those with cyclical hypercortisolism or in CRH-producing tumors, which may induce corticotroph hyperplasia.[6,34] False negative results can occur in the setting of poor catheter placement, petrosal sinus hypoplasia or anomalous venous drainage, or low peak inferior petrosal sinus ACTH levels.[52,54,55] There is little evidence that sampling from the cavernous sinuses is advantageous and is technically challenging.

BIOMARKERS

Calcitonin and plasma or urinary metanephrines have been shown to be the only biomarkers of specific diagnostic value in the EAS,[1,2] and they should be performed in all patients to exclude MTC or pheochromocytoma, respectively. Interestingly, serum calcitonin is the most frequently elevated tumor marker in the EAS regardless of tumor type and is elevated in 44% to 69% of EAS cases, including MTC, carcinoids, pheochromocytoma, gastrinomas, and occult tumors.[1,2,30] Fasting plasma gut hormones, most commonly gastrin, may be elevated in functioning pancreatic carcinoids, although in a recent series 8 out of 9 ACTH-secreting islet cell tumors were otherwise nonfunctioning.[10]

Although urinary 5-hydroxyindoleacetic acid (5-HIAA) levels are classically elevated in patients with well-differentiated midgut carcinoids (mainly in the presence of liver metastases), carcinoids arising from the foregut (such as lung, thymus, and pancreas) are usually deficient in the enzyme aromatic L-amino-acid decarboxylase and therefore produce less serotonin.[56] Nevertheless, high urinary 5-HIAA levels have been reported in up to 23% of foregut carcinoids with distant metastases,[56,57] and somatostatin analogues should be commenced before surgical or locoregional interventions to prevent carcinoid crisis.[58] Screening for carcinoid heart disease is also recommended.

PRO-OPIOMELANOCORTIN

Ectopic ACTH-secreting tumors typically do not process POMC efficiently, leading to increased prevalence of ACTH precursors in the circulation.[59] A higher POMC or pro-ACTH to ACTH ratio has been found in the EAS compared with Cushing's disease, and this may be a useful discriminative test in the future.[59]

IMMUNOHISTOCHEMISTRY

Tumor immunostaining for ACTH can be negative in up to 30% of ACTH-secreting tumors[1,10] and cannot be used to retrospectively validate biochemical tests. Although this finding has been attributed to the high secretory capacity of some tumors, negative ACTH immunostaining has also been reported in occult tumors with modest hormone secretion.[20] Other explanations for negative immunostaining include dedifferentiation of the tumor, the presence of ACTH precursors that do not react with the antibodies used, poor fixation during immunohistochemistry or, of course, that the identified tumor has been wrongly assumed to be the ectopic source.[10,20]

LOCALIZATION OF THE ADRENOCORTICOTROPIC HORMONE–SECRETING TUMOR AND STAGING

Localization of the source of ectopic ACTH secretion is crucial because it can avoid adrenalectomy and reduce the risk of metastatic disease. Although aggressive malignancies, like SCLC, are usually rapidly diagnosed, the localization of pulmonary carcinoids can be challenging because of their small size and usual location in the middle third of the lung adjacent to pulmonary vasculature from which they cannot readily be differentiated on computed tomography (CT) or MRI.[60]

Axial imaging with contrast-enhanced CT, MRI, and scintigraphic studies localize ACTH-secreting tumors in 70% to 90% of cases.[1,2] The introduction of functional imaging has greatly increased the capacity to diagnose NETs, including those causing the EAS (**Fig. 2**).[61] A systematic review, including 231 EAS cases (with only small numbers of SCLC), demonstrated that although approximately half of EAS sources are readily identified on cross-sectional imaging, extensive investigations are needed to discover elusive tumors in up to 30%.[19] In these patients, nuclear imaging identified 80% of tumors not seen on conventional imaging. Nineteen percent of ACTH-secreting tumors remained occult despite intensive investigation; however, in patients who underwent ^{68}Ga-DOTA-somatostatin analogue positron emission tomography (PET)/CT, no tumor remained occult, suggesting superiority over all other imaging techniques in which a significant number of tumors remained elusive. A role for ^{111}In-pentetreotide scintigraphy and ^{18}F-fluorodeoxyglucose (^{18}F-FDG) PET/CT in the detection of ACTH-secreting tumors was also demonstrated. ^{111}In-pentetreotide scintigraphy, with low false positive rate, was shown to be a good study to confirm abnormalities detected on CT or MRI. However, although ^{111}In-pentetreotide scintigraphy is considered a specific test (92%–100%) for the detection of carcinoid tumors, it is known to be considerably less sensitive (60%–80%) than ^{68}Ga-DOTA-somatostatin analogue PET/CT (88%–93%).[61] In addition, in those patients who had negative conventional and somatostatin receptor imaging,[19] the next best performing test to identify ACTH-secreting tumors was ^{18}F-FDG PET/CT; ^{18}F-FDG PET/CT has more utility in G3 and high G2 carcinoid tumors, which generally have higher glucose

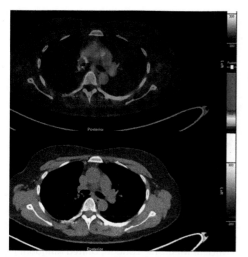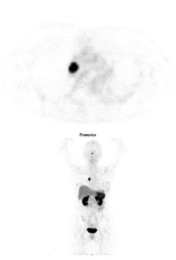

Fig. 2. Borderline enlarged right hilar lymph node (11 mm) with intense DOTATATE avidity on ^{68}Ga DOTATATE PET/CT in a 46-year-old woman with recurrence of EAS 19 years after right middle and upper lobectomy for a typical pulmonary carcinoid tumor. Patient remains in complete remission 3 years after repeat thoracotomy and resection of right hilar node (which confirmed metastatic typical pulmonary carcinoid). (*Courtesy of* Dr Shaunak Naval-kissoor, Department of Nuclear Medicine, Royal Free Hospital, London, United Kingdom.)

metabolism and less somatostatin receptor expression compared with low-grade carcinoid tumors.[61] Some EAS series have demonstrated a high proportion of patients with G2 and G3 carcinoid tumors,[10,15] and this may justify the use of ^{18}F-FDG PET/CT in patients with occult disease and negative somatostatin receptor imaging. Finally, some tumors may not express the somatostatin subtype-2 receptor in the presence of high circulating glucocorticoids, but these may be visualized when such levels are lowered medically.[62]

Apart from patients with typical pulmonary carcinoids, more than half of patients with ACTH-secreting carcinoid tumors present with metastatic disease.[15] Complete staging is therefore critical before consideration of surgery and requires a multimodality approach. CT imaging of liver metastases and pancreatic carcinoids is inferior to that of MRI,[61] and dynamic contrast-enhanced MRI is therefore the preferred modality for imaging of the pancreas and liver.[61] ^{68}Ga-DOTA-somatostatin analogue PET/CT provides high sensitivity (88%–93%) and specificity (88%–95%) for the diagnosis and staging of carcinoid tumors and is an important component of the preoperative assessment (**Fig. 3**).[61] It is more specific than conventional imaging in well-differentiated carcinoid tumors and will often diagnose lymph node and bone metastases not characterized on CT or MRI.[61]

MANAGEMENT OF THE ECTOPIC ADRENOCORTICOTROPIC HORMONE SYNDROME

The optimal treatment of the EAS is surgical resection of the tumor with curative intent. However, this relies on localization of the tumor before the development of distant metastases, and hence, is dependent on the underlying malignant potential of the disease. In the setting of well-differentiated carcinoid tumors, patients with limited lymph node involvement or small-volume hepatic metastases may be considered for metastasectomy or liver-directed therapies (eg, transarterial embolization, radiofrequency ablation) with the chance of cure.

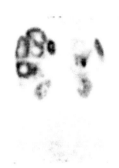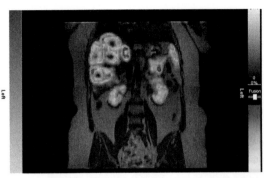

Fig. 3. ^{68}Ga DOTATATE PET/MRI in a 45-year-old woman who presented with slow onset of classical signs and symptoms of Cushing's syndrome. Scan demonstrates DOTATATE avid pancreatic tail neuroendocrine tumor and extensive bilobar liver metastases with central photopenia likely secondary to tumor necrosis. Liver biopsy confirmed a well-differentiated neuroendocrine tumor of intermediate grade (Ki-67 5%) with morphology consistent with pancreatic primary. (*Courtesy of* Dr Simon Wan, Institute of Nuclear Medicine, London, United Kingdom.)

Steroidogenesis inhibitors are the mainstay of treatment to gain control of hypercortisolemia and should be commenced promptly. Ketoconazole and metyrapone are favored for their efficacy and safety, and metyrapone is often used first line for its rapid therapeutic onset.[5,20] The new drug, osilodrostat, is pharmacologically related to metyrapone and is currently under trial. The glucocorticoid receptor antagonist, mifepristone, has been shown to be effective in small, retrospective EAS series,[63] although a major disadvantage compared with the steroidogenesis inhibitors is the lack of ability to follow cortisol levels to titrate treatment. Severe hypokalemia has also been reported as well as endometrial hyperplasia due to its antiprogestin activity.[63] Mitotane acts as an adrenolytic drug and is very slow in onset, but in view of its serious side effects (neurological and gastrointestinal), it is rarely used outside the setting of adrenocortical carcinoma.[6] Etomidate infusions have been used successfully when rapid control of hypercortisolism is required in the intensive care setting.[64] Steroidogenesis inhibitors should ideally be commenced before chemotherapy, but the dose may require downtitration or the addition of adequate steroid replacement once chemotherapy has commenced.

Therapy with steroidogenesis inhibitors can be continued for prolonged periods in patients with occult disease, allowing serial imaging over months to years in an attempt to identify the tumor. However, in the setting of indolent disease, it may take many years, sometimes decades, before the source is identified,[20] and bilateral adrenalectomy is often required to achieve biochemical cure. Other reasons for adrenalectomy include failed medical therapy, drug intolerance, and in patients with unresectable but indolent disease resulting in a presumptive prolonged survival. Rarely, bilateral adrenalectomy is performed in young women desiring pregnancy in whom steroidogenesis inhibitors are contraindicated. In 2 of the largest series,[1,2] 30% to 37% of EAS patients required bilateral adrenalectomy, and global experience with the less invasive laparoscopic approach has shown a dramatically decreased short-term morbidity of this procedure.[65,66] Patients treated with adrenalectomy require life-long glucocorticoid and mineralocorticoid replacement, and patient education is imperative to avoid acute episodes of adrenal insufficiency. In addition, patients with hypercortisolism controlled by any of the above measures may occasionally develop rebound thymic hyperplasia, which is important to recognize, especially in those patients with occult EAS, because it can be misinterpreted radiologically as tumor.[67]

Other potential treatment options to control hypercortisolemia in patients with unresectable or occult carcinoid tumors include somatostatin analogues and dopamine agonists, owing to frequent receptor coexpression.[68,69] These therapies may be useful, either alone or in combination, and complete responses have been described in small case series.[69,70] Treatment escapes, however, are frequent.[70,71]

For patients with unresectable or disseminated disease, tumor-directed therapy is guided by the underlying tumor histology and the fitness of the patient. SCLC requires an aggressive approach, often with concurrent platinum-based chemotherapy and thoracic radiotherapy, dependent on the stage of the disease. Antitumor therapy for carcinoid tumors encompasses a variety of treatments, including somatostatin analogues, peptide receptor radionuclide therapy, everolimus and sunitinib, cytotoxic chemotherapy, liver-directed therapies, and palliative hepatic debulking surgery. Given the impressive results of the NETTER-1 trial,[72] all patients with progressive, well-differentiated carcinoid tumors and adequate somatostatin receptor expression should be considered for peptide receptor radionuclide therapy. Promisingly, cases of remission of hypercortisolism after ^{177}Lu-DOTATATE have also been described in patients with ACTH-secreting carcinoid tumors.[15,73] In a multicenter, retrospective series by Davi and colleagues[15] (n = 110), 13 patients with EAS and adequate somatostatin receptor expression (6 pulmonary, 2 thymic, and 5 pancreatic carcinoids) were treated with peptide receptor radionuclide therapy of whom 10 (77%) obtained partial (>50% decrease in cortisol levels) or complete hormonal remission. Prospective studies are needed to validate these findings and characterize the durability of response.

PROGNOSIS

The prognosis of patients with the EAS is determined by both tumor histology and the severity of hypercortisolism, since both affect morbidity and mortality.[1,2,10,15] In all series, EAS patients with SCLC have the poorest survival with most patients dying within 12 months.[1,2] EAS has been demonstrated as a prognostic factor for early demise in SCLC patients. In a recent study of 383 patients with SCLC,[9] those with EAS (n = 23; 6%) had more extensive disease, greater weight loss, and a reduced objective response rate to first-line treatment (48% vs 71% in those with and without EAS, respectively). Median overall survival for those patients with SCLC and EAS was 6.6 months versus 13.1 months in patients without EAS or other paraneoplastic syndromes.

The presence of EAS also appears to shorten survival in patients with unresectable carcinoid tumors. Kamp and colleagues[10] reported a significantly shorter 5-year survival in 29 carcinoid patients with the EAS compared with 889 carcinoid patients without the EAS, despite a higher proportion of patients with distant metastatic disease in the non-EAS cohort (5-year survival 65% EAS vs 75% non-EAS, $P = .013$, log-rank test). In patients with the EAS, Kamp and colleagues[10] reported 8 deaths due to progression of metastatic disease and 5 deaths due to complications of hypercortisolism, including opportunistic infections, cardiac failure, and pulmonary embolism. Interestingly, this difference in survival between the EAS and non-EAS cohorts was no longer significant over complete duration of follow-up, and this may be explained by the proportion of EAS patients who successfully underwent curative surgery (7/29; 24%). Severity of hypercortisolism at diagnosis also appears to have a negative impact on prognosis. Davi and colleagues[15] demonstrated that those EAS patients with serum cortisol levels greater than 3-fold ($P<.001$, log-rank test) or urinary free cortisol greater than 5-fold ($P = .005$, log-rank test) had a significantly poorer 5-year survival compared with those patients with lower hormone levels.

Patients with carcinoid tumors and well-controlled hypercortisolism have prognoses determined by the underlying tumor pathological grade and stage of the disease, which are strongly linked.[74] Patients with typical pulmonary carcinoids tend to have the best prognosis.[1,2,15] In the previously mentioned study by Davi and colleagues,[15] ACTH-secreting typical pulmonary carcinoids had the lowest rates of distant metastases at 13% (followed by atypical pulmonary carcinoids 50%, pancreatic carcinoids 77%, thymic carcinoids 83%) and, therefore, the highest rates of curative surgery. Five-year survival for patients with ACTH-secreting pulmonary carcinoids (67% typical morphology; 27% atypical morphology) was 86%, and this parallels the general pulmonary carcinoid literature with documented 5-year survival of typical pulmonary carcinoids of 87% to 90%.[75,76] Furthermore, similar to the general carcinoid literature, Davi and colleagues[15] demonstrated a significantly worse 5-year survival in patients with G3 ACTH-secreting carcinoid tumors (G1 88%, G2 72%, G3 37%; $P = .007$, log-rank test) and in patients with distant metastases (47% vs 82% in patients without distant metastases; $P<.001$, log-rank test). Patients with an occult source of ACTH, most frequently a focal pulmonary carcinoid, tend to have a good prognosis, although this is dependent on effective control of hypercortisolism.[1] In most series, ACTH-secreting thymic carcinoids, pancreatic carcinoids, and MTCs tend to present with more aggressive disease and distant metastases, and consequently have poorer overall survival.[1,2,15]

Despite typical pulmonary carcinoids having an excellent 5-year survival, distant recurrences have been reported many years later, even following a radical resection of the primary tumor.[74,77,78] In the EAS series by Ilias and colleagues,[2] 3 patients with typical pulmonary carcinoids, who had successful curative resections and no lymph node involvement, relapsed after a mean of 10.7 years after surgery. Hence, long-term follow-up is recommended in all EAS patients, including those with presumed surgical cure, and surveillance is critical to detect surgically manageable recurrences.[58]

SUMMARY AND RECOMMENDATIONS

- Pulmonary carcinoid tumors are now recognized as the most frequent cause of the EAS.
- ACTH-secreting pulmonary carcinoids, like corticotroph tumors producing Cushing's disease, are often small and difficult to localize, and patients may present with a gradual onset of the classical signs and symptoms of Cushing's syndrome, indistinguishable from the presentation of Cushing's disease. All testing procedures should be considered to be probabilistic rather than algorithmic.
- Biochemical dynamic tests have variable sensitivity and specificity and have more discriminatory power when interpreted in combination. They should be interpreted cautiously, however, in patients with modestly elevated cortisol levels or in the setting of recent use of steroidogenesis inhibitors, because corticotroph cells may not be adequately suppressed and retain responsivity.
- BIPSS should be considered in those patients with ACTH-dependent Cushing's syndrome and an equivocal pituitary MRI (lesions <6 mm) or discordant dynamic tests.

- A positive BIPSS is a strong indicator of Cushing's disease. Although false positives can occur (the presence of a central-to-peripheral gradient in a patient with the EAS), they are rare. False negatives (the absence of a central-to-peripheral gradient in a patient with Cushing's disease) are, however, more common than previously appreciated, and a negative BIPSS does not necessarily exclude Cushing's disease.
- Localization of the source of ectopic ACTH secretion is crucial because it can avoid adrenalectomy and reduce the risk of metastatic disease.
- Most ACTH-secreting tumors are nowadays localized on CT, MRI, and/or scintigraphy.
- ^{68}Ga-DOTA-somatostatin analogue PET/CT has the highest sensitivity in localizing ACTH-secreting tumors not detected on initial investigation.
- In those patients with occult disease, repeat assessment should continue over lifelong follow-up in an attempt to identify the tumor.
- The lung remains the most likely location of an occult tumor.
- Prognosis is determined by both tumor histology and severity of hypercortisolism. Patients with typical pulmonary carcinoid tumors have the lowest rates of metastatic disease and best prognosis.
- For patients with carcinoid tumors not amenable to curative resection, a multidisciplinary approach should be adopted, including somatostatin analogue therapy, peptide receptor radionuclide therapy, chemotherapy, targeted therapies, and liver-directed therapies.

REFERENCES

1. Isidori AM, Kaltsas GA, Pozza C, et al. The ectopic adrenocorticotropin syndrome: clinical features, diagnosis, management, and long-term follow-up. J Clin Endocrinol Metab 2006;91(2):371–7.
2. Ilias I, Torpy DJ, Pacak K, et al. Cushing's syndrome due to ectopic corticotropin secretion: twenty years' experience at the National Institutes of Health. J Clin Endocrinol Metab 2005;90(8):4955–62.
3. Imura H, Matsukura S, Yamamoto H, et al. Studies on ectopic ACTH-producing tumors. II. Clinical and biochemical features of 30 cases. Cancer 1975;35(5): 1430–7.
4. Liddle G, Nicholson W, Island D, et al. Clinical and laboratory studies of ectopic humoral syndromes. Recent Prog Horm Res 1969;25:283–314.
5. Isidori AM, Lenzi A. Ectopic ACTH syndrome. Arq Bras Endocrinol Metabol 2007; 51(8):1217–25.
6. Lacroix A, Feelders RA, Stratakis CA, et al. Cushing's syndrome. Lancet 2015; 386(9996):913–27.
7. Bolland MJ, Holdaway IM, Berkeley JE, et al. Mortality and morbidity in Cushing's syndrome in New Zealand. Clin Endocrinol 2011;75(4):436–42.
8. Delisle L, Boyer MJ, Warr D, et al. Ectopic corticotropin syndrome and small-cell carcinoma of the lung: clinical features, outcome, and complications. Arch Intern Med 1993;153(6):746–52.
9. Nagy-Mignotte H, Shestaeva O, Vignoud L, et al. Prognostic impact of paraneoplastic Cushing's syndrome in small-cell lung cancer. J Thorac Oncol 2014;9(4): 497–505.
10. Kamp K, Alwani R, Korpershoek E, et al. Prevalence and clinical features of the ectopic ACTH syndrome in patients with gastroenteropancreatic and thoracic neuroendocrine tumors. Eur J Endocrinol 2016;174(3):271–80.

11. Barbosa SL-S, Rodien P, Leboulleux S, et al. Ectopic adrenocorticotropic hormone-syndrome in medullary carcinoma of the thyroid: a retrospective analysis and review of the literature. Thyroid 2005;15(6):618–23.

12. Jia R, Sulentic P, Xu J-M, et al. Thymic neuroendocrine neoplasms: biological behaviour and therapy. Neuroendocrinology 2017;105:105–14.

13. Ye L, Li X, Kong X, et al. Hypomethylation in the promoter region of POMC gene correlates with ectopic overexpression in thymic carcinoids. J Endocrinol 2005;185(2):337–43.

14. Newell-Price J, King P, Clark AJ. The CpG island promoter of the human proopiomelanocortin gene is methylated in nonexpressing normal tissue and tumors and represses expression. Mol Endocrinol 2001;15(2):338–48.

15. Davi MV, Cosaro E, Piacentini S, et al. Prognostic factors in ectopic Cushing's syndrome due to neuroendocrine tumors: a multicenter study. Eur J Endocrinol 2017;176(4):453–61.

16. Beuschlein F, Hammer GD. Ectopic pro-opiomelanocortin syndrome. Endocrinol Metab Clin North Am 2002;31(1):191–234.

17. Woo YS, Isidori AM, Wat WZ, et al. Clinical and biochemical characteristics of adrenocorticotropin-secreting macroadenomas. J Clin Endocrinol Metab 2005;90(8):4963–9.

18. Trott M, Farah G, Stokes V, et al. A thymic neuroendocrine tumour in a young female: a rare cause of relapsing and remitting Cushing's syndrome. Endocrinol Diabetes Metab case Rep 2016;2016:160018.

19. Isidori AM, Sbardella E, Zatelli MC, et al. Conventional and nuclear medicine imaging in ectopic Cushing's syndrome: a systematic review. J Clin Endocrinol Metab 2015;100(9):3231–44.

20. Grossman AB, Kelly P, Rockall A, et al. Cushing's syndrome caused by an occult source: difficulties in diagnosis and management. Nat Rev Endocrinol 2006;2(11):642.

21. Aron DC, Howlett TA. Pituitary incidentalomas. Endocrinol Metab Clin North Am 2000;29(1):205–21.

22. Newell-Price J, Bertagna X, Grossman AB, et al. Cushing's syndrome. Lancet 2006;367(9522):1605–17.

23. Liddle GW. Tests of pituitary-adrenal suppressibility in the diagnosis of Cushing's syndrome. J Clin Endocrinol Metab 1960;20(12):1539–60.

24. Strott CA, Nugent CA, Tyler FH. Cushing's syndrome caused by bronchial adenomas. Am J Med 1968;44(1):97–104.

25. Crapo L. Cushing's syndrome: a review of diagnostic tests. Metabolism 1979;28(9):955–77.

26. Hermus A, Pesman G, Benraad T, et al. The corticotropin-releasing-hormone test versus the high-dose dexamethasone test in the differential diagnosis of Cushing's syndrome. Lancet 1986;328(8506):540–4.

27. Grossman A, Howlett T, Perry L, et al. CRF in the differential diagnosis of Cushing's syndrome: a comparison with the dexamethasone suppression test. Clin Endocrinol 1988;29(2):167–78.

28. Dichek HL, Nieman LK, Oldfield EH, et al. A comparison of the standard high dose dexamethasone suppression test and the overnight 8-mg dexamethasone suppression test for the differential diagnosis of adrenocorticotropin-dependent Cushing's syndrome. J Clin Endocrinol Metab 1994;78(2):418–22.

29. Flack MR, Oldfield EH, Cutler GB, et al. Urine free cortisol in the high-dose dexamethasone suppression test for the differential diagnosis of the Cushing syndrome. Ann Intern Med 1992;116(3):211–7.

30. Howlett T, Drury P, Perry L, et al. Diagnosis and management of ACTH-dependent Cushing's syndrome: comparison of the features in ectopic and pituitary ACTH production. Clin Endocrinol 1986;24(6):699–713.
31. Tyrrell JB, Findling JW, Aron DC, et al. An overnight high-dose dexamethasone suppression test for rapid differential diagnosis of Cushing's syndrome. Ann Intern Med 1986;104(2):180–6.
32. Isidori AM, Kaltsas GA, Mohammed S, et al. Discriminatory value of the low-dose dexamethasone suppression test in establishing the diagnosis and differential diagnosis of Cushing's syndrome. J Clin Endocrinol Metab 2003;88(11): 5299–306.
33. Salgado LR, Fragoso MCBV, Knoepfelmacher M, et al. Ectopic ACTH syndrome: our experience with 25 cases. Eur J Endocrinol 2006;155(5):725–33.
34. Newell-Price J, Trainer P, Besser M, et al. The diagnosis and differential diagnosis of Cushing's syndrome and pseudo-Cushing's states. Endocr Rev 1998;19(5): 647–72.
35. Aron DC, Raff H, Findling JW. Effectiveness versus efficacy: the limited value in clinical practice of high dose dexamethasone suppression testing in the differential diagnosis of adrenocorticotropin-dependent Cushing's syndrome. J Clin Endocrinol Metab 1997;82(6):1780–5.
36. Nieman LK, Oldfield EH, Wesley R, et al. A simplified morning ovine corticotropin-releasing hormone stimulation test for the differential diagnosis of adrenocorticotropin-dependent Cushing's syndrome. J Clin Endocrinol Metab 1993;77(5):1308–12.
37. Newell-Price J, Morris D, Drake W, et al. Optimal response criteria for the human CRH test in the differential diagnosis of ACTH-dependent Cushing's syndrome. J Clin Endocrinol Metab 2002;87(4):1640–5.
38. Kaye T, Crapo L. The Cushing syndrome: an update on diagnostic tests. Ann Intern Med 1990;112:434–44.
39. Nieman L, Cutler G Jr, Oldfield E, et al. The ovine corticotropin-releasing hormone (CRH) stimulation test is superior to the human CRH stimulation test for the diagnosis of Cushing's disease. J Clin Endocrinol Metab 1989;69(1):165–9.
40. Nakahara M, Shibasaki T, Shizume K, et al. Corticotropin-releasing factor test in normal subjects and patients with hypothalamic-pituitary-adrenal disorders. J Clin Endocrinol Metab 1983;57(5):963–8.
41. Chrousos GP, Schulte HM, Oldfield EH, et al. The corticotropin-releasing factor stimulation test: an aid in the evaluation of patients with Cushing's syndrome. N Engl J Med 1984;310(10):622–6.
42. Luque R, Ibáñez-Costa A, López-Sánchez L, et al. A cellular and molecular basis for the selective desmopressin-induced ACTH release in Cushing disease patients: key role of AVPR1b receptor and potential therapeutic implications. J Clin Endocrinol Metab 2013;98(10):4160–9.
43. Tsagarakis S, Tsigos C, Vasiliou V, et al. The desmopressin and combined CRH-desmopressin tests in the differential diagnosis of ACTH-dependent Cushing's syndrome: constraints imposed by the expression of V2 vasopressin receptors in tumors with ectopic ACTH secretion. J Clin Endocrinol Metab 2002;87(4): 1646–53.
44. Newell-Price J. The desmopressin test and Cushing's syndrome: current state of play. Clin Endocrinol 1997;47(2):173.
45. Arlt W, Dahia P, Callies F, et al. Ectopic ACTH production by a bronchial carcinoid tumour responsive to desmopressin in vivo and in vitro. Clin Endocrinol 1997; 47(5):623–7.

46. Nieman L, Chrousos G, Oldfield E, et al. The ovine corticotropin-releasing hormone stimulation test and the dexamethasone suppression test in the differential diagnosis of Cushing's syndrome. Ann Intern Med 1986;105(6):862.

47. Invitti C, Giraldi FP, De Martin M, et al. Diagnosis and management of Cushing's syndrome: results of an Italian multicentre study. J Clin Endocrinol Metab 1999; 84(2):440–8.

48. Arnaldi G, Angeli A, Atkinson A, et al. Diagnosis and complications of Cushing's syndrome: a consensus statement. J Clin Endocrinol Metab 2003;88(12): 5593–602.

49. Kaltsas G, Giannulis M, Newell-Price J, et al. A critical analysis of the value of simultaneous inferior petrosal sinus sampling in Cushing's disease and the occult ectopic adrenocorticotropin syndrome. J Clin Endocrinol Metab 1999;84(2): 487–92.

50. Lopez J, Barcelo B, Lucas T, et al. Petrosal sinus sampling for diagnosis of Cushing's disease: evidence of false negative results. Clin Endocrinol 1996;45(2): 147–56.

51. Yamamoto Y, Davis DH, Nippoldt TB, et al. False-positive inferior petrosal sinus sampling in the diagnosis of Cushing's disease: report of two cases. J Neurosurg 1995;83(6):1087–91.

52. Swearingen B, Katznelson L, Miller K, et al. Diagnostic errors after inferior petrosal sinus sampling. J Clin Endocrinol Metab 2004;89(8):3752–63.

53. Findling JW, Raff H. Diagnosis and differential diagnosis of Cushing's syndrome. Endocrinol Metab Clin North Am 2001;30(3):729–47.

54. Doppman JL, Chang R, Oldfield EH, et al. The hypoplastic inferior petrosal sinus: a potential source of false-negative results in petrosal sampling for Cushing's disease. J Clin Endocrinol Metab 1999;84(2):533–40.

55. Wind JJ, Lonser RR, Nieman LK, et al. The lateralization accuracy of inferior petrosal sinus sampling in 501 patients with Cushing's disease. J Clin Endocrinol Metab 2013;98(6):2285–93.

56. Norheim I, Oberg K, Theodorsson-Norheim E, et al. Malignant carcinoid tumors. An analysis of 103 patients with regard to tumor localization, hormone production, and survival. Ann Surg 1987;206(2):115.

57. Ferolla P, Brizzi MP, Meyer T, et al. Efficacy and safety of long-acting pasireotide or everolimus alone or in combination in patients with advanced carcinoids of the lung and thymus (LUNA): an open-label, multicentre, randomised, phase 2 trial. Lancet Oncol 2017;18(12):1652–64.

58. Caplin ME, Baudin E, Ferolla P, et al. Pulmonary neuroendocrine (carcinoid) tumors: European Neuroendocrine Tumor Society expert consensus and recommendations for best practice for typical and atypical pulmonary carcinoids. Ann Oncol 2015;26(8):1604–20.

59. Oliver RL, Davis JR, White A. Characterisation of ACTH related peptides in ectopic Cushing's syndrome. Pituitary 2003;6(3):119–26.

60. Doppman J, Pass H, Nieman L, et al. Detection of ACTH-producing bronchial carcinoid tumors: MR imaging vs CT. AJR Am J Roentgenol 1991;156(1):39–43.

61. Sundin A, Arnold R, Baudin E, et al. ENETS consensus guidelines for the standards of care in neuroendocrine tumors: radiological, nuclear medicine and hybrid imaging. Neuroendocrinology 2017;105(2):212–44.

62. de Bruin C, Hofland L, Nieman L, et al. Mifepristone effects on tumor somatostatin receptor expression in two patients with Cushing's syndrome due to ectopic adrenocorticotropin secretion. J Clin Endocrinol Metab 2012;97(2):455–62.

63. Castinetti F, Conte-Devolx B, Brue T. Medical treatment of Cushing's syndrome: glucocorticoid receptor antagonists and mifepristone. Neuroendocrinology 2010;92(Suppl. 1):125–30.
64. Preda VA, Sen J, Karavitaki N, et al. Etomidate in the management of hypercortisolaemia in Cushing's syndrome: a review. Eur J Endocrinol 2012;167:137–43.
65. Thompson SK, Hayman AV, Ludlam WH, et al. Improved quality of life after bilateral laparoscopic adrenalectomy for Cushing's disease: a 10-year experience. Ann Surg 2007;245(5):790.
66. Ritzel K, Beuschlein F, Mickisch A, et al. Outcome of bilateral adrenalectomy in Cushing's syndrome: a systematic review. J Clin Endocrinol Metab 2013; 98(10):3939–48.
67. Tabarin A, Catargi B, Chanson P, et al. Pseudo-tumours of the thymus after correction of hypercortisolism in patients with ectopic ACTH syndrome: a report of five cases. Clin Endocrinol 1995;42(2):207–13.
68. de Bruin C, Feelders R, Lamberts S, et al. Somatostatin and dopamine receptors as targets for medical treatment of Cushing's syndrome. Rev Endocr Metab Disord 2009;10(2):91.
69. Pivonello R, Ferone D, de Herder W, et al. Dopamine receptor expression and function in corticotroph ectopic tumors. J Clin Endocrinol Metab 2007;92(1):65.
70. Pivonello R, Ferone D, Lamberts SW, et al. Cabergoline plus lanreotide for ectopic Cushing's syndrome. N Engl J Med 2005;352(23):2457–8.
71. Hofland LJ, Lamberts SW. The pathophysiological consequences of somatostatin receptor internalization and resistance. Endocr Rev 2003;24(1):28–47.
72. Strosberg J, El-Haddad G, Wolin E, et al. Phase 3 trial of 177Lu-Dotatate for midgut neuroendocrine tumors. N Engl J Med 2017;376(2):125–35.
73. Makis W, McCann K, Riauka TA, et al. Ectopic corticotropin-producing neuroendocrine tumor of the pancreas treated with 177Lu DOTATATE induction and maintenance peptide receptor radionuclide therapy. Clin Nucl Med 2016;41(1):50–2.
74. Yao JC, Hassan M, Phan A, et al. One hundred years after "carcinoid": epidemiology of and prognostic factors for neuroendocrine tumors in 35,825 cases in the United States. J Clin Oncol 2008;26(18):3063–72.
75. Travis W, Rush W, Flieder D, et al. Survival analysis of 200 pulmonary neuroendocrine tumors with clarification of criteria for atypical carcinoid and its separation from typical carcinoid. Am J Surg Pathol 1998;22(8):934.
76. Fink G, Krelbaum T, Yellin A, et al. Pulmonary carcinoid: presentation, diagnosis, and outcome in 142 cases in Israel and review of 640 cases from the literature. Chest 2001;119(6):1647–51.
77. Lou F, Sarkaria I, Pietanza C, et al. Recurrence of pulmonary carcinoid tumors after resection: implications for postoperative surveillance. Ann Thorac Surg 2013; 96(4):1156–62.
78. Perez EA, Koniaris LG, Snell SE, et al. 7201 carcinoids: increasing incidence overall and disproportionate mortality in the elderly. World J Surg 2007;31(5): 1022–30.

Medical Therapy for Cushing's Syndrome in the Twenty-first Century

Nicholas A. Tritos, MD, DSc[a],*, Beverly M.K. Biller, MD[b]

KEYWORDS

- Cushing's syndrome • Cushing's disease • Ketoconazole • Metyrapone • Mitotane
- Etomidate • Cabergoline • Pasireotide

KEY POINTS

- Medical therapy is useful as adjunct treatment in the management of Cushing's syndrome.
- Available medications include steroidogenesis inhibitors, centrally acting agents, and glucocorticoid receptor antagonists.
- The choice between medical treatment options is empiric and requires a careful assessment of risks and benefits of each therapeutic option for an individual patient.
- Several investigational agents are currently under study as potential therapies for Cushing's syndrome.
- Novel medical therapies may be developed as a consequence of better understanding of the pathogenesis of the tumors underlying Cushing's syndrome.

INTRODUCTION

Prompt control of hypercortisolism is needed to reverse clinical and biochemical manifestations and decrease excess morbidity and mortality in patients with endogenous Cushing's syndrome (CS).[1–4] Resection of the underlying tumor is currently the mainstay of treatment of CS.[3] After trans-sphenoidal pituitary surgery, persistent or recurrent hypercortisolism may occur in, respectively, 10% to 20% and 20% to 30% of patients with pituitary corticotroph adenomas (ie, Cushing's disease [CD]), which

Disclosure Statement: Dr N.A. Tritos has received institution-directed research support from Ipsen, Novartis, Novo Nordisk, and Pfizer. Dr B.M.K. Biller has received institution-directed research support from Cortendo and Novartis and occasional consulting honoraria from Cortendo, Novartis, Novo Nordisk, Sandoz, and Pfizer.

[a] Neuroendocrine Unit, Neuroendocrine Clinical Center, Massachusetts General Hospital, Harvard Medical School, 100 Blossom Street, Cox 1, Suite 140, Boston, MA 02114, USA; [b] Neuroendocrine Unit, Massachusetts General Hospital, Harvard Medical School, 55 Fruit Street, Bulfinch 4, Boston, MA 02114, USA
* Corresponding author.
E-mail address: ntritos@mgh.harvard.edu

underlies approximately 70% of all cases of CS.[3,4] In other patients, the underlying tumor may be difficult to localize or can be unresectable, including in some patients with corticotroph macroadenomas, metastatic neuroendocrine tumors or advanced adrenocortical carcinomas.

The role of medical therapy in CS/CD is currently adjunctive.[3] Medications are often used to control hypercortisolism in patients with CD who have failed trans-sphenoidal pituitary surgery and have received radiation therapy to the sella.[5,6] In these patients, it may take several years for the salutary effects of radiation therapy to develop. In addition, medical therapy may be advised to stabilize the condition of acutely ill patients with CS/CD, who are not fit to undergo definitive surgery immediately. Medical therapy can also be recommended in patients whose surgery has been deferred for various reasons or those whose tumor location is uncertain. Patients with unresectable or metastatic tumors may also benefit from medical therapy to control hypercortisolism. The care of patients with CS/CD generally requires a multimodality approach involving experienced physicians from several disciplines (surgery, neurosurgery, endocrinology, radiation oncology, and medical oncology).

The aims of the present article are to outline current and novel medical therapies for patients with CS/CD. To retrieve pertinent articles, electronic literature searches were conducted using the keyword, CS, CD, medical therapy, treatment, ketoconazole, metyrapone, mitotane, etomidate, cabergoline, pasireotide, and mifepristone. Articles cited in this review were included based on the authors' judgment.

The primary goal of medical therapy is to control hypercortisolism, thereby ameliorating symptoms and signs of CS. Most studies of medical therapies have used 24-hour urine-free cortisol (UFC) as the primary endpoint for efficacy.[3] In addition, some studies have examined the effect of medical therapies on late-night salivary cortisol, a measure of nadir cortisol levels in patients with typical sleep wakefulness cycles, third shift workers thus being excluded.[7] All medications used to treat CS/CD have the potential to decrease cortisol levels and/or mitigate cortisol action below normal, leading to potentially life-threatening hypoadrenalism.[3] Therefore, all patients receiving medical therapy for CS/CD require close follow-up and regular monitoring to establish clinical effectiveness, avert hypoadrenalism, and detect and manage other adverse effects.[5,8]

As shown in **Fig. 1**, medications for CS can be categorized depending on their site of action, including steroidogenesis inhibitors (which inhibit 1 or several enzymes involved in cortisol biosynthesis), centrally acting agents (which interfere with corticotropin release from pituitary corticotroph tumors), and glucocorticoid receptor (GR) antagonists (which inhibit cortisol action).[3] With the exception of pasireotide and mifepristone, agents discussed in this article have not been specifically labeled by the United States Food and Drug Administration (FDA) as therapies for CS/CD. Pasireotide, ketoconazole, and metyrapone are licensed by the European Medicines Agency for CS/CD.

STEROIDOGENESIS INHIBITORS

Steroidogenesis inhibitors in use in CS include ketoconazole, metyrapone, mitotane, and etomidate (**Table 1**).[3] Currently available drugs in this group have been studied in case series but not in controlled clinical trials. Investigational steroidogenesis inhibitors that are in clinical development include osilodrostat (LCI699) (clinicaltrials. gov: NCT02468193 and clinicaltrials.gov: NCT02697734) and levoketoconazole (clinicaltrials.gov: NCT01838551). Steroidogenesis inhibitors have been studied and

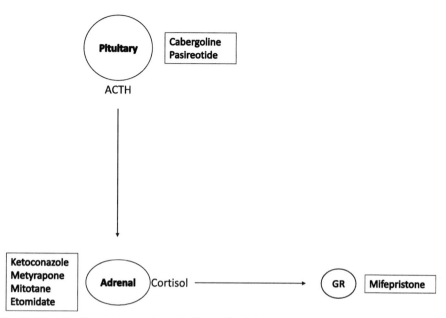

Fig. 1. Site of action of currently available medical therapies for CS. With the exception of pasireotide and mifepristone, available agents are currently used off-label in the United States. ACTH, corticotropin.

can be effective in patients with CS of diverse etiologies because they decrease adrenal secretion of cortisol regardless of the source of cortisol excess.

Steroidogenesis inhibitors are usually titrated to normal 24-hour UFC while monitoring for the development of hypoadrenalism and assuring drug tolerance.[3] Alternatively, these agents can be used in a block and replace regimen, aiming at completely suppressing endogenous cortisol secretion (usually based on 24-h UFC values), while glucocorticoid replacement is being administered to prevent the development of hypoadrenalism. This latter regimen can be particularly helpful in patients with intermittent (cyclic) CS/CD. Caution is advised in using a block and replace regimen, however, because it is possible for these patients to remain hypercortisolemic as a consequence of incompletely suppressed endogenous cortisol secretion and/or to receive excessive exogenous replacement. Because tachyphylaxis may occur over time in some patients receiving steroidogenesis inhibitors (sometimes termed, escape), all patients under treatment require regular long-term monitoring.

Ketoconazole

Ketoconazole is an imidazole derivative that was originally developed as an orally active antifungal agent. In addition, ketoconazole was found to inhibit multiple enzymes involved in adrenal steroidogenesis, thus decreasing cortisol biosynthesis and secretion.[9] It has also been suggested that ketoconazole may modulate corticotropin synthesis and release from the pituitary corticotrophs but this has not been convincingly demonstrated.[3] Several small studies have established its effectiveness in patients with Cushing's syndrome of various etiologies.[10] As monotherapy, ketoconazole administration leads to normalization in 24-hour UFC levels in approximately 50% of patients.[9] Escape from its salutary effects, however, may occur.

Table 1
Medical therapies currently used for Cushing's syndrome

Medication	Mechanism of Action	Remarks	Dose Range
Ketoconazole	Steroidogenesis inhibitor	• Often preferred in women • Potentially hepatotoxic	200–600 mg po bid–tid
Metyrapone	Steroidogenesis inhibitor	• Often preferred in men • Seems safe during pregnancy	250–1000 mg po tid–qid
Mitotane	Steroidogenesis inhibitor	• Adrenolytic in high doses • Mostly used in adrenocortical carcinoma • Abortifacient and teratogenic	0.5–3.0 g po tid
Etomidate	Steroidogenesis inhibitor	• Very rapid onset of action • Potential to induce sedation/anesthesia	0.03 mg/kg IV as a bolus, followed by continuous infusion (0.1–0.3 mg/kg/h)
Cabergoline	Centrally acting agent (D2R agonist)	• Higher doses than those used to treat hyperprolactinemia often needed	0.5–7.0 mg po weekly
Pasireotide	Centrally acting agent (SSTR agonist)	• May achieve pituitary tumor control • Diabetes mellitus may develop	0.3–0.9 mg SC bid
Mifepristone	GR antagonist	• Labeled for use in patients with hyperglycemia/diabetes mellitus who have failed surgery or are not surgical candidates • Dose titration based on clinical criteria only • Abortifacient	300–1200 mg po daily

Pasireotide and mifepristone are the only agents that are currently approved by the FDA as therapies for subgroups of patients who have failed surgery or are not surgical candidates. Mitotane is currently approved by the FDA for treatment of adrenocortical carcinoma. Ketoconazole and metyrapone are approved by the European Medicines Agency for the treatment of CS. Pasireotide is approved by the European Medicines Agency for the treatment of CD.

Abbreviations: bid, twice daily; D2R, dopamine 2 receptor; IV, intravenously; po, by mouth; qid, 4 times daily; SC, subcutaneously; tid, 3 times daily.

Hypochlorhydria may decrease the effectiveness of ketoconazole, which requires gastric acid for absorption. Therefore, ketoconazole may not be effective in patients taking medications to decrease gastric acid secretion or in those with achlorhydria.

Hypogonadism often results in men as a consequence of inhibition of testosterone steroidogenesis in testes.[11] Other adverse effects associated with ketoconazole use include headache, nausea, skin rash, and hepatotoxicity. Transaminitis may occur in approximately 15% of patients after ketoconazole administration and usually improves after a dose decrease.[5,11] In addition, idiosyncratic, potentially life-threatening hepatotoxicity may occur in approximately 1 of 15,000 patients treated with ketoconazole.[12] The FDA has inserted a black box warning in the ketoconazole label to caution patients and prescribers of the drug's potential to cause serious hepatotoxicity. Therefore, patient education regarding this risk and regular monitoring of liver chemistries is essential in patients treated with ketoconazole. It is advisable to decrease or discontinue the medication if serum liver enzymes exceed 3 times the upper end of normal.[5,11]

Ketoconazole has the potential for interactions with many commonly used medications metabolized through the cytochrome P450 3A4 pathway.[13] Thus, prescribers need to thoroughly evaluate concomitant therapies used in patients with CS who are considered for ketoconazole therapy.

Metyrapone

Metyrapone primarily acts by inhibiting 11β-hydroxylase, thereby leading to a decrease in cortisol biosynthesis and an increase in several precursor molecules, including 11-deoxycortisol and 11-deoxycorticosterone, which have mineralocorticoid activity, as well as androgenic steroids.[3] Assays specific for cortisol (such as those based on tandem mass spectrometry) are recommended to monitor its effects, because 11-deoxycortisol often cross-reacts with cortisol in immunoassays. Metyrapone has a rapid onset of action and controls hypercortisolism in 50% to 75% of treated patients.[14,15] Metyrapone has been used successfully in pregnancy and seems safe for the fetus; however, the drug is not specifically labeled for use during gestation.[16,17] Tachyphylaxis may occur in some patients with CD treated with metyrapone as a consequence of the decrease in feedback inhibition on corticotropin secretion that results from enzymatic blockade of cortisol secretion.

The accumulation of androgenic precursors may result in hirsutism or acne in women.[14] In addition, the accumulation of precursors with mineralocorticoid activity may result in hypertension, edema, or hypokalemia. Blood pressure and serum potassium levels need to be monitored in treated patients. Other possible adverse effects include nausea and dizziness.[3,14]

Mitotane

Mitotane (o,p'-DDD) is structurally related to an older insecticide (dichorodiphenyltrichloroethane [DDT]) and inhibits several enzymatic steps in adrenal steroidogenesis.[3] It is also adrenolytic with prolonged use in higher doses. Its onset of action is slow, but mitotane therapy eventually controls hypercortisolism in approximately 70% to 85% of patients.[18,19] Mitotane may also prolong recurrence-free survival in subgroups of patients with adrenocortical carcinoma, wherein it has been used either as adjuvant therapy or as treatment of metastatic disease.[20–23]

Mitotane use is associated with serious potential toxicities, which have limited its use to patients with adrenocortical carcinoma; it is rarely used as treatment of CD in the United States. Adverse effects that may occur in patients treated with mitotane include gastrointestinal, hepatic, hematologic, urologic, ophthalmic, metabolic, skin, and neurologic manifestations.[22,23] Hypoadrenalism is generally anticipated in patients on mitotane therapy as a consequence of its enzymatic and adrenolytic effects and can be permanent with long-term use. In addition, the drug leads to accelerated cortisol clearance, thus necessitating the administration of higher than usual hydrocortisone replacement doses in treated patients.[3] Mitotane raises serum levels of cortisol-binding globulin, thus potentially confounding the interpretation of serum cortisol levels. Mitotane is abortifacient and teratogenic and is extensively stored in adipose tissue. As a consequence of its delayed clearance and potent teratogenicity, it is advisable that women avoid pregnancy for a minimum of 5 years after mitotane discontinuation.[5,17]

Etomidate

Etomidate is an intravenous sedative and anesthetic agent, which also acts primarily by inhibiting 11β-hydroxylase, leading to a decrease in cortisol synthesis.[24] Etomidate is effective in rapidly decreasing serum cortisol levels after administration in lower doses than those required to induce anesthesia.[24,25] The drug has been used to control severe, potentially life-threatening hypercortisolism and its complications (including sepsis, severe hypertension, and psychosis) and can be helpful as a bridge to definitive therapy. Close monitoring in an intensive care unit is required to detect and manage sedation in treated patients.[3] Nausea, vomiting, dystonia, or myoclonus may also occur in patients treated with etomidate.

Osilodrostat

Osilodrostat (LCI699) is an investigational agent that is being studied as potential treatment of patients with CS.[11] Osilodrostat potently inhibits 11β-hydroxylase and aldosterone synthase, thereby decreasing both cortisol and aldosterone biosynthesis. In a phase II study of patients with CD, osilodrostat administration normalized 24-hour UFC in 92% of 12 patients.[26] In a 22-week extension study, 24-hour UFC normalization was reported in 79% of 19 patients.[27] Whether tachyphylaxis may occur with long-term use remains to be established.

Similarly to metyrapone, osilodrostat administration results in accumulation of precursor steroids with mineralocorticoid or androgenic activity, which may lead to corresponding adverse effects, including hypertension, edema, hypokalemia or hirsutism, and acne.[11] Phase III studies of osilodrostat are currently under way (clinicaltrials. gov: NCT02468193 and clinicaltrials.gov: NCT02697734).

Levoketoconazole

Levoketoconazole (COR-003) is a ketoconazole enantiomer (2S,4R) that is being investigated as potential therapy for CS.[5,11,28] Levoketoconazole is more potent in inhibiting several adrenal steroidogenic enzymes than its enantiomer (2R,4S) or the racemic mixture.[28] In addition, preliminary data suggest that the risk of developing transaminitis after levoketoconazole administration may be lower than the corresponding risk associated with the racemic mixture. A phase III clinical trial of levoketoconazole is currently in progress (clinicaltrials.gov: NCT01838551).

Abiraterone Acetate

Abiraterone acetate inhibits 17α-hydroxylase and 17,20 lyase, which results in decreased testosterone biosynthesis.[29,30] Abiraterone acetate is used as therapy in patients with advanced prostate cancer.[29] Because abiraterone acetate also inhibits cortisol synthesis, it may have a role in the management of patients with CS.[30] The use of abiraterone acetate was reported in a single case study of a patient with severe hypercortisolism secondary to adrenocortical carcinoma refractory to mitotane therapy, who showed a beneficial, short-term clinical and biochemical response to this medication.[31] The drug is currently under investigation in patients with adrenocortical carcinoma (clinicaltrials.gov: NCT03145285).

CENTRALLY ACTING AGENTS

Centrally acting agents act by inhibiting corticotropin release in patients with CD (see **Table 1**).[3,5,32] In addition, some agents may have some role in maintaining tumor control. Cyproheptadine and ketanserin were previously used with limited success in CD but are not currently recommended because of limited effectiveness. Cabergoline and pasireotide are dopamine receptor and somatostatin receptor (SSTR) agonists, respectively, and are the only drugs in their respective class that are effective in subgroups of patients with CD (see **Table 1**).[3,5,32] Their clinical effectiveness is predicated by the presence of dopamine receptors and SSTRs in the majority (80%–85%) of corticotroph adenomas.[3,5,32]

Cabergoline

Cabergoline is a dopamine receptor agonist that shows selectivity for the D2 receptor isoform. Cabergoline is approved by the FDA for patients with hyperprolactinemia.[33] Published data suggest that cabergoline may lead to 24-hour UFC normalization in up to 40% of patients with CD.[34–36] Tachyphylaxis may occur, however, in some patients over time. Cabergoline doses that are needed to control hypercortisolism are generally higher (1–7 mg/wk) than those typically used in hyperprolactinemic patients (0.5–2 mg/wk).

Adverse effects associated with cabergoline use most commonly include nausea, vomiting, and orthostatic dizziness.[33] These may improve over time in some patients and can be minimized by gradual dose titration and administration at bedtime with a snack. Less common adverse effects may include headache, nasal congestion, constipation, and digital vasospasm (Raynaud phenomenon). Infrequent but potentially serious adverse effects include anxiety, depression or psychosis.[33] A variety of impulsivity disorders have been reported in rare cases and may reflect effects of cabergoline on dopamine receptors in central reward pathways, leading to increased impulsivity.[37–39] Patients need to be warned about these rare but potentially serious adverse effects and instructed to discontinue the drug if they develop. High-dose cabergoline therapy has been associated with increased risk of cardiac valvulopathy in patients with Parkinson disease and may reflect cabergoline activation of serotonin (5-hydroxytryptamine receptor 2B [5HT2B]) receptors.[40,41] Several studies have reported that cabergoline therapy in doses typically used to treat hyperprolactinemia does not seem associated with cardiac valvulopathy.[42] The potential risk of cardiac valvulopathy, however, has not been specifically studied in patients with CD who may be receiving higher cabergoline doses over prolonged intervals. Periodic echocardiography can be considered as surveillance for valvulopathy in such patients; however, the cost-effectiveness of this approach has not been systematically evaluated.

Pasireotide

Pasireotide is an SSTR agonist, which engages multiple receptor isoforms, including SSTR 1, 2, 3, and 5.[43] In particular, activation of SSTR5 is considered central to the effectiveness of pasireotide in CD. Pasireotide administration leads to 24-hour UFC normalization in 20% to 25% of patients with CD.[44,45] Patients with less severe hypercortisolism at baseline are more likely to achieve 24-hour UFC normalization with pasireotide therapy. In addition, this medication can normalize late-night salivary cortisol in some patients with CD.[7] Pasireotide therapy may also lead to beneficial effects on body weight, blood pressure, and serum lipids in patients with CD.[45,46] Tumor escape from the drug's salutary effects may infrequently occur.[28] Pasireotide may decrease tumor size in up to 44% of patients with CD.[45] In 2012, twice-daily subcutaneous pasireotide was approved by the FDA as therapy in patients with CD who have failed pituitary surgery or are not surgical candidates. A long-acting formulation of pasireotide (pasireotide long acting release [LAR]) has also been developed and studied as monthly therapy in CD, wherein it leads to 24-hour UFC normalization in approximately 40% of patients.[28,47,48] This agent has been reported to decrease the size of a corticotroph tumor in a patient with Nelson syndrome.[49] The long-acting pasireotide formulation is not currently approved by the FDA for use in CD.

Pasireotide administration is associated with several adverse effects common to other SSTR agonists, including gastrointestinal toxicity (nausea, abdominal pain, diarrhea, and gallstones), bradycardia, QT prolongation, hair loss, and vitamin B_{12} deficiency.[45] Hypoadrenalism may develop in a minority of treated patients. In addition, diabetes mellitus may develop in approximately 48% of patients, thus predicating recommendations for glucose monitoring during pasireotide therapy.[45,50] Lower degrees of hyperglycemia are even more common in patients treated with pasireotide. Activation of SSTR5 likely inhibits insulin and incretin secretion in these patients.[50] Metformin, incretin-based therapies, and insulin have been proposed as therapies of choice for hyperglycemia/diabetes mellitus in patients treated with pasireotide.[5,32]

Retinoic Acid

Retinoic receptor activation by retinoic acid inhibits pro-opiomelanocortin expression, corticotropin release and corticotroph tumor growth in preclinical models.[51] In addition, the effectiveness of isotretinoin, a 13-cis-retinoic acid isomer, in patients with CD was suggested by the findings of several small studies.[52,53] Additional data from clinical trials are needed to further characterize the efficacy and safety of retinoic acid in CD.

Other Potential Pharmacologic Approaches

Peroxisome proliferator-activated receptor gamma agonists, including rosiglitazone, showed early promise as therapy in patients with CD.[54] The efficacy of rosiglitazone seems, however, limited in CD based on more recent data.[55,56]

R-roscovitine inhibits cyclin-dependent kinase and cyclin E and has shown promise in preclinical studies.[57] Available data suggest that r-roscovitine decreases corticotropin secretion and tumor growth in animal models.[58] A phase II study of r-roscovitine in patients with CD is currently in progress (clinicaltrials.gov: NCT02160730). Gefitinib, an inhibitor of epidermal growth factor receptor tyrosine kinase, also inhibits corticotropin secretion and tumor growth in preclinical models.[59] Recent studies have identified activating mutations in ubiquitin-specific peptidase 8 in approximately 33% of corticotroph adenomas.[60] These observations suggest that ubiquitin-specific peptidase 8 may constitute an important molecular target for pharmacotherapy in CD.[60,61] Similarly, the expression of vasopressin and growth hormone secretagogue receptors in corticotroph adenomas suggests that these may also be meaningful molecular targets for drug development.[62,63]

Selective peptide antagonists of the melanocortin 2 receptor, which mediates corticotropin action on adrenal steroidogenesis, have been developed and have shown useful activity inhibiting glucocorticoid secretion in preclinical models, but clinical data are currently lacking.[28]

GLUCOCORTICOID RECEPTOR ANTAGONISTS

Mifepristone is currently the only available agent in this class.[64] In 2012, the drug was approved by the FDA for use in patients with CS (regardless of underlying etiology) and hyperglycemia or diabetes mellitus, who have either failed surgery or are not surgical candidates. Mifepristone potently binds to the GR as well as the progesterone receptor with high affinity, thereby inhibiting their respective downstream signaling pathways.[64] Mifepristone administration leads to several beneficial effects in patients with CS, including a decrease in body weight, blood glucose, and blood pressure as well as global clinical improvement.[65,66] Mifepristone therapy must be titrated based on clinical criteria because there are currently no biomarkers of cortisol action available to guide therapy.[67] There are studies in progress that are aiming at identifying such biomarkers. The drug can interact with several agents metabolized through the cytochrome P450 3A4 pathway, thus necessitating care in evaluating all medications taken by patients who are considered for mifepristone therapy.[67]

Blood pressure may increase in a subgroup of patients with CS treated with mifepristone because of unopposed activation of the mineralocorticoid receptor by endogenous cortisol present in high concentrations, which often exceed the capacity of inactivating enzymes (11β-hydroxysteroid dehydrogenase type 2) in patients with CS.[66] Severe hypokalemia may also occur in patients on mifepristone therapy as a result of mineralocorticoid receptor activation by excess cortisol. All patients receiving mifepristone require regular blood pressure and potassium monitoring.

Headache, nausea, dizziness, and arthralgias have been reported in patients on mifepristone and may signify the presence of hypoadrenalism.[66] In these patients, adrenal insufficiency may occur as an extension of mifepristone's pharmacologic actions on the GR and must be diagnosed based only on clinical criteria. Both cortisol and corticotropin levels generally increase in comparison with baseline levels among patients with CD treated with mifepristone, so serum cortisol levels cannot be used to confirm the presence of adrenal insufficiency.[68] Patients who develop symptoms suggestive of hypoadrenalism can be rescued by dexamethasone administration in higher than replacement doses for several days, whereas mifepristone is held to allow for endogenous clearance mechanisms to bring about a decrease in mifepristone levels.

Inhibition of progesterone receptor by mifepristone terminates pregnancy and also may result in endometrial thickening and irregular vaginal bleeding; however, premalignant endometrial hyperplasia has not been reported.[66,69] A novel investigational agent is currently being developed, which inhibits the GR but does not interact with the PR, and may, therefore, lack endometrial adverse effects.[28] Other adverse effects associated with mifepristone use include dyslipidemia and reversible elevations in thyrotropin levels. Corticotroph tumor progression or regression has been reported in treated patients.[68] Periodic pituitary imaging is prudent in patients with CD who are treated with mifepristone.

COMBINATION THERAPY

In addition to monotherapy, there may be a role for combination therapy in some patients, including those with severe hypercortisolism. Published data suggest an additive effect of agents used in combination, including ketoconazole plus metyrapone with or without mitotane, ketoconazole plus cabergoline, or pasireotide plus cabergoline and ketoconazole.[70–73]

In 1 study of 11 patients with severe corticotropin-dependent CS, the combination of ketoconazole, metyrapone, and mitotane therapy led to a rapid decline in 24-hour UFC within 48 hours of treatment initiation.[73] In another study of 14 patients with severe ectopic corticotropin syndrome and 8 patients with adrenocortical carcinoma, ketoconazole plus metyrapone therapy was administered and led to a dramatic decrease in 24-hour UFC within 1 week from onset of therapy.[71] These data suggest that combination therapy that involves several steroidogenesis inhibitors can be rapidly effective in controlling life-threatening hypercortisolism in patients with severe CS of various etiologies.

Combination therapy that includes both steroidogenesis inhibitors and centrally acting agents may also be effective in patients with CD. In a study of 17 patients with CD who were treated with 1 to 3 agents (pasireotide alone, together with cabergoline, or together with cabergoline plus ketoconazole), 24-hour UFC normalization was reported in the majority (88%) of cases.[72] In another study of 14 patients with CD, the combination of ketoconazole plus cabergoline led to 24-hour UFC normalization in 79% of treated patients.[70]

These data are encouraging and suggest a potential role of combination therapy, particularly for patients with severe hypercortisolism. Randomized clinical trials, however, evaluating the efficacy of combination therapy have not yet been published.

SUMMARY

Several agents are available as adjunctive therapies in CS, including steroidogenesis inhibitors, centrally acting agents, and GR antagonists. Medical therapy is currently indicated in patients who have failed surgical management or are not surgical candidates or in occasional patients who need to be bridged to surgery. Choice of medical therapy is individualized based on several variables, including disease severity, tumor size and location, comorbidities, concurrent medications, anticipated adherence to therapy, and cost (**Box 1**).

Several pharmaceutical agents are currently in development as potential treatments of CS. It is anticipated that the elucidation of novel molecular targets may eventually culminate in the development of additional, more effective therapies for treatment of patients with this potentially devastating syndrome.

Box 1
Factors that may influence the choice between medical therapies for Cushing's syndrome

Disease severity/urgency of treatment
  Steroidogenesis inhibitors, alone or in combination, are preferred in patients with severe disease; mifepristone may also be considered.

Tumor size
  Pasireotide may be considered in patients with larger pituitary tumors (macroadenomas).

Patient demographics
  Ketoconazole is often preferred in women; metyrapone is often preferred in men.

Comorbidities
  Mifepristone may be considered in patients with hyperglycemia or diabetes mellitus. Ketoconazole may be avoided in patients with achlorhydria.

Concurrent medications
  Caution is advised with ketoconazole or mifepristone use, since both have significant potential for drug-drug interactions.

Anticipated difficulty with adherence to therapy
  Caution with use of medications that require multiple doses in a 24-hour period.

Pregnancy
  Metyrapone is often preferred.

Cost
  Pasireotide and mifepristone are currently more expensive than other available agents.

REFERENCES

1. Cushing H. The basophil adenomas of the pituitary body and their clinical manifestations (pituitary basophilism). Bull Johns Hopkins Hosp 1932;50: 137–95.
2. Cushing H. The basophil adenomas of the pituitary body. Ann R Coll Surg Engl 1969;44:180–1.
3. Nieman LK, Biller BM, Findling JW, et al. Treatment of Cushing's syndrome: an endocrine society clinical practice guideline. J Clin Endocrinol Metab 2015; 100:2807–31.
4. Swearingen B, Biller BM, Barker FG 2nd, et al. Long-term mortality after trans-sphenoidal surgery for Cushing disease. Ann Intern Med 1999;130:821–4.
5. Tritos NA, Biller BM. Medical management of Cushing's disease. J Neurooncol 2014;117:407–14.
6. Tritos NA, Biller BM, Swearingen B. Management of Cushing disease. Nat Rev Endocrinol 2011;7:279–89.
7. Findling JW, Fleseriu M, Newell-Price J, et al. Late-night salivary cortisol may be valuable for assessing treatment response in patients with Cushing's disease: 12-month, Phase III pasireotide study. Endocrine 2016;54:516–23.
8. Tritos NA, Biller BM. Advances in medical therapies for Cushing's syndrome. Discov Med 2012;13:171–9.
9. Castinetti F, Guignat L, Giraud P, et al. Ketoconazole in Cushing's disease: is it worth a try? J Clin Endocrinol Metab 2014;99:1623–30.
10. Engelhardt D, Weber MM. Therapy of Cushing's syndrome with steroid biosynthesis inhibitors. J Steroid Biochem Mol Biol 1994;49:261–7.
11. Fleseriu M, Petersenn S. Medical therapy for Cushing's disease: adrenal steroidogenesis inhibitors and glucocorticoid receptor blockers. Pituitary 2015;18: 245–52.
12. McCance DR, Ritchie CM, Sheridan B, et al. Acute hypoadrenalism and hepato-toxicity after treatment with ketoconazole. Lancet 1987;1:573.
13. Nieman LK. Update in the medical therapy of Cushing's disease. Curr Opin Endocrinol Diabetes Obes 2013;20:330–4.
14. Daniel E, Aylwin S, Mustafa O, et al. Effectiveness of metyrapone in treating Cushing's Syndrome: a retrospective multicenter study in 195 patients. J Clin Endocrinol Metab 2015;100(11):4146–54.
15. Verhelst JA, Trainer PJ, Howlett TA, et al. Short and long-term responses to metyrapone in the medical management of 91 patients with Cushing's syndrome. Clin Endocrinol (Oxf) 1991;35:169–78.
16. Gormley MJ, Hadden DR, Kennedy TL, et al. Cushing's syndrome in pregnancy—treatment with metyrapone. Clin Endocrinol (Oxf) 1982;16:283–93.
17. Lindsay JR, Jonklaas J, Oldfield EH, et al. Cushing's syndrome during pregnancy: personal experience and review of the literature. J Clin Endocrinol Metab 2005;90:3077–83.
18. Luton JP, Cerdas S, Billaud L, et al. Clinical features of adrenocortical carcinoma, prognostic factors, and the effect of mitotane therapy. N Engl J Med 1990;322: 1195–201.
19. Luton JP, Mahoudeau JA, Bouchard P, et al. Treatment of Cushing's disease by O,p'DDD. Survey of 62 cases. N Engl J Med 1979;300:459–64.
20. Baudry C, Coste J, Bou Khalil R, et al. Efficiency and tolerance of mitotane in Cushing's disease in 76 patients from a single center. Eur J Endocrinol 2012; 167:473–81.

21. Hermsen IG, Fassnacht M, Terzolo M, et al. Plasma concentrations of o,p'DDD, o,p'DDA, and o,p'DDE as predictors of tumor response to mitotane in adrenocortical carcinoma: results of a retrospective ENS@T multicenter study. J Clin Endocrinol Metab 2011;96:1844–51.

22. Mauclere-Denost S, Leboulleux S, Borget I, et al. High-dose mitotane strategy in adrenocortical carcinoma: prospective analysis of plasma mitotane measurement during the first 3 months of follow-up. Eur J Endocrinol 2012;166:261–8.

23. Terzolo M, Angeli A, Fassnacht M, et al. Adjuvant mitotane treatment for adrenocortical carcinoma. N Engl J Med 2007;356:2372–80.

24. Schulte HM, Benker G, Reinwein D, et al. Infusion of low dose etomidate: correction of hypercortisolemia in patients with Cushing's syndrome and dose-response relationship in normal subjects. J Clin Endocrinol Metab 1990;70:1426–30.

25. Preda VA, Sen J, Karavitaki N, et al. Etomidate in the management of hypercortisolaemia in Cushing's syndrome: a review. Eur J Endocrinol 2012;167:137–43.

26. Bertagna X, Pivonello R, Fleseriu M, et al. LCI699, a potent 11beta-hydroxylase inhibitor, normalizes urinary cortisol in patients with Cushing's disease: results from a multicenter, proof-of-concept study. J Clin Endocrinol Metab 2014;99: 1375–83.

27. Fleseriu M, Pivonello R, Young J, et al. Osilodrostat, a potent oral 11beta-hydroxylase inhibitor: 22-week, prospective, Phase II study in Cushing's disease. Pituitary 2016;19(2):138–48.

28. Cuevas-Ramos D, Lim DST, Fleseriu M. Update on medical treatment for Cushing's disease. Clin Diabetes Endocrinol 2016;2:16.

29. Berruti A, Pia A, Terzolo M. Abiraterone and increased survival in metastatic prostate cancer. N Engl J Med 2011;365:766 [author reply: 767–8].

30. Fiorentini C, Fragni M, Perego P, et al. Antisecretive and antitumor activity of abiraterone acetate in human adrenocortical cancer: a preclinical study. J Clin Endocrinol Metab 2016;101:4594–602.

31. Claps M, Lazzari B, Grisanti S, et al. Management of severe Cushing syndrome induced by adrenocortical carcinoma with abiraterone acetate: a case report. AACE Clin Case Rep 2016;2:e337–41.

32. Fleseriu M, Petersenn S. New avenues in the medical treatment of Cushing's disease: corticotroph tumor targeted therapy. J Neurooncol 2013;114:1–11.

33. Klibanski A. Clinical practice. Prolactinomas. N Engl J Med 2010;362:1219–26.

34. Burman P, Eden-engstrom B, Ekman B, et al. Limited value of cabergoline in Cushing's disease: a prospective study of a 6-week treatment in 20 patients. Eur J Endocrinol 2016;174:17–24.

35. Godbout A, Manavela M, Danilowicz K, et al. Cabergoline monotherapy in the long-term treatment of Cushing's disease. Eur J Endocrinol 2010;163:709–16.

36. Pivonello R, De Martino MC, Cappabianca P, et al. The medical treatment of Cushing's disease: effectiveness of chronic treatment with the dopamine agonist cabergoline in patients unsuccessfully treated by surgery. J Clin Endocrinol Metab 2009;94:223–30.

37. Bancos I, Nannenga MR, Bostwick JM, et al. Impulse control disorders in patients with dopamine agonist-treated prolactinomas and nonfunctioning pituitary adenomas: a case-control study. Clin Endocrinol (Oxf) 2014;80:863–8.

38. Bancos I, Nippoldt TB, Erickson D. Hypersexuality in men with prolactinomas treated with dopamine agonists. Endocrine 2017;56:456–7.

39. Barake M, Evins AE, Stoeckel L, et al. Investigation of impulsivity in patients on dopamine agonist therapy for hyperprolactinemia: a pilot study. Pituitary 2014; 17:150–6.

40. Schade R, Andersohn F, Suissa S, et al. Dopamine agonists and the risk of cardiac-valve regurgitation. N Engl J Med 2007;356:29–38.

41. Zanettini R, Antonini A, Gatto G, et al. Valvular heart disease and the use of dopamine agonists for Parkinson's disease. N Engl J Med 2007;356:39–46.

42. Valassi E, Klibanski A, Biller BM. Clinical review: potential cardiac valve effects of dopamine agonists in hyperprolactinemia. J Clin Endocrinol Metab 2010;95: 1025–33.

43. Ben-Shlomo A, Schmid H, Wawrowsky K, et al. Differential ligand-mediated pituitary somatostatin receptor subtype signaling: implications for corticotroph tumor therapy. J Clin Endocrinol Metab 2009;94:4342–50.

44. Boscaro M, Bertherat J, Findling J, et al. Extended treatment of Cushing's disease with pasireotide: results from a 2-year, Phase II study. Pituitary 2014;17:320–6.

45. Colao A, Petersenn S, Newell-price J, et al. A 12-month phase 3 study of pasireotide in Cushing's disease. N Engl J Med 2012;366:914–24.

46. Schopohl J, Gu F, Rubens R, et al. Pasireotide can induce sustained decreases in urinary cortisol and provide clinical benefit in patients with Cushing's disease: results from an open-ended, open-label extension trial. Pituitary 2015;18:604–12.

47. Lacroix A, Gu F, Gallardo W, et al. Efficacy and safety of once-monthly pasireotide in Cushing's disease: a 12 month clinical trial. Lancet Diabetes Endocrinol 2018; 6(1):17–26.

48. Petersenn S, Bollerslev J, Arafat AM, et al. Pharmacokinetics, pharmacodynamics, and safety of pasireotide LAR in patients with acromegaly: a randomized, multicenter, open-label, phase I study. J Clin Pharmacol 2014;54:1308–17.

49. Katznelson L. Sustained improvements in plasma ACTH and clinical status in a patient with Nelson's syndrome treated with pasireotide LAR, a multireceptor somatostatin analog. J Clin Endocrinol Metab 2013;98:1803–7.

50. Henry RR, Ciaraldi TP, Armstrong D, et al. Hyperglycemia associated with pasireotide: results from a mechanistic study in healthy volunteers. J Clin Endocrinol Metab 2013;98:3446–53.

51. Castillo V, Giacomini D, Paez-Pereda M, et al. Retinoic acid as a novel medical therapy for Cushing's disease in dogs. Endocrinology 2006;147:4438–44.

52. Pecori Giraldi F, Ambrogio AG, Andrioli M, et al. Potential role for retinoic acid in patients with Cushing's disease. J Clin Endocrinol Metab 2012;97:3577–83.

53. Vilar L, Albuquerque JL, Lyra R, et al. The role of isotretinoin therapy for Cushing's disease: results of a prospective study. Int J Endocrinol 2016;2016:8173182.

54. Ambrosi B, Dall'asta C, Cannavo S, et al. Effects of chronic administration of PPAR-gamma ligand rosiglitazone in Cushing's disease. Eur J Endocrinol 2004; 151:173–8.

55. Morcos M, Fohr B, Tafel J, et al. Long-term treatment of central Cushing's syndrome with rosiglitazone. Exp Clin Endocrinol Diabetes 2007;115:292–7.

56. Pecori Giraldi F, Scaroni C, Arvat E, et al. Effect of protracted treatment with rosiglitazone, a PPARgamma agonist, in patients with Cushing's disease. Clin Endocrinol (Oxf) 2006;64:219–24.

57. Liu NA, Jiang H, Ben-shlomo A, et al. Targeting zebrafish and murine pituitary corticotroph tumors with a cyclin-dependent kinase (CDK) inhibitor. Proc Natl Acad Sci U S A 2011;108:8414–9.

58. Liu NA, Araki T, Cuevas-ramos D, et al. Cyclin E-mediated human proopiomelanocortin regulation as a therapeutic target for cushing disease. J Clin Endocrinol Metab 2015;100:2557–64.

59. Fukuoka H, Cooper O, Ben-shlomo A, et al. EGFR as a therapeutic target for human, canine, and mouse ACTH-secreting pituitary adenomas. J Clin Invest 2011; 121:4712–21.

60. Reincke M, Sbiera S, Hayakawa A, et al. Mutations in the deubiquitinase gene USP8 cause Cushing's disease. Nat Genet 2015;47:31–8.

61. Theodoropoulou M, Reincke M, Fassnacht M, et al. Decoding the genetic basis of Cushing's disease: USP8 in the spotlight. Eur J Endocrinol 2015;173:M73–83.

62. Dahia PL, Ahmed-Shuaib A, Jacobs RA, et al. Vasopressin receptor expression and mutation analysis in corticotropin-secreting tumors. J Clin Endocrinol Metab 1996;81:1768–71.

63. Korbonits M, Jacobs RA, Aylwin SJ, et al. Expression of the growth hormone secretagogue receptor in pituitary adenomas and other neuroendocrine tumors. J Clin Endocrinol Metab 1998;83:3624–30.

64. Fleseriu M, Biller BM, Findling JW, et al. Mifepristone, a glucocorticoid receptor antagonist, produces clinical and metabolic benefits in patients with refractory Cushing syndrome: results from the study of the efficacy and safety of mifepristone in the treatment of endogenous Cushing syndrome (SEISMIC). Endocr Rev 2011;32:OR09-5.

65. Castinetti f, Fassnacht M, Johanssen S, et al. Merits and pitfalls of mifepristone in Cushing's syndrome. Eur J Endocrinol 2009;160:1003–10.

66. Fleseriu M, Biller BM, Findling JW, et al. Mifepristone, a glucocorticoid receptor antagonist, produces clinical and metabolic benefits in patients with Cushing's syndrome. J Clin Endocrinol Metab 2012;97:2039–49.

67. Fleseriu M, Molitch ME, Gross C, et al. A new therapeutic approach in the medical treatment of Cushing's syndrome: glucocorticoid receptor blockade with Mifepristone. Endocr Pract 2013;19:313–26.

68. Fleseriu M, Findling JW, Koch CA, et al. Changes in plasma ACTH levels and corticotroph tumor size in patients with Cushing's disease during long-term treatment with the glucocorticoid receptor antagonist mifepristone. J Clin Endocrinol Metab 2014;99:3718–27.

69. Mutter GL, Bergeron C, Deligdisch L, et al. The spectrum of endometrial pathology induced by progesterone receptor modulators. Mod Pathol 2008;21:591–8.

70. Barbot M, Albiger N, Ceccato F, et al. Combination therapy for Cushing's disease: effectiveness of two schedules of treatment: should we start with cabergoline or ketoconazole? Pituitary 2014;17:109–17.

71. Corcuff JB, Young J, Masquefa-Giraud P, et al. Rapid control of severe neoplastic hypercortisolism with metyrapone and ketoconazole. Eur J Endocrinol 2015;172: 473–81.

72. Feelders RA, de Bruin C, Pereira AM, et al. Pasireotide alone or with cabergoline and ketoconazole in Cushing's disease. N Engl J Med 2010;362:1846–8.

73. Kamenicky P, Droumaguet C, Salenave S, et al. Mitotane, metyrapone, and ketoconazole combination therapy as an alternative to rescue adrenalectomy for severe ACTH-dependent Cushing's syndrome. J Clin Endocrinol Metab 2011;96: 2796–804.

Pregnancy in Patients with Cushing's Syndrome

Marcio Carlos Machado, MD, PhD[a,b,c],
Maria Candida Barisson Vilares Fragoso, MD, PhD[a],
Marcello Delano Bronstein, MD, PhD[a],*

KEYWORDS

- Cushing's syndrome • Pregnancy • Hypercortisolism

KEY POINTS

- Despite high prevalence of Cushing's syndrome in women of reproductive age, pregnancy rarely occurs due to hypogonadotrophic hypogonadism secondary to cortisol and androgens excess.
- Causes of Cushing's syndrome in pregnancy are adrenal disorders (in particular adenomas) in 60% cases, Cushing's disease in 33%, and 7% ectopic Cushing's syndrome.
- Although cortisol levels can be high, the circadian rhythm of cortisol secretion is preserved during normal pregnancy.
- Uncontrolled Cushing's syndrome during pregnancy is associated with a high rate of maternal and fetal complications. The rates of preeclampsia and premature delivery are increased even in patients with treated hypercortisolism.
- Surgery in the second trimester is the main treatment option in pregnant Cushing's syndrome patients.

INTRODUCTION

Cushing's syndrome (CS) is one of the endocrine conditions that often impair ovulation and, consequently, fertility. De novo CS during pregnancy is challenging to diagnose due to shared clinical features and impact on normal gestation on testing. Untreated CS during pregnancy significantly increases the risk for complications for mother and fetus. This review intends to bring insights both in diagnosis and treatment of CS in pregnancy.

Disclosure Statement: The authors have nothing to disclose.
[a] Neuroendocrine Unit, Division of Endocrinology and Metabolism, Hospital das Clínicas, University of São Paulo Medical School, Avenida Enéas de Carvalho Aguiar, n° 155, 8° andar, bloco 03, São Paulo, São Paulo 05403-000, Brazil; [b] Endocrinology Service, AC Camargo Cancer Center, Rua Prof. Antonio Prudente n° 211, São Paulo, SP 01509-010, Brazil; [c] Laboratory for Endocrinology Cellular and Molecular – LIM25, University of São Paulo Medical School, Av. Dr. Arnaldo, 455, 4° andar, São Paulo, SP 01246-903, Brazil
* Corresponding author.
E-mail address: mdbronstein@uol.com.br

Endocrinol Metab Clin N Am 47 (2018) 441–449
https://doi.org/10.1016/j.ecl.2018.02.004
0889-8529/18/© 2018 Elsevier Inc. All rights reserved.

endo.theclinics.com

HYPOTHALAMIC-PITUITARY-ADRENAL AXIS CHANGES DURING PREGNANCY

Pregnancy is considered a physiologic state of hypercortisolism due to an activation of the hypothalamic-pituitary-adrenal axis (HPA) (**Fig. 1**). Nevertheless, albeit sharing some clinical features with CS, normal pregnancy usually is not accompanied by specific clinical manifestations of CS, such as large purple striae, proximal muscle weakness, and cutaneous atrophy/easy bruising.

The corticotropin-releasing hormone (CRH) is synthetized in the hypothalamus but has also been detected in thecal and in stromal cells as well as in cells of the ovarian corpora luteum.[1] The epithelial cells of the endometrium have shown CRH receptors,[2,3] which mediate CRH effects on maturation of the fetal adrenal, fetal-placental unit circulation, and placenta itself. The placental CRH has an identical molecular structure to the hypothalamic form.[4]

During pregnancy, CRH and corticotropin levels increase in the first trimester due to CRH and corticotropin secretion by the placenta. CRH-binding protein levels also increase.[5] Due to corticotropin stimulation, maternal adrenal glands gradually become hypertrophic during pregnancy. The result is a small rise of cortisol levels (serum,

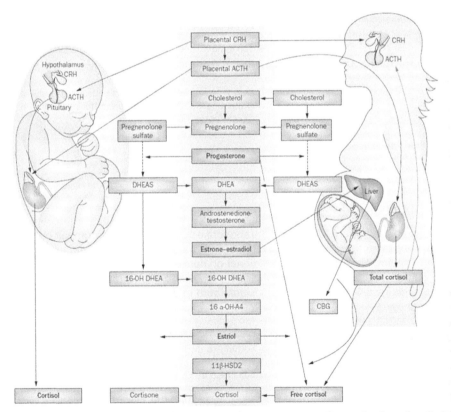

Fig. 1. The physiologic activation of the HPA axis during pregnancy. The production of cortisol linked to CBG is increased, as is the free fraction. The concentration of corticotropin is high, and the adrenal cortex is responsible for stimulus. 16 a-OH-4A, 16α-hydroxyandrostenedione. 16'OH, 16α-Hydroxydehydroepiandrosterone; 16α-OH-A4, 16α-hydroxyandrostenedione; DHEA, dehydroepiandrosterone; HSD2, 11β-hydroxysteroid dehydrogenase type 2. (*From* Bronstein MD, Paraiba DB, Jallad RS. Management of pituitary tumors in pregnancy. Nat Rev Endocrinol 2011;7:306; with permission.)

salivary, and urinary), which becomes more important as pregnancy advances. The cortisol secretion, however, maintains a pulsatile and circadian rhythm.[6]

The corticosteroid-binding globulin (CBG) production increases due to high levels of estradiol in pregnancy, reaching highest levels at the end of pregnancy. This causes an overestimation of serum total cortisol measured by commercial assays.[7] Serum free cortisol, however, also increases approximately 1.6-fold by the 11th week of pregnancy due to the pregnancy-induced HPA activation.[6] Consequently, urinary free cortisol increases up to 3-fold the normal range.[8] The placenta expresses 11β-hydroxysteroid dehydrogenase type 2, which converts cortisol to cortisone, thereby protecting the fetus from the high maternal cortisol levels.[9]

Response of corticotropin and cortisol to dynamic tests changes during pregnancy. Administration of exogenous 1-μg/kg human CRH during pregnancy does not cause a significant rise in corticotropin and cortisol levels.[10] Nevertheless, administration of higher doses of human CRH (2 μg/kg) can produce an elevation of corticotropin and cortisol starting from the third trimester.[11] Finally, the suppression of cortisol to low-dose dexamethasone suppression test is attenuated compared with the nonpregnant state.[9]

The circulating fetal CRH is almost exclusively of placental origin and corticotropin can be detectable in fetal plasma at 12 weeks of gestation.[10] The CRH-binding protein is elevated in the first 2 trimesters of pregnancy and decreases considerably in the last trimester, with consequent elevation of bioavailable plasmatic CRH. The increase of CRH plays a role in the labor and fetal lung maturation.[12] Fetal adrenals are enormous compared with the adult adrenal glands, and the major steroid produced is dehydroepiandrosterone sulfate (DHEAS), in contrast to the preponderance of cortisol detected in the fetal circulation, which seems to come from maternal source.[13] In addition, the fetal adrenal converts placental progesterone to cortisol. Another origin of cortisol is the amniotic fluid where cortisone is converted into cortisol by the choriodecidua.

At approximately the fourth day postpartum, maternal CRH, corticotropin, and cortisol gradually return to prepregnancy levels, and the response to CRH recovers few weeks after delivery. The adrenal glands are suppressed in a similar fashion as in early stages of successfully operated patients with Cushing's disease (CD) and gradually return to prepregnancy state by 12 weeks after delivery.[13] This transient period of adrenal suppression might be related to mood disorders and autoimmune diseases frequently observed in postpartum women.

PREGNANCY IN PATIENTS WITH CUSHING'S SYNDROME

There are significant differences regarding etiology of CS that occurs in pregnant and nonpregnant women. In pregnancy, the prevalence of adrenal disorders (particularly adenomas) is higher (60%) than prevalence of CD (33%). In contrast, nonpregnant patients have higher prevalence of CD (70%) than adrenal adenomas (15%).[1] This difference is probably related to the higher impact on fertility of the mixed secretion of cortisol and androgens by the adrenal glands in CD, whereas adrenal adenomas frequently only produce cortisol.[14,15] Lindsay and Nieman,[1] reviewing 136 pregnancies in 122 women with CS, described the following causes: adrenal adenoma (n: 56); CD (n: 40); adrenal carcinoma (n: 12); ectopic corticotropin secretion (n: 4); and corticotropin-independent hyperplasia (n: 4)—possibly due to atypical receptor stimulation and Carney complex (n: 1).

DIAGNOSIS OF CUSHING'S SYNDROME DURING PREGNANCY

The diagnosis of CS during pregnancy is challenging. Three patient categories can be encountered: (1) pregnancy in context of known CS; (2) de novo development of CS during pregnancy, and (3) development of clinical features and complications similar with CS during pregnancy (striae, arterial hypertension, and diabetes mellitus). Presence of muscular weakness, deep purple striae (especially outside of abdomen), and osteoporosis is worrisome for CS. Hirsutism is rare in de novo CS during pregnancy because most cases are due to benign adrenal adenomas without hyperandrogenism.[16] Despite these helpful clinical clues, the diagnosis should be supported by laboratory and imaging procedures.

Laboratory diagnosis of CS during pregnancy is hampered by changes in serum and urinary cortisol levels and abnormal dynamic testing that can occur in normal pregnancy[4,17] (**Table 1**). Total serum cortisol increases due to estrogen-induced production of CBG, which causes false-positive results on low-dose dexamethasone suppression test.[1] High urinary free cortisol 1 to 3 times the upper limit of normal range can be encountered during the second and third trimesters of pregnancy.[8] The evaluation of circadian rhythm of cortisol secretion is recommended, because it is usually preserved during normal pregnancy despite higher serum and urinary cortisol levels. A recent study assessed nocturnal salivary cortisol and identified the following thresholds: first trimester 0.25 μg/dL (6.9 nmol/L), second trimester 0.26 μg/dL (7.2 nmol/L), and third trimester 0.33 μg/dL (9.1 nmol/L) (**Fig. 2**). The upper reference value for nocturnal salivary cortisol of nonpregnant adults for this ELISA (Salimetrics [Salimetrics, LLC, State College, PA, USA]) method was 0.12 μg/dL (3.3 nmol/L).[18]

After confirmation of diagnosis of CS, the next step is measuring corticotropin levels. These may not be suppressed in patients, however, with cortisol-secreting adrenal adenomas, probably due to pituitary corticotropin stimulation by placental CRH or by placental corticotropin itself.[17,19] Patients with CD diagnosed during pregnancy present corticotropin levels in the upper the normal range or even higher.[17]

High-dose dexamethasone suppression test correctly identified practically all reported cases of CD using the 50% cortisol decrease threshold, and stimulation with 100-μg intravenous CRH induced the expected corticotropin and cortisol responses in CD patients.[20] Bilateral and inferior petrosal sinus sampling has been performed in a few pregnant women with suspected CD.[21] This test should be used carefully to avoid unnecessary radiation and possible thromboembolic events.[17] Nongadolinium MRI may not identify small microadenomas.[1,22] Additionally, the physiologic enlargement of the pituitary gland during pregnancy may mask a small tumor.[1] Imaging without gadolinium should be performed only if surgery is planned prior to birth, and adrenal CT scans should be avoided. Adrenal imaging by ultrasound is safe during pregnancy. When interpreting imaging tests, the issue of pituitary and adrenal incidentaloma should be considered.

MATERNOFETAL COMPLICATIONS OF CUSHING'S SYNDROME

A recent systematic review of published cases reported 214 cases of pregnancy and active CS. Patients were classified in 2 groups: (1) active CS during pregnancy and (2)

Table 1 Laboratory methods for diagnosis of Cushing's syndrome during pregnancy	
Method	**Observation for Cushing's Syndrome Diagnosis**
Low-dose dexamethasone suppression test	False positive due to CBG estrogen-induced
24-h urinary free cortisol	Consider more than >3× ULNR in the second/third trimester
Late night salivary cortisol	Consider more than >2–3× ULNR

Abbreviation: ULNR, upper limit of normal range.

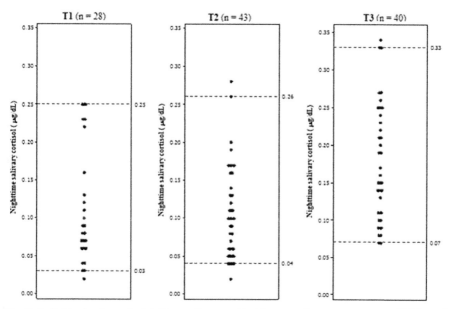

Fig. 2. Individual values of nighttime salivary cortisol in normal pregnancy group (2.5th and 97.5th percentiles; to convert to nmol/L, multiply by 27.6). T1, first trimester of pregnancy; T2, second trimester of pregnancy; T3, third trimester of pregnancy. (*From* Lopes LM, Francisco RP, Galletta MA, et al. Determination of nighttime salivary cortisol during pregnancy: comparison with values in non-pregnancy and Cushing's disease. Pituitary 2016;19:34; with permission.)

history of CS treated and controlled before pregnancy. This study included some patients who delivered within the 12 months prior to CS diagnosis in the first category.[23]

The most common described maternal morbidities were hypertension (40%–68%), diabetes or glucose intolerance (25%–37%), preeclampsia (14%–27%), osteoporosis and fractures (5%), psychiatric disorders (4%), cardiac failure (3%), wound infections (2%), and maternal death (2%).[17,23]

Concerning newborns, a tendency for higher live birth rate was encountered in women treated during pregnancy. The most frequent fetal morbidity was prematurity seen in approximately 43% to 66% of pregnancies.[17,23] Other described complications are intrauterine growth retardation (15%–21%), spontaneous abortion or intrauterine death (5%–24%), respiratory distress (14%), stillbirths (6%), and hypocortisolism (2%).[17,23]

TREATMENT OF CUSHING'S SYNDROME IN THE PREGNANCY

Not all pregnant patients with active CS reported in the literature underwent treatment of hypercortisolism. Cases discovered at the end of pregnancy were managed conservatively by treatment of comorbidities, such as hypertension and diabetes mellitus.

Similarly to nonpregnant women, surgery is the first line of treatment option in pregnant CS patients.[1,17,24,25] Radiotherapy and mitotane are contraindicated during pregnancy due to the delayed results and potential harmful or teratogenic effects.[26]

In patients with CD and pregnancy, 42.5% were not submitted to specific treatment of hypercortisolism.[17] The treated cases underwent transsphenoidal pituitary surgery, medical treatment or bilateral adrenalectomy. Pituitary surgery performed between

Table 2
Reports of medications used during pregnancy in patients with active Cushing's syndrome

Medication	n = 33	Percentage	Dose	Observations
Metyrapone[17,30,31,34,37,41,42]	17	52	0.5–3.0 g/d	Hypertension worsening and preeclampsia increase
Ketoconazole[17,34–37]	7	21	0.6–1.0 g/d	Teratogenic (only in animals)
Cabergoline[35,38–40]	4	12	2.0–3.5 mg/wk	Only direct drug to tumor
Cyproheptadine[17]	3	9	—	Lack of efficacy
Aminoglutethimide[17]	1	3	2.5 g/d	Fetal masculinization
Mitotane[17]	1	3	—	Teratogenic

the end of first trimester and early second trimester (12–29 weeks of gestation) has been associated with a lower rate of maternal and fetal complications. Several factors influence surgical decision, such as severity of hypercortisolism, trimester of gestation, and therapeutic risk-benefit for the maternal-fetal outcomes.[25,27]

Unilateral adrenalectomy for adrenal adenomas and carcinomas was performed with good results both on cortisol status and birth rate.[24,28,29] Bilateral adrenalectomy for refractory CD or severe ectopic corticotropin syndrome cases is sometimes indicated.

Medical therapy, usually initiated during the second or third trimester, is generally the second line of treatment option after surgery. Treatment with steroidogenesis inhibitors was the most frequent option, particularly with metyrapone[30] (**Table 2**). This drug achieved control of hypercortisolism in most cases, with 1 report of adrenal insufficiency.[17,31] The most troublesome side effect of metyrapone is the increase of precursors, such as 11-deoxycorticosterone, which can worsen the hypertension and increase the risk for preeclampsia. Although metyrapone crosses the placental membrane in animal studies, no neonatal abnormalities have been reported in human patients.[32,33] Ketoconazole, one of the most used steroidogenesis inhibitors in nonpregnant CS patients, has been rarely used in pregnancy due to potential side effects, such as antiandrogenic effect and teratogenicity (only in animal studies).[17,34,35] Some recent case reports treated with ketoconazole, however, had good results.[36,37]

Other adrenal steroidogenesis blockers, such as aminoglutethimide and mitotane, were rarely used, because aminoglutethimide and mitotane can induce fetal masculinization and teratogenicity, respectively.[16] Only 3 cases of CD treated with cabergoline during pregnancy were reported to date.[35,38–40] They achieved control of hypercortisolism and maternal-fetal outcomes at doses of 2.0 mg/wk to 3.5 mg/wk. To date, no reports of pasireotide use during pregnancy in CS were published.

In summary, hypercortisolism in patients with known CS should be controlled before pregnancy occurs. Pregnant women with active disease must be carefully evaluated. Normocortisolism can be achieved by pituitary or adrenal surgery preferably during the second trimester. Among medical treatments, most experience has accumulated with metyrapone, followed by ketoconazole.

SUMMARY

Despite its rarity, pregnancy in patients with CS is a challenging situation due to maternofetal complications, especially in nontreated cases. Surgery and medical treatment aimed at restoring the cortisol balance reduce maternal and fetal morbidity and mortality in women with CS.

REFERENCES

1. Lindsay JR, Nieman LK. The hypothalamic-pituitary-adrenal axis in pregnancy: challenges in disease detection and treatment. Endocr Rev 2005;26:775–9.
2. Sehringer B, Zahradnik HP, Simon M, et al. mRNA expression profiles for corticotrophin-releasing hormone, urocortin, CRH-binding protein and CRH receptors in human term gestational tissues determined by real-time quantitative RT-PCR. J Mol Endocrinol 2004;32:339–48.
3. Wetzka B, Sehringer B, Schafer WR, et al. Expression patterns of CRH, CRH receptors, and CRH binding protein in human gestational tissue at term. Exp Clin Endocrinol Diabetes 2003;111:154–61.
4. Carr BR, Parker CR Jr, Madden JD, et al. Maternal plasma adrenocorticotropin and cortisol relationships throughout human pregnacy. Am J Obstet Gynecol 1981;139:416–22.
5. Behan DP, Linton EA, Lowry PJ. Isolation of the human plasma corticotrophin-releasing factor-binding protein. J Endocrinol 1989;122:23–31.
6. Demey-Ponsart E, Foidart JM, Sulon J, et al. Serum CBG, free and total cortisol and circadian patterns of adrenal function in normal pregnancy. J Steroid Biochem 1982;16:165–9.
7. Nolten WE, Lindheimer MD, Rueckert PA, et al. Diurnal patterns and regulation of cortisol secretion in pregnancy. J Clin Endocrinol Metab 1980;51:466–72.
8. Jung C, Ho JT, Torpy DJ, et al. A longitudinal study of plasma and urinary cortisol in pregnancy and postpartum. J Clin Endocrinol Metab 2011;96:1533–40.
9. Odagiri E, Ishiwatari N, Abe Y, et al. Hypercortisolism and the resistance to dexamethasone suppression during gestation. Endocrinol Jpn 1988;35:685–90.
10. Schulte HM, Weisner D, Allolio B. The corticotrophin releasing hormone test in late pregnancy: lack of adrenocorticotrophin and cortisol response. Clin Endocrinol 1990;33:99–106.
11. Suda T, Iwashita M, Ushiyama T, et al. Responses to corticotropin-releasing hormone and its bound and free forms in pregnant and nonpregnant women. J Clin Endocrinol Metab 1989;69:38–42.
12. Linton EA, Perkins AV, Woods RJ, et al. Corticotropin releasing hormone-binding protein (CRH-BP): plasma levels decrease during the third trimester of normal human pregnancy. J Clin Endocrinol Metab 1993;76:260–2.
13. Pivonello R, De Martino MC, Auriemma RS, et al. Pituitary tumors and pregnancy: the interplay between a pathologic condition and a physiologic status. J Endocrinol Invest 2014;37:99–112.
14. Prebtani AP, Donat D, Ezzat S. Worrisome striae in pregnancy. Lancet 2000;355: 1692.
15. Abdelmannan D, Aron DC. Adrenal disorders in pregnancy. Endocrinol Metab Clin North Am 2011;40:779–94.
16. McClamrock HD, Adashi EY. Gestational hyperandrogenism. Fertil Steril 1992;57: 257–74.
17. Lindsay JR, Jonklaas J, Oldfield EH, et al. Cushing's syndrome during pregnancy: personal experience and review of the literature. J Clin Endocrinol Metab 2005;90:3077–83.

18. Lopes LM, Francisco RP, Galletta MA, et al. Determination of nighttime salivary cortisol during pregnancy: comparison with values in non-pregnancy and Cushing's disease. Pituitary 2016;19:30–8.

19. Arnaldi G, Angeli A, Atkinson AB, et al. Diagnosis and complications of Cushing's syndrome: a consensus statement. J Clin Endocrinol Metab 2003;88:5593–602.

20. Nieman LK, Biller BM, Findling JW, et al. The diagnosis of Cushing's syndrome: an endocrine society clinical practice guideline. J Clin Endocrinol Metab 2008; 93:1526–40.

21. Pinette MG, Pan YQ, Oppenheim D, et al. Bilateral inferior petrosal sinus corticotropin sampling with corticotropin-releasing hormone stimulation in a pregnant patient with Cushing's syndrome. Am J Obstet Gynecol 1994;171:563–4.

22. Cabezon C, Bruno OD, Cohen M, et al. Twin pregnancy in a patient with Cushing's disease. Fertil Steril 1999;72:371–2.

23. Caimari F, Valassi E, Garbayo P, et al. Cushing's syndrome and pregnancy outcomes: a systematic review of published cases. Endocrine 2017;55:555–63.

24. Vilar L, Freitas Mda C, Lima LH, et al. Cushing's syndrome in pregnancy: an overview. Arq Bras Endocrinol Metabol 2007;51:1293–302.

25. Bronstein MD, Paraiba DB, Jallad RS. Management of pituitary tumors in pregnancy. Nat Rev Endocrinol 2011;7:301–10.

26. Leiba S, Weinstein R, Shindel B, et al. The protracted effect of o,p'-DDD in Cushing's disease and its impact on adrenal morphogenesis of young human embryo. Ann Endocrinol (Paris) 1989;50:49–53.

27. Abbassy M, Kshettry VR, Hamrahian AH, et al. Surgical management of recurrent Cushing's disease in pregnancy: a case report. Surg Neurol Int 2015;6:S640–5.

28. Martínez García R, Martínez Pérez A, Domingo del Pozo C, et al. Cushing's syndrome in pregnancy. Laparoscopic adrenalectomy during pregnancy: the mainstay treatment. J Endocrinol Invest 2016;39:273–6.

29. Andreescu CE, Alwani RA, Hofland J, et al. Adrenal Cushing's syndrome during pregnancy. Eur J Endocrinol 2017;177:K13–20.

30. Lim WH, Torpy DJ, Jeffries WS. The medical management of Cushing's syndrome during pregnancy. Eur J Obstet Gynecol Reprod Biol 2013;168:1–6.

31. Blanco C, Maqueda E, Rubio JA, et al. Cushing's syndrome during pregnancy secondary to adrenal adenoma: metyrapone treatment and laparoscopic adrenalectomy. J Endocrinol Metab 2006;29:164–7.

32. Hana V, Dokoupilova M, Marek J, et al. Recurrent ACTH-independent Cushing's syndrome in multiple pregnancies and its treatment with metyrapone. Clin Endocrinol 2001;54:277–81.

33. Connell JM, Cordiner J, Davies DL, et al. Pregnancy complicated by Cushing's syndrome: potential hazard of metyrapone therapy. Case report. Br J Obstet Gynaecol 1985;92:1192–5.

34. Boronat M, Marrero D, Lopez-Plasencia Y, et al. Successful outcome of pregnancy in a patient with Cushing's disease under treatment with ketoconazole during the first trimester of gestation. Gynecol Endocrinol 2011;27:675–7.

35. Berwaerts J, Verhelst J, Mahler C, et al. Cushing's syndrome in pregnancy treated by ketoconazole: case report and review of the literature. Gynecol Endocrinol 1999;13:175–82.

36. Costenaro F, Rodrigues TC, de Lima PB, et al. A successful case of Cushing's disease pregnancy treated with ketoconazole. Gynecol Endocrinol 2015;31: 176–8.

37. Zieleniewski W, Michalak R. A successful case of pregnancy in a woman with ACTH-independent Cushing's syndrome treated with ketoconazole and metyrapone. Gynecol Endocrinol 2017;33:349–52.
38. Woo I, Ehsanipoor RM. Cabergoline therapy for Cushing disease throughout pregnancy. Obstet Gynecol 2013;122:485–7.
39. Nakhleh A, Saiegh L, Reut M, et al. Cabergoline treatment for recurrent Cushing's disease during pregnancy. Hormones (Athens) 2016;15:453–8.
40. Sek KS, Deepak DS, Lee KO. Use of cabergoline for the management of persistent Cushing's disease in pregnancy. BMJ Case Rep 2017.
41. Mundra V, Solorzano CC, DeSantis P. Cushing syndrome: a rare ocurrence in pregnancy. Endocrinologist 2010;20(4):165–7.
42. Achong N, D'Emden M, Fagermo N, et al. Pregnancy-induced Cushing's syndrome in recurrent pregnancies: case report and literature review. Aust N Z J Obstet Gynaecol 2012;52:96–100.

Cushing's Syndrome in Pediatrics: An Update

Maya B. Lodish, MD, MHSc, Margaret F. Keil, PhD, CRNP*,
Constantine A. Stratakis, MD, D(Med)Sci

KEYWORDS

- Cushing's syndrome • Pituitary tumors • Adrenal cortex • Carney complex
- Adrenocortical hyperplasia • Adrenal cancer

KEY POINTS

- Cushing's syndrome in childhood results mostly from the exogenous administration of glucocorticoids; endogenous Cushing's syndrome is a rare disease.
- In childhood, lack of height gain concomitant with weight gain is the most common presentation of Cushing's syndrome.
- The first step in the diagnosis of Cushing's syndrome is documentation of hypercortisolism with the 24-hour urinary free cortisol, late-night salivary cortisol, or a low-dose dexamethasone-suppression test.
- In children older than the age of 6 years, Cushing's syndrome is most commonly caused by a corticotropin-secreting pituitary tumor, in children less than 6 years old, adrenal causes are more common etiologic factors of Cushing's syndrome.
- When the diagnosis of Cushing's syndrome is confirmed, algorithms for testing to distinguish corticotropin-dependent disease from the corticotropin-independent syndrome are available. Surgery is the first-line treatment intervention.

EPIDEMIOLOGY AND ETIOLOGIC FACTORS

Endogenous Cushing's syndrome (CS) is a rare multisystem disorder that results from overproduction of the glucocorticoid hormone cortisol, whether due to corticotropin-dependent or corticotropin-independent cause. In contrast, exogenous or iatrogenic CS occurs when glucocorticoids in the form of medications, such as prednisone, which are commonly used for inflammatory disorders, are given in high enough doses for prolonged periods of time. The overall incidence of endogenous CS is 0.7 to 2.4 per million people per year.[1] Only approximately 10% of the new cases

The authors have nothing to disclose.
Section on Endocrinology and Genetics, *Eunice Kennedy Shriver* National Institute of Child Health and Human Development (NICHD), National Institutes of Health (NIH), NIH-Clinical Research Center, 10 Center Drive, Building 10, Room 1E-3330, MSC1103, Bethesda, MD 20892, USA
* Corresponding author.
E-mail address: keilm@mail.nih.gov

Endocrinol Metab Clin N Am 47 (2018) 451–462
https://doi.org/10.1016/j.ecl.2018.02.008
endo.theclinics.com

each year occur in children. In both adults and children, CS is most commonly caused by a corticotropin-secreting pituitary tumor.

Under normal conditions cortisol is secreted from the cortical cells of the adrenal glands under the control of the pituitary hormone corticotropin (adrenocorticotropic hormone). Corticotropin-releasing hormone (CRH) is synthesized in the hypothalamus and carried to the anterior pituitary in the portal system. CRH stimulates adrenocorticotropic hormone (corticotropin) release from the anterior pituitary, which in turn stimulates the adrenal cortex to secrete cortisol (hypothalamic-pituitary-adrenal [HPA] axis).[2,3] Cortisol primarily inhibits the secretion of CRH and, secondarily, corticotropin in a negative feedback regulation system. In CS, the HPA axis has lost its ability for self-regulation owing to excessive secretion of either corticotropin or cortisol, and the loss of the negative feedback function. Diagnostic tests, on the other hand, take advantage of the tight regulation of the HPA axis in the normal state and its disturbance in CS to guide therapy toward the primary cause of this disorder.[4,5]

Cushing's disease (CD) results from overproduction of corticotropin by a pituitary adenoma, which in turn results in overproduction of cortisol from the adrenal cortex and a state of hypercortisolism. Other forms of CS are due to autonomous production of cortisol from adrenal cortical tumors, or ectopic corticotropin syndrome (overproduction of corticotropin from a nonpituitary tumor). CD and the ectopic corticotropin syndrome are often referred to as corticotropin-dependent CS, whereas adrenal cortical tumors cause corticotropin-independent CS. Approximately 75% to 90% of CS cases in children are due to CD. CD is uncommon in children under 6 years of age; adrenal causes of CS (adenoma, carcinoma, or bilateral hyperplasia) are the typical etiologic factors in younger children.

Autonomous secretion of cortisol from the adrenal glands, or corticotropin-independent CS, accounts for approximately 15% of all the cases of CS in childhood. CS is a manifestation of approximately one-third of all adrenal tumors. In adrenal cancer, adrenal adenomas, bilateral micronodular adrenal hyperplasia, and primary bilateral macronodular adrenocortical hyperplasia, a spectrum of tumor growth exists as a result of a variety of genetic defects that have been recently identified. (See discussion of the genetics of pituitary and adrenal tumors associated with CS, in this issue.)

The annual incidence of pediatric adrenocortical carcinoma (ACC) according to the Surveillance, Epidemiology, and End Results (SEER) database from 1973 through 2008 was 0.21 per million.[6] ACC has a bimodal age distribution, with a peak in early childhood at 3 years,[7] and a peak in adulthood in the 40s and 50s.[8] These tumors are characterized by poor survival, especially in the context of distant metastases, large tumor volume, and older age.[9] Adrenocortical cancers in childhood may be associated with the Li-Fraumeni or Beckwith-Wiedemann syndromes, and rarely with adenomatous polyposis coli and other rare genetic conditions.

Defects in cyclic adenosine monophosphate (cAMP) signaling underlie most cortisol-producing adrenal hyperplasia and tumors.[10] McCune Albright syndrome, in which a somatic mutation of the GNAS1 gene leads to constitutive activation of the Gsa protein, may be associated with infantile CS.[11] Primary pigmented adrenocortical nodular disease (PPNAD) is a genetic disorder usually associated with Carney complex, a syndrome of multiple endocrine gland abnormalities in addition to myxomas and lentigines.[12] The adrenal glands in PPNAD are characterized by multiple pigmented nodules that autonomously secrete cortisol and are surrounded by an atrophic cortex. Children and adolescents with PPNAD frequently have periodic or cyclical CS. The underlying genetic defect in most forms of PPNAD is mutations of the *PRKAR1A* gene coding for the regulatory type I-alpha subunit of protein kinase A (PKA).[13]

Ectopic corticotropin production occurs rarely in young children, accounting for less than 1% of the cases of CS in adolescents.[14] Sources of ectopic corticotropin include carcinoid tumors in the bronchus, pancreas, or thymus; medullary carcinomas of the thyroid; small cell carcinoma of the lung; pheochromocytomas; and other pancreatic and gastrointestinal neuroendocrine tumors. Ectopic corticotropin-CRH cosecreting tumors are also extremely rare in children and adolescents. The diagnosis of this condition is frequently missed and is sometimes confused with CD due to the effect of CRH on the pituitary.[15]

CLINICAL PRESENTATION

In most children, the onset of CS is insidious.[2-4] The most common presenting symptom is weight gain. In childhood, lack of height gain concomitant with weight gain is the most common presentation of CS. A growth chart typical for a child with CS is shown in **Fig. 1**. Other common presenting signs and symptoms of CS in children are listed in **Table 1**.[2,16-19]

DIAGNOSTIC GUIDELINES

Accurate diagnosis and classification of CS is crucial for determining the appropriate therapeutic intervention. The clinical evaluation and medical history, especially review of growth data, are important to make the initial diagnosis. On suspicion of CS, laboratory and imaging confirmations are necessary. An algorithm of the diagnostic process is presented in **Fig. 2**. The Endocrine Society published guidelines on the diagnostic workup of CS in 2008.[5]

The first step in the diagnosis of CS is documentation of hypercortisolism, typically with 24-hour urinary free cortisol (UFC) with at least 2, preferably 3, consecutive collections (correct for body surface area); late-night salivary cortisol; and/or a low-dose dexamethasone-suppression test (DST) (1 mg overnight or 2 mg/d over 48 hours). None of these tests has 100% diagnostic accuracy, each test has its own limitations, and multiple tests are usually needed to establish the diagnosis. In some studies, late-night salivary cortisol has been shown to have superior diagnostic performance to UFC, and it has been shown to be a simple, accurate way to screen for hypercortisolism in children[20-22]; however, there is much variation in laboratory performance of this test. Recently, hair cortisol has been used as an additional measure of evaluating patients with suspected CS.[23] UFC measurements over 24 hours can be challenging and false-positive elevations can be caused due to pseudo-Cushing's states, including physical and emotional stress, chronic and severe obesity, pregnancy, chronic exercise, depression, poor diabetes control, alcoholism, anorexia, narcotic withdrawal, anxiety, malnutrition, and high water intake. Conversely, inadequate collection of urine may lead to falsely low UFC levels. Measuring cortisol at midnight with an indwelling intravenous tube is the gold standard for documenting hypercortisolemia. A midnight cortisol value of greater than 4.4 mg/dL has a high sensitivity and specificity for CS.[4] However, diurnal testing requires an inpatient stay and its use as a routine screening test is limited.

When the diagnosis of CS is confirmed, there are several tests to distinguish the corticotropin-dependent from the corticotropin-independent disease. A spot morning plasma corticotropin of greater than or equal to 29 pg/mL in children with confirmed CS has a sensitivity of 70% in identifying children with an corticotropin-dependent form of the syndrome.[4] The standard high-dose DST (or Liddle test) is used to differentiate CD from ectopic corticotropin secretion and adrenal causes of CS. In this test, 120 mg/kg

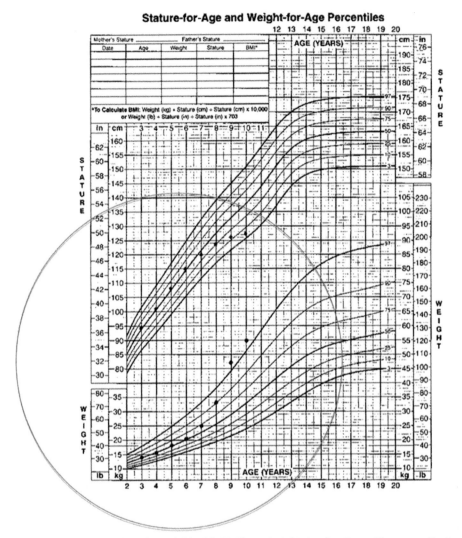

Fig. 1. Typical growth chart for a child with CS. Linear height deceleration with concomitant weight gain starting at age 8 years. (*From* Stratakis CA. Cushing syndrome in pediatrics. Endocrinol Metab Clin North Am 2012;41(4):796; with permission.)

Table 1	
Presenting signs and symptoms of Cushing's syndrome in children	
Dermatologic	Facial plethora, acne, acanthosis nigricans, easy bruising, supratemporal and supraclavicular fat pads, moon facies, fungal infection, hirsutism, fine downy hair, violaceous striae (unusual in children <7 y age)
Neurologic	Headaches
Cardiovascular	Hypertension, coagulopathy
Growth	Growth deceleration with concomitant weight gain, central obesity
Gonadal	Amenorrhea, virilization, gynecomastia
Other	Nephrolithiasis, bone fractures, impaired glucose tolerance, type 2 diabetes
Psychological	Depression, anxiety, mood swings, irritability, fatigue

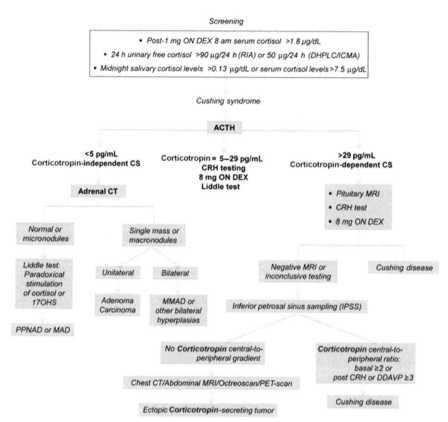

Fig. 2. Diagnostic algorithm in CS. Screening for hypercortisolemia includes 1 mg overnight (ON) dexamethasone (DEX), 24-hour urine free cortisol, or midnight salivary cortisol. The corticotropin level is used to differentiate corticotropin-independent versus corticotropin-independent CS and appropriate testing to confirm the cause of CS. CT, computed tomography; DDAVP, desmopressin; DHPLC, denaturing high-performance liquid chromatography; ICMA, immunochemiluminometric assay; IPSS, inferior petrosal sinus sampling; MAD, microdnodular adrenal disease; MMAD, massive macronodular adrenal disease; OHS, hydroxy-steroid; RIA, radioimmunoassay. (*From* Stratakis CA. Cushing's syndrome in pediatrics. Endocrinol Metab Clin North Am 2012;41(4):797; with permission.)

(maximum dose 8 mg) of dexamethasone is administered at 11 PM and plasma cortisol is measured at 9 AM the morning before and the morning following the dexamethasone. In children, a 20% cortisol suppression from baseline had sensitivity and specificity of 97.5% and 100%, respectively, with the high-dose DST for differentiating patients with CD from those with adrenal tumors.[4] An ovine-corticotropin-releasing hormone (oCRH) stimulation test may also be obtained for the differentiation of CD from ectopic corticotropin secretion and/or adrenal lesions. The criterion for diagnosis of CD is a mean increase of 20% above baseline for cortisol values at 30 and 45 minutes, and an increase in the mean corticotropin concentrations of at least 35% higher than the basal value at 15 and 30 minutes after CRH administration.[24] If bilateral adrenocortical hyperplasia is suspected, the classic Liddle test (low-dose dexamethasone of 30 μg/kg/dose; maximum 0.5 mg/dose) every 6 hours for 8 doses; followed by the high-dose dexamethasone (120 μg/kg/dose, maximum 2 mg/dose) every 6 hours for 8 doses may be used. This test shows a paradoxic stimulation of cortisol secretion in PPNAD.[25]

Diagnostic imaging is another important tool in the localization and characterization of CS:

- Pituitary MRI in thin sections (1–2 mm) with high resolution and with contrast (gadolinium)
- High-resolution 18F-fluorodeoxyglucose (^{18}FDG) PET for detection of small functioning corticotrophs adenomas[26]
- Adrenal computed tomography (CT) scan is useful in the distinction between CD and adrenal causes of CS
- CT or MRI scan of the neck, chest, abdomen, and pelvis may be used for the detection of an ectopic source of corticotropin production
- Labeled octreotide scanning, PET, and/or gallium 68 (68Ga)-dodecanetetraacetic acid tyrosine-3-octreotate (DOTATATE) PET-CT may help in the localization of an ectopic corticotropin source
- If the biochemical workup is not definitive for a pituitary source and/or if a lesion is not visible on pituitary MRI, bilateral inferior petrosal sinus sampling has been used for the localization of a pituitary microadenoma.[27]

TREATMENT

In 2015, the Endocrine Society published clinical practice guidelines for treating CS; however, they are not specific for children.[24] Transsphenoidal surgical (TSS) resection of the corticotropin-secreting pituitary tumor remains the first-line therapeutic intervention in CD. In specialized centers with experienced neurosurgeons, the success rate of the first TSS is close to or even higher than 90%.[28,29] Pituitary surgery may not be successful and disease may recur years after initial surgery. The success rate of repeat TSS is lower than the initial surgery, closer to 60%. Postoperative complications include diabetes insipidus, syndrome of inappropriate antidiuretic hormone secretion, central hypothyroidism, hypogonadism, growth hormone (GH) deficiency, bleeding, infection, and pituitary apoplexy. The mortality rate is extremely low, at less than 1%. For those patients not achieving an initial remission or developing recurrence after an initial remission, therapeutic options are limited.

Pituitary radiotherapy (RT) often used in adults is generally avoided in children, especially those who are prepubertal, owing to complications of radiation (cerebral cortex toxicity, hypopituitarism). However, in children, conventional RT without adjunctive medical treatment should take effect more rapidly than in adults.[30] Unfortunately, hypopituitarism is a common complication of RT and pituitary function requires frequent assessment.[31] The traditional dose of RT is 4500 to 5000 cGy given over a 6-week period. However, innovative types of stereotactic RT are now available for the treatment of CD, including linear particle accelerator (LINAC), gamma knife stereotactic radiosurgery (SRS), and proton beam therapy. Although large pediatric studies are not available, literature from adults shows that SRS provides an effective and tolerated treatment option for patients with pituitary adenomas. SRS offers the benefit of more rapid treatment and the potential for reduced side effects. In a recent retrospective review of 262 patients treated with SRS, tumor control rate was 89%; higher margin radiation dose to the adenoma and suprasellar extension were 2 independent predictors of SRS-induced hypopituitarism.[32] In a long-term study of radiation therapy in pituitary adenomas, including individuals as young as age 10 years, radiation therapy was seen to increase the quality of life in 95% of subjects, and local progression-free survival following radiation therapy was 90% at 2 years.[33] It is important to realize that SRS may lead to radiation-induced optic neuropathy and associated blindness when the dose to the anterior visual pathway is greater than 8 Gy.[34]

Currently, medical therapy for CD serves primarily in an adjunctive role after unsuccessful pituitary surgery. There are 3 mechanisms of action for drugs used in medical therapy: modulation of corticotropin release, inhibition of adrenal steroidogenesis, and glucocorticoid receptor blockade. Until recently there had been no medications approved by the US Food and Drug Administration for use in CD, which led to off-label use of some drugs, most commonly ketoconazole. **Table 2** lists current options for medical therapy.[24,35] There is very limited experience using ketoconazole or other therapeutics in the medical treatment of pediatric patients with CS.

Benign adrenal tumors are best treated with surgical resection. In the case of bilateral micronodular or macronodular adrenal disease, bilateral total adrenalectomy is the preferred treatment. Treatment guidelines for children with adrenal cancer are lacking because of the rarity of this disease. A recent Children's Oncology Group trial evaluating cisplatin, etoposide, and doxorubicin combined with surgery showed an excellent outcome for stage III ACC, but poor outcome with stage IV ACC.[36]

Adrenalectomy is an option for refractory CD or corticotropin-dependent CS. Early bilateral adrenalectomy in patients with uncontrolled CS may improve adverse events.[37] However, a potential complication after bilateral adrenalectomy in patients with CD is growth of the corticotropinoma, elevated corticotropin levels, and hyperpigmentation (Nelson syndrome). Recent approximations from 2 systematic reviews in adults found that Nelson syndrome occurred in 21% to 24% of the patients.[38] Adrenal crisis is another lifelong risk in these individuals.

GLUCOCORTICOID REPLACEMENT

After the completion of successful TSS in CD, or excision of an autonomously functioning adrenal adenoma, there will be a period of adrenal insufficiency while the hypothalamic

Table 2
Medical treatment of Cushing's syndrome

	Mechanism of Action	Side Effects	US Food and Drug Administration (FDA) or European Medicines Agency (EMA) Approval
Ketoconazole	Antifungal azole inhibits steroidogenesis	Gastrointestinal side effects, hepatotoxicity, breakthrough requiring dose escalation, adrenal insufficiency	EMA for adults
Mitotane	Adrenolytic	Gastrointestinal side effects, fatigue, dermatologic changes	FDA approval for treatment of adrenal cancer
Pasireotide	Somatostatin analogue	Adrenal insufficiency, hyperglycemia, bradycardia, gastrointestinal side effects, hepatotoxicity, fatigue, headache	FDA approval for adults with CS who are not surgical candidates
Mifepristone	Glucocorticoid receptor blocker	Hypokalemia, adrenal insufficiency, endometrial thickening	FDA approval for adults with CS with diabetes or glucose intolerance who are not surgical candidates

pituitary adrenal axis is recovering. During this period, glucocorticoid should be replaced at the suggested physiologic replacement dosage (12–15 mg/m^2/d 2 or 3 times daily).[39] In the immediate postoperative period, stress doses of cortisol should be initiated. This should be weaned relatively rapidly to a physiologic replacement dose and followed every few months. The adrenocortical function should be periodically assessed with a 1-hour corticotropin test (normal response is a cortisol level greater than 18 μg/dL at 30 or 60 minutes after corticotropin stimulation)[39] and the glucocorticoid dose tapered. Average time to recovery of the HPA axis post-TSS in children is 12.6 plus or minus 3 months; early recovery of HPA axis (<6 months) is associated with recurrence.[39]

After bilateral adrenalectomy, patients require lifetime replacement with both glucocorticoids (as described previously) and mineralocorticoids (fludrocortisone 0.1–0.3 mg/d). These patients also need stress doses of glucocorticoids in the immediate postoperative period and should be weaned to physiologic replacement relatively quickly.

In addition, stress dosing for acute illness, trauma, or surgical procedures is required for both temporary and permanent adrenal insufficiency.[24] Adrenal crisis, which is associated with increased morbidity and mortality,[40,41] highlights the importance of ongoing patient and caregiver education.[41,42]

MEDICAL, PSYCHOSOCIAL, AND COGNITIVE OUTCOMES

CS in childhood has the potential for long-term adverse medical outcomes due to prolonged exposure of the body to high levels of glucocorticoids, as well as morbidity associated with surgical or radiation treatment.[7,9,17,31,43] **Table 2** lists treatment and long-term clinical effects of CS in childhood.[2,9,17,31,44–46] Disparities related to delayed diagnosis and treatment in nonwhites that was associated with higher risk for persistent CD or recurrent CD after surgery.[47] Posttreatment challenges for the child or adolescent treated for CS include optimizing growth and pubertal development, normalizing body composition, and promoting psychological health and cognitive development.[48] Systolic hypertension persisted in 16% of CD and 21% of corticotropin-independent CS cases, and diastolic hypertension was noted in approximately 4% of all pediatric patients 1 year after cure.[49] Adverse effects of abdominal adiposity, insulin resistance, hypertension, and cardiovascular dysfunction may persist after cure of CS.[18] Studies of final height and catchup growth after treatment of CS have shown conflicting results; children with poorer than expected catchup growth should be tested to confirm ongoing remission of hypercortisolemia and evaluation of GH axis recovery.[45,50,51]

CS has been associated with multiple psychiatric and psychological disturbances, most commonly emotional lability, depression, and/or anxiety[2,51–53] (**Table 3**). Significant psychopathology may remain after remission of hypercortisolism and even after recovery of the HPA axis.[52,54] Children with CS may experience a decline in cognitive and school performance 1 year after surgical cure, without any associated psychopathology, with younger age at first evaluation associated with greater deterioration in IQ scores.[53,55] Also, active CS, particularly in younger children, was associated with impaired quality of life scores and, despite improvement from before to 1 year after cure, residual impairment remained.[55] Although most self-reported CS symptoms showed improvement after cure, forgetfulness, unclear thinking, and decreased attention span did not improve.[55]

Suicidal ideation in adults (~17%) with active CS and suicidal ideation was present in approximately 6% of children after surgical cure of CS.[52,56] Normalization of the HPA axis may unveil or trigger psychopathological manifestations not precipitated by hypercortisolemia or vice versa. This highlights the importance of screening for

Table 3
Long-term effects of Cushing's syndrome in childhood

	Comorbidity
Treatment-related	
Transsphenoidal surgery	Panhypopituitarism (partial or complete), pseudotumor cerebri, recurrence of CS
Pituitary irradiation	Panhypopituitarism (partial or complete), cranial neuropathies, radiation-induced tumors, cognitive decrement
Adrenalectomy	Adrenal insufficiency, Nelson syndrome
Pharmacologic therapy	Recurrence of CS, hepatotoxicity, hypertension, hypokalemia, endometrial hyperplasia
Long-term clinical effects	
Growth	Compromised final height
Metabolic	Increased body mass index, visceral obesity, impaired glucose metabolism, hyperlipidemia
Cardiovascular	Hypertension, increased arterial rigidity
Neuropsychiatric	Cerebral atrophy, amygdala and hippocampus dysfunction, behavioral changes, panic disorder, suicidal ideation, schizophrenia, obsessive-compulsive symptomology, psychosis, irritability, impaired self-esteem, distorted body image
Cognitive	cognitive decrement, memory and concentration impairment, decreased attention span, forgetfulness
Quality of life	Residual deficit in physical and psychological scores

risk factors for suicide and suicide ideation in children before and after treatment of CS. Patients and their caregivers should be advised that they may experience changes in mood, behavior, cognitive function, and quality of life for months or years after surgical cure of CS. Early recognition of CS in children is imperative; late diagnosis is associated with significant morbidity and mortality.[43,47,48]

REFERENCES

1. Sharma ST, Nieman LK, Feelders RA. Cushing's syndrome: epidemiology and developments in disease management. Clin Epidemiol 2015;7:281–93.
2. Magiakou MA, Mastorakos G, Oldfield EH, et al. Cushing's syndrome in children and adolescents. Presentation, diagnosis, and therapy. N Engl J Med 1994; 331(10):629–36.
3. Orth DN. Cushing's syndrome. N Engl J Med 1995;332(12):791–803.
4. Batista DL, Riar J, Keil M, et al. Diagnostic tests for children who are referred for the investigation of Cushing syndrome. Pediatrics 2007;120(3):e575–86.
5. Nieman LK, Biller BM, Findling JW, et al. The diagnosis of Cushing's syndrome: an Endocrine Society Clinical Practice Guideline. J Clin Endocrinol Metab 2008;93(5):1526–40.
6. McAteer JP, Huaco JA, Gow KW. Predictors of survival in pediatric adrenocortical carcinoma: a Surveillance, Epidemiology, and End Results (SEER) program study. J Pediatr Surg 2013;48(5):1025–31.
7. Michalkiewicz E, Sandrini R, Figueiredo B, et al. Clinical and outcome characteristics of children with adrenocortical tumors: a report from the International Pediatric Adrenocortical Tumor Registry. J Clin Oncol 2004;22(5):838–45.

8. Ng L, Libertino JM. Adrenocortical carcinoma: diagnosis, evaluation and treatment. J Urol 2003;169(1):5–11.

9. Cecchetto G, Ganarin A, Bien E, et al. Outcome and prognostic factors in high-risk childhood adrenocortical carcinomas: a report from the European Cooperative Study Group on Pediatric Rare Tumors (EXPeRT). Pediatr Blood Cancer 2017;64(6).

10. Zilbermint M, Stratakis CA. Protein kinase A defects and cortisol-producing adrenal tumors. Curr Opin Endocrinol Diabetes Obes 2015;22(3):157–62.

11. Brown RJ, Kelly MH, Collins MT. Cushing syndrome in the McCune-Albright syndrome. J Clin Endocrinol Metab 2010;95(4):1508–15.

12. Almeida MQ, Stratakis CA. Carney complex and other conditions associated with micronodular adrenal hyperplasias. Best Pract Res Clin Endocrinol Metab 2010; 24(6):907–14.

13. Stratakis CA. Genetics of adrenocortical tumors: carney complex. Ann Endocrinol (Paris) 2001;62(2):180–4.

14. More J, Young J, Reznik Y, et al. Ectopic ACTH syndrome in children and adolescents. J Clin Endocrinol Metab 2011;96(5):1213–22.

15. Karageorgiadis AS, Papadakis GZ, Biro J, et al. Ectopic adrenocorticotropic hormone and corticotropin-releasing hormone co-secreting tumors in children and adolescents causing Cushing syndrome: a diagnostic dilemma and how to solve it. J Clin Endocrinol Metab 2015;100(1):141–8.

16. Rahman SH, Papadakis GZ, Keil MF, et al. Kidney stones as an underrecognized clinical sign in pediatric Cushing disease. J Pediatr 2016;170:273–7.e1.

17. Lodish MB, Hsiao HP, Serbis A, et al. Effects of Cushing disease on bone mineral density in a pediatric population. J Pediatr 2010;156(6):1001–5.

18. Keil MF, Graf J, Gokarn N, et al. Anthropometric measures and fasting insulin levels in children before and after cure of Cushing syndrome. Clin Nutr 2012; 31(3):359–63.

19. Afshari A, Ardeshirpour Y, Lodish MB, et al. Facial plethora: modern technology for quantifying an ancient clinical sign and its use in Cushing syndrome. J Clin Endocrinol Metab 2015;100(10):3928–33.

20. Elias PC, Martinez EZ, Barone BF, et al. Late-night salivary cortisol has a better performance than urinary free cortisol in the diagnosis of Cushing's syndrome. J Clin Endocrinol Metab 2014;99(6):2045–51.

21. Manetti L, Rossi G, Grasso L, et al. Usefulness of salivary cortisol in the diagnosis of hypercortisolism: comparison with serum and urinary cortisol. Eur J Endocrinol 2013;168(3):315–21.

22. Gafni RI, Papanicolaou DA, Nieman LK. Nighttime salivary cortisol measurement as a simple, noninvasive, outpatient screening test for Cushing's syndrome in children and adolescents. J Pediatr 2000;137(1):30–5.

23. Hodes A, Lodish MB, Tirosh A, et al. Hair cortisol in the evaluation of Cushing syndrome. Endocrine 2017;56(1):164–74.

24. Nieman LK, Biller BM, Findling JW, et al. Treatment of Cushing's syndrome: an endocrine society clinical practice guideline. J Clin Endocrinol Metab 2015; 100(8):2807–31.

25. Louiset E, Stratakis CA, Perraudin V, et al. The paradoxical increase in cortisol secretion induced by dexamethasone in primary pigmented nodular adrenocortical disease involves a glucocorticoid receptor-mediated effect of dexamethasone on protein kinase A catalytic subunits. J Clin Endocrinol Metab 2009;94(7):2406–13.

26. Chittiboina P, Montgomery BK, Millo C, et al. High-resolution(18)F-fluorodeoxyglu-cose positron emission tomography and magnetic resonance imaging for pituitary adenoma detection in Cushing disease. J Neurosurg 2015;122(4):791–7.

27. Oldfield EH, Doppman JL, Nieman LK, et al. Petrosal sinus sampling with and without corticotropin-releasing hormone for the differential diagnosis of Cushing's syndrome. N Engl J Med 1991;325(13):897–905.

28. Lonser RR, Wind JJ, Nieman LK, et al. Outcome of surgical treatment of 200 children with Cushing's disease. J Clin Endocrinol Metab 2013;98(3):892–901.

29. Storr HL, Drake WM, Evanson J, et al. Endonasal endoscopic transsphenoidal pituitary surgery: early experience and outcome in paediatric Cushing's disease. Clin Endocrinol (Oxf) 2014;80(2):270–6.

30. Acharya SV, Gopal RA, Goerge J, et al. Radiotherapy in paediatric Cushing's disease: efficacy and long term follow up of pituitary function. Pituitary 2010;13(4): 293–7.

31. Chan LF, Storr HL, Plowman PN, et al. Long-term anterior pituitary function in patients with paediatric Cushing's disease treated with pituitary radiotherapy. Eur J Endocrinol 2007;156(4):477–82.

32. Xu Z, Lee Vance M, Schlesinger D, et al. Hypopituitarism after stereotactic radiosurgery for pituitary adenomas. Neurosurgery 2013;72(4):630–7, 636–7.

33. Rieken S, Habermehl D, Welzel T, et al. Long term toxicity and prognostic factors of radiation therapy for secreting and non-secreting pituitary adenomas. Radiat Oncol 2013;8:18.

34. Leavitt JA, Stafford SL, Link MJ, et al. Long-term evaluation of radiation-induced optic neuropathy after single-fraction stereotactic radiosurgery. Int J Radiat Oncol Biol Phys 2013;87(3):524–7.

35. Castinetti F, Guignat L, Giraud P, et al. Ketoconazole in Cushing's disease: is it worth a try? J Clin Endocrinol Metab 2014;99(5):1623–30.

36. Rodriguez-Galindo C, Pappo AS, Krailo MD, et al. Treatment of childhood adrenocortical carcinoma (ACC) with surgery plus retroperitoneal lymph node dissection (RPLND) and multiagent chemotherapy: results of the Children's Oncology Group ARAR0332 protocol. J Clin Oncol 2016;34(15).

37. Morris LF, Harris RS, Milton DR, et al. Impact and timing of bilateral adrenalectomy for refractory adrenocorticotropic hormone-dependent Cushing's syndrome. Surgery 2013;154(6):1174–83 [discussion: 1183–4].

38. Ritzel K, Beuschlein F, Mickisch A, et al. Clinical review: outcome of bilateral adrenalectomy in Cushing's syndrome: a systematic review. J Clin Endocrinol Metab 2013;98(10):3939–48.

39. Lodish M, Dunn SV, Sinaii N, et al. Recovery of the hypothalamic-pituitary-adrenal axis in children and adolescents after surgical cure of Cushing's disease. J Clin Endocrinol Metab 2012;97(5):1483–91.

40. Hahner S, Spinnler C, Fassnacht M, et al. High incidence of adrenal crisis in educated patients with chronic adrenal insufficiency: a prospective study. J Clin Endocrinol Metab 2015;100(2):407–16.

41. Shulman DI, Palmert MR, Kemp SF, et al. Adrenal insufficiency: still a cause of morbidity and death in childhood. Pediatrics 2007;119(2):e484–94.

42. Bornstein SR, Allolio B, Arlt W, et al. Diagnosis and treatment of primary adrenal insufficiency: an endocrine society clinical practice guideline. J Clin Endocrinol Metab 2016;101(2):364–89.

43. Gkourogianni A, Lodish MB, Zilbermint M, et al. Death in pediatric Cushing syndrome is uncommon but still occurs. Eur J Pediatr 2015;174(4):501–7.

44. Tirosh A, Lodish M, Lyssikatos C, et al. Coagulation profile in patients with different etiologies for Cushing syndrome: a prospective observational study. Horm Metab Res 2017;49(5):365–71.

45. Magiakou MA, Mastorakos G, Chrousos GP. Final stature in patients with endogenous Cushing's syndrome. J Clin Endocrinol Metab 1994;79(4):1082–5.

46. Birdwell L, Lodish M, Tirosh A, et al. Coagulation profile dynamics in pediatric patients with Cushing syndrome: a prospective, observational comparative study. J Pediatr 2016;177:227–31.

47. Gkourogianni A, Sinaii N, Jackson SH, et al. Pediatric Cushing disease: disparities in disease severity and outcomes in the Hispanic and African-American populations. Pediatr Res 2017;82(2):272–7.

48. Keil MF. Quality of life and other outcomes in children treated for Cushing syndrome. J Clin Endocrinol Metab 2013;98(7):2667–78.

49. Lodish MB, Sinaii N, Patronas N, et al. Blood pressure in pediatric patients with Cushing syndrome. J Clin Endocrinol Metab 2009;94(6):2002–8.

50. Lodish MB, Gourgari E, Sinaii N, et al. Skeletal maturation in children with Cushing syndrome is not consistently delayed: the role of corticotropin, obesity, and steroid hormones, and the effect of surgical cure. J Pediatr 2014;164(4):801–6.

51. Devoe DJ, Miller WL, Conte FA, et al. Long-term outcome in children and adolescents after transsphenoidal surgery for Cushing's disease. J Clin Endocrinol Metab 1997;82(10):3196–202.

52. Starkman MN. Neuropsychiatric findings in Cushing syndrome and exogenous glucocorticoid administration. Endocrinol Metab Clin North Am 2013;42(3):477–88.

53. Merke DP, Giedd JN, Keil MF, et al. Children experience cognitive decline despite reversal of brain atrophy one year after resolution of Cushing syndrome. J Clin Endocrinol Metab 2005;90(5):2531–6.

54. Dorn LD, Cerrone P. Cognitive function in patients with Cushing syndrome: a longitudinal perspective. Clin Nurs Res 2000;9(4):420–40.

55. Keil MF, Merke DP, Gandhi R, et al. Quality of life in children and adolescents 1-year after cure of Cushing syndrome: a prospective study. Clin Endocrinol (Oxf) 2009;71(3):326–33.

56. Keil MF, Zametkin A, Ryder C, et al. Cases of psychiatric morbidity in pediatric patients after remission of Cushing syndrome. Pediatrics 2016;137(4) [pii: e20152234].

Moving?

Make sure your subscription moves with you!

To notify us of your new address, find your **Clinics Account Number** (located on your mailing label above your name), and contact customer service at:

Email: journalscustomerservice-usa@elsevier.com

800-654-2452 (subscribers in the U.S. & Canada)
314-447-8871 (subscribers outside of the U.S. & Canada)

Fax number: 314-447-8029

Elsevier Health Sciences Division
Subscription Customer Service
3251 Riverport Lane
Maryland Heights, MO 63043

*To ensure uninterrupted delivery of your subscription, please notify us at least 4 weeks in advance of move.

Printed and bound by CPI Group (UK) Ltd, Croydon, CR0 4YY

11/05/2025

01866586-0001